P9-DWH-910

Anatomy of Love

Anatomy of Love

The Natural History of Monogamy, Adultery, and Divorce

Helen E. Fisher, Ph.D.

W·W· Norton and Company • New York London

Lines by Samuel Hoffenstein reprinted from *A Treasury of Humorous Verse* by Samuel Hoffenstein, by permission of Liveright Publishing Corporation. Copyright 1946 by Liveright Publishing Corporation. Copyright renewed 1974 by Liveright Publishing Corporation.

Excerpt from "Little Gidding" in *Four Quartets,* copyright 1943 by T. S. Eliot and renewed 1971 by Esme Valerie Eliot, reprinted by permission of Harcourt Brace Jovanovich, Inc. and Faber and Faber Ltd.

Copyright © 1992 by Helen E. Fisher

All rights reserved
Printed in the United States of America
First Edition

The text of this book is composed in 11/13.5 Avanta with display set in Lucian
Composition and manufacturing by the Haddon Craftsmen, Inc.
Book design by Guenet Abraham

Library of Congress Cataloging-in-Publication Data

Fisher, Helen E.
Anatomy of love : the natural history of monogamy, adultery, and divorce / by Helen E. Fisher.
p.   cm.
Includes bibliographical references and index.
1. Marriage.   2. Adultery,   3. Divorce.   4. Sex customs.
I. Title.
HQ728.F454   1992
306.7—dc20   92-4809

ISBN 0-393-03423-2

W.W. Norton & Company, Inc.
500 Fifth Avenue, New York, N.Y. 10110

W.W. Norton & Company Ltd.
10 Coptic Street, London WC1A 1PU

1 2 3 4 5 6 7 8 9 0

FOR RAY CARROLL

Contents

To the Reader

A "Way of Seeing"

I am an identical twin. By the time I was four or five, I had begun to notice grown-ups staring at my twin sister and me as they asked us questions. Did I know when Lorna was in trouble? Did we like the same toys? Did I ever think I was Lorna? I remember sitting in the backseat of the family car and comparing hands. We laughed alike and still do. We both like risk, although we display it very differently. She is a hot-air-balloon pilot in Colorado, whereas I discuss emotionally charged issues such as adultery and divorce on television and the podium. She is also an artist. She paints large canvases with tiny brushstrokes, whereas I move tiny words across hundreds of manuscript pages. Both are jobs that require patience and attention to details. And we both work alone.

So as a child I started, quite unconsciously, to weigh my behavior: How much of it was inherited? How much of it was learned?

Then, in graduate school, I discovered the "nature/nurture" debate. John Locke's concept of the "tabula rasa," or empty tablet, was particularly troubling. Was every infant really a blank sheet of paper on which culture inscribed personality? I didn't believe it.

Then I read Jane Goodall's book *In the Shadow of Man,* about the wild chimpanzees of Tanzania. These creatures had different personalities, and they made friends, held hands, kissed, gave one another gifts of leaves and twigs, and mourned when a companion died. I was overcome by the emotional continuity between man and beast. And I became convinced that some of my behavior was biological in origin.

So this book is about the *innate* aspects of sex and love and marriage, those mating traits and tendencies that we *inherited* from our past. Human behavior is a complex mixture of environmental and hereditary forces and I do not wish to minimize the power of culture in influencing human action. But it is the genetic contributions to behavior that have always intrigued me.

The book began on a New York subway. I was pouring over American marriage statistics and I noticed some peculiar patterns to divorce. I wondered if these same patterns might appear in other cultures. So I looked at divorce data on sixty-two societies contained in the demographic yearbooks of the United Nations; there I found some similar curious designs. Then I examined data on adultery in forty-two cultures. And when I compared these worldwide figures on human bonding with patterns of monogamy, "cheating," and desertion in birds and nonhuman mammals, I found some similarities so compelling that they led me to a general theory for the evolution of human sex and family life.

Why do we marry? Why are some of us adulterous? Why do human beings divorce? Why do we remarry and try our luck again? The book begins with chapters on the *nature* of courting, infatuation, monogamy, adultery, and divorce. Then, starting in chapter 6, I dial back to the beginning of human social life and trace the evolution of our sexuality from its inception on the grasslands of East Africa some four million years ago, through life among the cave painters of Ice Age Europe and on into contemporary times, both in the West and more "exotic" places.

In the course of presenting my theories, I examine why we fall in love with one person rather than another, the experience of love at first sight, the physiology of attachment and philandering, why men have large penises and women display permanently enlarged breasts, gender differences in the brain, the evolution of "women, men, and power," the genesis of teenage, the origin of our conscience, and many other creations of our human sexual impulse. Finally, in the last chapter, I use all these data to make some predictions about "relationships" tomorrow and, if we survive as a species, millennia from now.

But first a few caveats. Along the way I make many generalizations. Neither your behavior nor mine fits all of the patterns I will describe. Why should it? There is no reason to expect a tight correlation between all human actions and general rules of human nature. I focus on the predominant patterns, rather than on the exceptions.

Moreover, I make no effort to be "politically correct." Nature designed men and women to work together. But I cannot pretend that they are alike. They are not alike. And I have given evolutionary and biological explanations for their differences where I find them appropriate.

I have also resisted some fads in anthropology. It is at present unpopular, for example, to use the !Kung Bushmen of southern Africa as a model for reconstructing life in our hunting-gathering past. My reasons for continuing to use their society as a model are laid out in one of many endnotes that I hope you will have time to read.

Most alarming to some readers, I discuss the possible genetic components and adaptive features of complicated, controversial, and often highly painful social behaviors such as adultery and divorce. I am certainly *not advocating* infidelity or desertion; rather, I am trying to understand these disturbing facts of human life.

Last, I am an ethologist, one who is interested in the genetic aspects of behavior. Ethologists have, as Margaret Mead once said of the anthropological perspective, a "way of seeing." In my view, human beings have a common nature, a set of shared *unconscious* tendencies or potentialities that are encoded in our DNA and that evolved because they were of use to our forebears millions of years ago. We are not aware of these predispositions, but they still motivate our actions.

I do not think, however, that we are puppets of our genes, that our DNA *determines* our behavior. On the contrary, culture sculpts innumerable and diverse traditions from our common human genetic material; then individuals respond to their environment and heredity in idiosyncratic ways that philosophers have long attributed to "free will."

In our drive to understand ourselves, we first studied the sun and moon and stars, then the plants and animals around us. Only in the past two centuries have we scientifically examined our social networks and our minds. Victorians put books by male and female authors on separate shelves. Sex researcher Alfred Kinsey made his pioneering studies of American sexuality as recently as the 1950s. And academics have only just begun to inspect the genetic undercurrents of human mating practices. So this book is an attempt to explore the *nature* of our romantic lives.

There is magic to love—as poets and sweethearts know. I don't pretend to penetrate this sanctum. But our sexual imperatives are tangible, knowable. And I firmly believe that the better we come to understand our human heritage, the greater will be our power over it and the stronger our free will.

Helen E. Fisher

Acknowledgments

Thank you Ray Carroll, Florine and Gene Katz, and Helen Fisher, my mother, for your wonderful encouragement. Thank you Judy Andrews and Sue Carroll, for your fine research assistance.

I am enormously grateful to Mary Cunnane, my editor at W. W. Norton, as well as William Rusin, Fran Rosencrantz, Jeannie Luciano, Patricia Anthonyson, Caroline Crawford, and the rest of the Norton staff for their invaluable efforts on behalf of this book.

I also thank Amanda Urban, my agent, for her expert guidance, Lynn Goldberg and Louise Brockett for their sound advice, Nancy Crampton for taking my picture, Michael Rothman for drawing the illustration in the book, Otto Sonntag for copyediting the book, and Sydney Cohen for preparing the index.

I am indebted to my colleagues Robert Alford, Laura Betzig, Vern Bullough, Robert Carneiro, Ray Carroll, Andrew Cherlin, Ceciley Collins, Ellen Dissanayake, Perry Faithorn, Stan Freed, David Givens, Terry Harrison, Sarah Hrdy, Albin Jones, Florine Katz, Warren Kinzey, Laura Klein, Peter Lacey, Michael Liebowitz, Richard Milner, Merry Muraskin, Barbara Pillsbury, Carolyn Reynolds, Alice Rossi, Lionel Tiger, Wenda Trevathan, Michael Trupp, Randall White, and Milford Wolpoff for their good counsel or important comments on various sections of the manuscript.

Last, I thank my friends and family for their patience and good humor during the several years of writing this book.

Know then thyself, presume not God to scan;
The proper study of mankind is man.
Placed on this isthmus of a middle state,
A being darkly wise and rudely great:
With too much knowledge for the Sceptic side,
With too much weakness for the Stoic's pride,
He hangs between, in doubt to act or rest;
In doubt to deem himself a God or beast;
In doubt his mind or body to prefer;
Born but to die, and reas'ning but to err;
Alike in ignorance, his reason such,
Whether he thinks too little or too much;
Chaos of thought and passion, all confused;
Still by himself abused or disabused;
Created half to rise, and half to fall;
Great lord of all things, yet a prey to all;
Sole judge of truth, in endless error hurled;
The glory, jest, and riddle of the world.

—Alexander Pope

1
Courting
Games People Play

Moved by the force of love,
fragments of the world seek out one another
so that a world may be.

—*Pierre Teilhard de Chardin*

In an apocryphal story, a colleague once turned to the great British geneticist J. B. S. Haldane, and said, "Tell me, Mr. Haldane, knowing what you do about nature, what can you tell me about God?" Haldane replied, "He has an inordinate fondness for beetles." Indeed, the world contains over 300,000 species of beetles. I would add that "God" loves the human mating game, for no other aspect of our behavior is so complex, so subtle, or so pervasive. And although these sexual strategies differ from one individual to the next, the essential choreography of human courtship, love, and marriage has myriad designs that seem etched into the human psyche, the product of time, selection, and evolution.

They begin the moment men and women get within courting range—with the way we flirt.

Body Talk

In the 1960s Irenaus Eibl-Eibesfeldt, a German ethologist,[1] noticed a curious pattern to women's flirting behavior. Eibl-Eibesfeldt had used a camera with a secret lens so that when he directed the camera straight ahead, he was actually taking pictures to the side. This way he could focus on local sights and catch on film the unstaged facial expressions of people near him. In his travels to Samoa, Papua, France, Japan, Africa, and Amazonia, he recorded numerous flirting sequences. Then, back in his laboratory at the Max Planck Institute for Behavioral Physiology, near Munich, Germany, he carefully examined each courting episode, frame by frame.

A universal pattern of female flirting emerged. Women from places as different as the jungles of Amazonia, the salons of Paris, and the highlands of New Guinea apparently flirt with the same sequence of expressions.

First, the woman smiles at her admirer and lifts her eyebrows in a swift, jerky motion as she opens her eyes wide to gaze at him. Then she drops her eyelids, tilts her head down and to the side, and looks away. Frequently she also covers her face with her hands, giggling nervously as she retreats behind her palms. This sequential flirting gesture is so distinctive that Eibl-Eibesfeldt is convinced it is innate, a human female courtship ploy that evolved eons ago to signal sexual interest.

Other gambits people use may also come from our primeval past. The coy look is a gesture in which a woman cocks her head and looks up shyly at her suitor. A female possum does this too, turning toward her suitor, cocking her snouty jaw, and looking straight into his eyes. Animals frequently toss their heads in order to solicit attention. Courting women do it regularly; they raise their shoulders, arch their backs, and toss their locks in a single sweeping motion. Albatross toss their heads and snap their bills between bouts of nodding, bowing, and rubbing bills together. Mud turtles extend and retract their heads, almost touching noses. Women are not the only creatures who use their heads to flirt.[2]

Men also employ courting tactics similar to those seen in other species. Have you ever walked into the boss's office and seen him leaning back in his chair, hands clasped behind his head, elbows high, and chest thrust out? Perhaps he has come from behind his desk, walked up to you, smiled, arched his back, and thrust his upper body in your direction? If so, watch out. He may be subconsciously announcing his dominance over you. If you are a woman, he may be courting you instead.

The "chest thrust" is part of a basic postural message used across the animal kingdom—"standing tall." Dominant creatures puff up. Codfish bulge their heads and thrust out their pelvic fins. Snakes, frogs, and toads inflate their bodies. Antelope and chameleons turn broadside to emphasize their bulk. Mule deer look askance to show their antlers. Cats bristle. Pigeons swell. Lobsters raise themselves onto the tips of their walking legs and extend their open claws. Gorillas pound their chests. Men just thrust out their chests.

When confronted by a more dominant animal, many creatures shrink. People turn in their toes, curl their shoulders, and hang their heads. Wolves tuck their tails between their legs and slink. Subordinate lobsters crouch. And many species bow. A bullied codfish curls its body downward. Lizards move their whole bodies up and down. Deferential chimpanzees nod their heads so rapidly and repeatedly that primatologists call it bobbing.

These "crouch" and "loom" positions seen in a host of creatures are often manifest in courtship too. I recall a cartoon in a European magazine. In the first box a man in swimming trunks stands alone on an empty beach—his head sags, his stomach protrudes, his chest is concave. In the next box, an attractive woman is shown walking along the beach past the man; now his head is erect, his stomach sucked in, his chest inflated. In the last box, the woman is gone and he has resumed his normal, sad-sack pose. It is not uncommon to see men and women swell and shrink in order to signal importance, defenselessness, and approachability.

The "Copulatory" Gaze

The gaze is probably the most striking human courting ploy. Eye language. In Western cultures, where eye contact between the sexes is permitted, men and women often stare intently at a potential mate for about two to three seconds during which their pupils may dilate—a sign of extreme interest. Then the starer drops his or her eyelids and looks away.[3]

No wonder the custom of the veil has been adopted in so many cultures. Eye contact seems to have an immediate effect. The gaze triggers a primitive part of the human brain, calling forth one of two basic emotions—approach or retreat. You cannot ignore the eyes of another fixed on you; you must respond. You may smile and start conversation. You may look away and edge toward the door. But first you will probably tug at an earlobe, adjust your sweater, yawn, fidget with your eyeglasses, or perform some other meaningless movement—a "displacement gesture"—to alleviate anxiety while you make up your mind how to acknowledge this invitation, whether to flee the premises or stay and play the courting game.

This look, known to ethologists as the copulatory gaze, may well be embedded in our evolutionary psyche. Chimpanzees and other primates gaze at enemies to threaten them; they look deeply into the eyes of one another in order to reconcile after a battle too. The gaze is also employed before coitus, as seen among "pygmy" chimpanzees—apes closely related to the common chimp but smaller and perhaps smarter. Several of these almost human creatures live in the San Diego Zoo, where males and females copulate regularly. But just before intercourse the couple spend several moments staring deeply into each other's eyes.[4]

Baboons gaze at each other during courtship too. These animals may have branched off of our human evolutionary tree more than nineteen million years ago, yet this similarity in wooing persists. As anthropologist Barbara Smuts has said of a budding baboon courtship on the Eburru cliffs of Kenya, "It looked like watching two novices in a singles bar."[5]

The affair began one evening when a female baboon, Thalia, turned and caught a young male, Alex, staring at her. They were about fifteen feet apart. He glanced away immediately. So she stared at him—until he turned to look at her. Then she intently fiddled with her toes. On it went. Each time she stared at him, he looked away; each time he stared at her, she groomed her feet. Finally Alex caught Thalia gazing at him—the "return gaze."

Immediately he flattened his ears against his head, narrowed his eyelids, and began to smack his lips, the height of friendliness in baboon society. Thalia froze. Then, for a long moment, she looked him in the eye. Only after this extended eye contact had occurred did Alex approach her, at which point Thalia began to groom him— the beginning of a friendship and sexual liaison that was still going strong six years later, when Smuts returned to Kenya to study baboon friendships.

Perhaps it is the eye—not the heart, the genitals, or the brain— that is the initial organ of romance, for the gaze (or stare) often triggers the human smile.

"There is a smile of love / And there is a smile of deceit," wrote the poet William Blake. Actually human beings have at least eighteen distinctive types of smiles,[6] only some of which we use while court- ing. Both men and women use the "simple smile," a closed-mouth gesture, when they greet a familiar passerby. In this expression, the lips are closed but stretched, and no teeth are showing; the gesture is often combined with a nod to express acknowledgment. People who smile at you like this will probably not pause to get acquainted.

The human "upper smile" signals stronger interest. In this expres- sion, you expose your upper teeth to show your positive intentions. The upper smile is often combined with a one-sixth-of-a-second eye- brow flash, in which the eyebrows are raised, then quickly dropped. Eibl-Eibesfeldt has seen this upper smile among Europeans, Bali- nese, Amazonian Indians, and Bushmen of southern Africa, and he reports that it is used in all sorts of friendly contacts—including flirting. Chimps and gorillas use this half smile when they play. But they show their bottom teeth rather than their top ones. In this way they conceal their daggerlike upper fangs, canine teeth with which they threaten one another.

The "open smile," in which the lips are completely drawn back and both upper and lower teeth are fully exposed, is what we often use to "pick up" one another. Former President Jimmy Carter's smile is a remarkable example. Carter was courting our minds, our votes, our opinions; had he coupled this "super smile" with the sequential flirt, the coy look, the head toss, the chest thrust, or the gaze, his intentions would have been unmistakably sexual instead.

The "nervous social smile," another type of human grin, plays a distinctly negative role in courtship. It stems from an ancient mammalian practice to bare one's teeth when cornered. I once saw a marvelous example of it during a television appearance. My host was being verbally assailed by her other guest. She could not be impolite or leave the set. So she pulled her lips back and exposed both rows of firmly clenched teeth. Then she froze, holding this nervous grin.

Chimpanzees employ the nervous social smile, the "bared teeth" display, when confronted by a superior. They use it to express a combination of fear, friendliness, and appeasement. We make the nervous social smile in difficult social situations too, but never when courting. So if a potential lover grins at you with clenched teeth, you can be fairly sure that he or she is thinking less of wooing than of surviving the introduction.

Universal Courting Cues

Despite the obvious correlations between the courting gestures of humans and those of other animals, it has taken over a century of investigation to prove that human beings around the world actually do share many of the same nonverbal cues. Darwin was the first to wonder about the heritability of human facial expressions and body postures. To confirm his suspicion that all men and women use the same gestures and poses to express basic human emotions, he sent a query to colleagues in remote areas of the Americas, Africa, Asia, and Australia in 1867.

Among his many questions about the aboriginals were these: "When a man is indignant or defiant does he frown, hold his body and head erect, square his shoulders and clench his fists?" "Is disgust shown by the lower lip being turned down, the upper lip slightly raised, with a sudden expiration?" "When in good spirits do the eyes sparkle, with the skin a little wrinkled round and under them, and with the mouth a little drawn back at the corners?"[7]

Scientists, journalists, missionaries, and friends from around the world replied yes to Darwin's queries, and he became convinced that joy, sorrow, happiness, surprise, fear, and many other human feelings were expressed in panhuman gestural patterns inherited from a common evolutionary past. These nonverbal cues included the human smile. As he later wrote in his book *The Expression of the Emotions in Man and Animals* (1872), "With all the races of man the expression of good spirit appears to be the same, and is easily recognized."

More than a hundred years later psychologist Paul Ekman and his colleagues confirmed Darwin's conviction that the same basic facial postures are used by various peoples around the world. When he showed pictures of American faces to Fore tribesmen of New Guinea, Sadong villagers of Sarawak, Brazilians, and Japanese and asked them to identify the expressions, these diverse men and women easily recognized the expressions of sorrow, surprise, disgust, fear, and anger—as well as the American grin.[8]

Smiling, it seems, we were born to do. Some infants begin to imitate their mother's smile within thirty-six hours after birth, and all babies begin social smiling at about three months of age.[9] Even children born blind and deaf burst into radiant grins, although they have never seen this facial gesture in those around them.

Like the smile, the sequential flirt, the coy look, the head toss, the chest thrust, and the gaze are probably all part of a standard human repertoire of gestures that, used in certain contexts, evolved to attract a mate.

Could these courting cues be part of a larger human mating dance?

David Givens, an anthropologist, and Timothy Perper, a biologist, think so. Both scientists have spent several hundred hours in American cocktail lounges watching men and women pick each other up. Givens did his work in the pubs around the University of Washington campus in Seattle. Perper sipped his beer, stared at young singles, and took notes in the Main Brace Lounge, The Homestead, and other bars in New Jersey, New York, and eastern Canada. Both scientific voyeurs found the same general pattern to the courting process.[10]

According to these investigators, American singles-bar courtship has several stages, each with distinctive escalation points. I shall divide them into five. The first is the "attention getting" phase. Young men and women do this somewhat differently. As soon as they enter the bar, both males and females typically establish a territory—a seat, a place to lean, a position near the jukebox or dance floor. Once settled, they begin to attract attention to themselves.

Tactics vary. Men tend to pitch and roll their shoulders, stretch, stand tall, and shift from foot to foot in a swaying motion. They also exaggerate their body movements. Instead of simply using the wrist to stir a drink, men often employ the entire arm, as if stirring mud. The normally smooth motion necessary to light a cigarette becomes a whole-body gesture, ending with an elaborate shaking from the elbow to extinguish the match. And the whole body is employed in hearty laughter—made loud enough to attract a crowd. Thus simple gestures are embellished, overdone.

Then there is the swagger with which young men often move to and fro. Male baboons on the grasslands of East Africa also swagger when they foresee a potential sexual encounter. A male gorilla walks back and forth stiffly as he watches a female out of the corner of his eye. This parading gait is known to primatologists as bird-dogging. Males of many species also preen. Human males pat their hair, adjust their clothes, tug their chins, or perform other self-clasping or grooming movements that diffuse nervous energy and keep the body moving.

Older men often use different props, advertising their availability with expensive jewelry, clothing, and other accoutrements that spell success. But all of these signals can be reduced to one basic, three-part message: "I am here; I am important; I am harmless." What a difficult mixture of signals to give out simultaneously—importance *and* approachability. Yet men succeed; women regularly court men.

"It is better to be looked over than overlooked," Mae West once said. And women know it. Young women begin the attention-getting phase with many of the same maneuvers that men use—smiling, gazing, shifting, swaying, preening, stretching, moving in their territory to draw attention to themselves. Often they incorporate a battery of feminine moves as well. They twist their curls, tilt their heads, look up coyly, giggle, raise their brows, flick their tongues, lick their upper lips, blush, and hide their faces in order to signal, "I am here."

Some women also have a characteristic walk when courting; they arch their backs, thrust out their bosoms, sway their hips, and strut. No wonder many women wear high-heeled shoes. This bizarre Western custom, invented by Catherine de Medici in the 1500s, unnaturally arches the back, tilts the buttocks, and thrusts the chest out into a female come-hither pose. The clomping noise of their spiky heels helps draw attention too.

With this high-heeled gait, puckered lips, batting eyes, dancing brows, upturned palms, pigeoned toes, rocking bodies, swaying skirts, and gleaming teeth, women signal approachability to men.

Grooming Talk

Stage two, the "recognition" stage, starts when eyes meet eyes; then one or the other potential lover acknowledges the demarche with a smile or slight body shift, and the couple move into talking range.[11] This can be the beginning of the romance.

But it is nowhere near as risky as the next major escalation point: stage three—talk. This idle, often meaningless conversation, which Desmond Morris calls grooming talk, is distinctive because voices often become higher, softer, and more singsongy—tones one also uses to express affection to children and concern for those in need of care.

Grooming talk starts with such benign statements as "I like your watch" or "How's the food?" The icebreakers are as varied as the human imagination, but the best leads are either compliments or questions, since both require a response. Moreover, *what* you say often matters less than *how* you say it. This is critical. The moment you open your mouth and speak, you give away your intentions with your inflection and intonation. A high-pitched, gentle, mellifluous "hello" is often a sign of sexual interest, whereas a clipped, low, matter-of-fact, or perfunctory "hi" rarely leads to love. If a prospective mate laughs somewhat more than the situation calls for, she or he is probably flirting too.

Talking is dangerous for an important reason. The human voice is like a second signature that reveals not only your intentions but also your background, education, and intangible idiosyncrasies of character that can attract or repel a potential mate in moments. Actors, public speakers, diplomats, and habitual liars know the power of vocal tones, so they regularly modulate their voices. Movie actors raise their voices almost an octave to adopt sweet, flowing tones when "flirting" on the set. And smart liars avoid fibbing on the telephone, a purely auditory medium where subtle inconsistencies in emphasis and intonation are easily discerned. We are taught from childhood to control our facial expressions, as when our parents tell us to "smile for grandma," but most of us are unconscious of the power of the voice.

Both Givens and Perper saw many potential love affairs go astray soon after conversation started.[12] But if a couple weather this perceptual onslaught—and each begins to listen *actively* to the other—they often move to stage four: touch.[13]

Touching begins with "intention cues"—leaning forward, resting one's arm toward the other's on the table, moving one's foot closer if both persons are standing or stroking one's own arm as if to stroke the other's. Then the climax—one person touches the other on the shoulder, the forearm, the wrist, or some other socially available body part. Normally the woman touches first, grazing her hand along her suitor's body in the most casual but calculated manner.

How insignificant this touching looks, yet how important this touching is. Human skin is like a field of grass, each blade a nerve ending so sensitive that the slightest graze can etch into the human brain a memory of the moment. The receiver notices this message instantly. If he flinches, the pickup is over. If he withdraws, even barely, the sender may never try to touch again. If he ignores the overture, she may touch once more. But if he leans toward her, smiles, or returns the gesture with his own deliberate touch, they have surmounted a major barrier well known in the animal community.

Most mammals caress when courting. Blue whales rub each other with their flippers. Male butterflies stroke and rub their mate's abdomens as they couple. Dolphins nibble. Moles rub noses. Dogs lick.

Chimpanzees kiss, hug, pat, and hold hands. Mammals generally stroke, groom, or nuzzle prior to copulation.

Touch has been called the mother of the senses. No doubt this is true, for every human culture has codes that indicate who may touch whom and when, where, and how. Imaginative and resourceful in their variety, these touching games are basic to human courting too. So if our pair continue to talk and touch—bobbing, tilting, gazing, smiling, swaying, flirting—they usually achieve the last stage of the courtship ritual: total body synchrony.

Keeping Time

Body synchrony is the final and most intriguing component of the pickup. As potential lovers become comfortable, they pivot or swivel until their shoulders become aligned, their bodies face-to-face. This rotation toward each other may start before they begin to talk or hours into conversation, but after a while the man and woman begin to move in tandem. Only briefly at first. When he lifts his drink, she lifts hers. Then they desynchronize. In time, however, they mirror each other more and more. When he crosses his legs, she crosses hers; as he leans left, she leans left; when he smooths his hair, she smoothes hers. They move in perfect rhythm as they gaze deeply into each other's eyes.

This beat of love, of sex, of eternal human reproduction, may be interrupted at any moment. But if the two are to pass on the thread of human life, they will resume their tempo and continue their mating dance. Couples that reach total body synchrony often leave the bar together.

Is the five-part pickup universal to men and women? We do not know. Certainly not everybody in the world exhibits all of the behavior patterns that Givens and Perper found in American singles joints. People in most societies do not meet in bars. Many do not even court one another openly; instead, their marriages are arranged. And few anthropologists have studied the postures, gestures, and expressions that men and women in other cultures use when they interact. But there is a great deal of ancillary evidence to suggest that some of these patterns are universal to humankind.

In Borneo, for example, a Dusun woman often cocks her head and gazes at a potential lover. When she passes him the rice wine at a party, she casually touches him on the hands as well.[14] In fact, most travelers know that you do not have to speak the local language to flirt successfully. The gaze, the smile, the gentle touch seem to be integral to wooing everywhere.

There is even more evidence that body synchrony is universal to human courtship. In every society where men and women are allowed to choose their lovers, singles meet at parties or festivals and dance. And what is dancing but rhythmic gestures, tandem body movement?

The Medlpa of New Guinea have even ritualized this mimicry. Among these people unmarried girls meet potential spouses in a *tanem het*, a common-room in their parents' house. Several potential spouses, dressed from head to toe in finery, assemble and sit in pairs. The "head rolling" festivities begin as couples sing. Then potential partners sway their heads, rub foreheads and noses, and bow to each other repeatedly, all to a throbbing beat. To the Medlpa, synchrony is harmony. They say that the better one partner keeps the other's time, the more likely the couple are suited to each other.[15]

Actually, body synchrony is basic to many social interactions—courtship being only one. In the 1960s a student of anthropologist Edward Hall took a camera to a playground in the American Midwest and, crouching behind an abandoned car to watch and tape, he caught on film the children's movements as they interacted during recess. Carefully studying the filmed sequences, Hall noticed in the children's body motions a uniform, synchronized rhythm. Apparently all of the children played in tandem, to a beat. Moreover, one very active little girl skipped around the playground—and set the pace. Every other child unconsciously kept her time.[16]

Called interactional synchrony, this human mirroring begins in infancy. By the second day of life, a newborn has begun to synchronize its body movements with the rhythmic patterns of the human voice. And it is now well established that people in many other cultures get into rhythm when they feel comfortable together. Photographs and slow-motion films of people in cafés, railroad stations, supermarkets, cocktail parties, and other public places in diverse societies illustrate this human tendency to adopt one another's postures.

And the beat goes on. When friends are hooked up to electro-encephalographs, which measure brain activity, the resulting tracings show that even brain waves get "in sync" when two people have a harmonious conversation. In fact, if you sit at the dinner table and watch carefully, you can conduct the conversation with your hand as family members talk and eat. Stressed syllables usually keep the beat. But even silences are rhythmic; as one person pats her mouth, another reaches for the salt—right on cue. Rests and syncopations, voices lowered, elbows raised, these mark the pulse of living as well as of love.[17]

Our need to keep each other's time reflects a rhythmic mimicry common to many other animals. On a number of occasions primatologist Wolfgang Kohler entered the chimp enclosure in a primate research center to find a group of males and females trotting in "a rough approximate rhythm" around and around a pole. Kohler said the animals wagged their heads as they swung along, each leading with the same foot. Chimps sometimes sway from side to side as they stare into one another's eyes just prior to copulation too. In fact, nothing is more basic to courtship in animals than rhythmic movement. Cats circle. Red deer prance. Howler monkeys court with rhythmic tongue movements. Stickleback fish do a zigzag jig. From bears to beetles, courting couples perform rhythmic rituals to express their amorous intentions.

To dance is natural. So I think it reasonable to suggest that body synchrony is a universal stage of the human courting process: as we become attracted to each other, we begin to keep a common beat.

Wooing Runs on Messages

Human courtship has other similarities to courtship in "lower" animals. Normally people woo each other slowly. Caution during courtship is also characteristic of spiders. The male wolf spider, for example, must enter the long, dark entrance of a female's compound in order to court and copulate. This he does slowly. If he is overeager, she devours him.

Men and women who are too aggressive at the beginning of the courting process also suffer unpleasant consequences. If you come too close, touch too soon, or talk too much, you will probably be repelled. Like wooing among wolf spiders, baboons, and many other creatures, the human pickup runs on messages. At every juncture in the ritual each partner must respond correctly, otherwise the courtship fails.

In fact, Perper began to see a curious division of labor in this exchange of signals. American women generally initiate the courting sequence—starting with subtle nonverbal cues such as a slight shift in body weight, a smile, or gaze. Women began two-thirds of all the pickups that Perper witnessed. And the women he later interviewed were quite conscious of having coaxed a potential lover into conversation, touching him carefully here or there, enticing him ever forward with coquettish looks, questions, compliments, and jokes.

Female forwardness is not, of course, a purely American phenomenon. In the 1950s Clellan Ford and Frank Beach, well-known tabulators of cross-cultural sex practices, confirmed that although most peoples think men are supposed to take the initiative in sexual advances, in practice women around the world actively begin sexual liaisons. This is still the case. Men and women in seventy-two of ninety-three societies surveyed in the 1970s maintained that both sexes demonstrated a roughly equal sex drive.[18]

The strong human female sex drive mirrors behavior in other parts of the animal kingdom. All female mammals come into "heat," and as estrus emerges they actively solicit males, behavior known as female proceptivity.

A wild female chimpanzee in estrus, for instance, will stroll up to a male, tip her buttocks toward his nose, and pull him to his feet to copulate. When he has finished, she copulates with almost every other male in the community. In one laboratory environment, captive female chimps initiated up to 85 percent of all matings.[19] Captive male orangutans tend to fall asleep after coitus, but at the height of estrus a female will pester a male to stay awake for a second round. And if you have not seen the aggressive sexuality of female apes, surely you have observed the antics of female dogs. You have to bar the door if you want a bitch in heat to remain chaste.

This female sexual persistence makes biological sense. As Darwin pointed out, those who breed survive. Thus it is to a female's genetic advantage to seek sex.

In fact, it is curious that Westerners cling to the concept that men are the seducers and women the coy, submissive recipients of male overtures. This false notion is probably a relic of our long agricultural past, when women were pawns in elaborate property exchanges at marriage and their value depended on their "purity." Hence girls were strictly chaperoned, and their sex drive was denied. Today, however, Western women have regained their sexual freedom. Released from the world of arranged betrothals and sexual subservience, they are often pursuers too.

Eventually, however, the man must respond to the woman's overtures if the liaison is to proceed. As one woman reported to Perper, "At some point the man should get the hint and take it from there."

Men seem to sense this shift in leadership, a shift that Perper calls initiative transfer. It normally occurs just after the couple have left the bar. Now the male must begin his "moves"—put his arm around the woman, kiss her, woo her into the mood for coitus. And it is interesting how well men know their role. When Perper asked thirty-one of his male informants to describe the pickup sequence, all but three skipped over the initial parts—those directed by the woman. Only one man could recall the details of who spoke first, who touched whom when, or how either partner began to express interest in the other. But all thirty-one men spoke at length about their own duties, how they started to kiss, pet, and maneuver the woman into bed.

Who, then, is the hunter, who the prey, who the seducer, who the bewitched? Clearly both partners play essential roles. If one or the other misses an important cue, the pickup ends. When all the signals are received and each responds correctly, the beat continues. But, like other animals engaged in courtship, human partners must play on time for the pickup to succeed.

American singles bars in a peculiar way resemble the singles clubs of certain birds—the lek. *Lek* is a Swedish ornithological term for a piece of ground where male and female birds meet, mix, and match. Not many avian species copulate at a leking ground, but among them is the North American sage grouse. In early March male sage grouse appear at locations ranging from eastern California to Montana and Wyoming. There, on specific patches of open meadow used yearly for mating, each male establishes a tiny "display" territory where he proceeds, for several hours after dawn for about six weeks, to propagandize—strutting, preening, "booming," and puffing to advertise his importance to passing females.[20]

Female sage grouse migrate to the leking ground after the males are settled. First a female struts through the property boundaries of these male establishments and surveys the occupants, a process that may take her two or three days. Then she rests inside the territory of an individual she finds appealing. Shortly both resident and guest begin their courting dance, adapting to each other's rhythms, parading to show their affection before they mate.

Are the antics at cocktail parties, church socials, office luncheons, bars, or after-hours clubs fundamentally different from the cavorting on a leking ground? As an anthropologist, I find it difficult to ignore the fact that people and sage grouse both set up display territories, both exhibit mannerisms designed to pick the other up, and both move in synchrony before they mate. Apparently nature has a few basic rules of courtship.

The Dinner Date

Two more universal features of wooing are less subtle—food and song. Probably no single ritual is more common to Western would-be lovers than the "dinner date." If the man is courting, he pays— and a woman almost instinctively knows her partner is wooing her. In fact, there is no more widespread courtship ploy than offering food in hopes of gaining sexual favors in exchange. Around the world men give women presents prior to lovemaking. A fish, a piece of meat, sweets, and beer are among the countless delicacies men have invented as offerings.[21]

This ploy is not exclusive to men. Black-tipped hang flies often catch aphids, daddy longlegs, or houseflies on the forest floor. When a male has felled a particularly juicy prey, he exudes secretions from an abdominal scent gland that catch the breeze, announcing a successful hunting expedition. Often a passing female hang fly stops to enjoy the meal—but not without copulating while she eats. Male birds feed potential lovers too. The male common tern often brings a little fish to his beloved. The male roadrunner presents a little lizard. Male chimpanzees living along Lake Tanganyika, in eastern Africa, offer a morsel of baby gazelle, hare, or some other animal they have caught and killed. The estrous female consumes the gift, then copulates with the donor.[22]

"The way to a man's heart is through his stomach," the adage says.

Perhaps. A few female mammals do feed their lovers; women are among them. But around the world courting women feed men with nowhere near the regularity that men feed women.[23] And where food is impractical or unfashionable, men give their girlfriends tobacco, jewelry, cloth, flowers, or some other small but prized gifts as tokens of their affection and as a mild enticement for a tryst.

"Courtship feeding," as this custom is called, probably predates the dinosaurs, because it has an important reproductive function. By providing food to females, males show their abilities as hunters, providers, and worthy procreative partners.

"If music be the food of love, play on." Shakespeare elegantly played tribute to the last primeval courting lure—melody. Singing or playing a musical instrument to attract a mate is a common practice around the world. Among the Hopi Indians of the American Southwest, men traditionally sang a complex love song to an intended. So did men among the Samoans of the western Pacific, the Chiricahua of the American Southwest, and the Sanpoil of what is today the eastern part of the state of Washington. An Apache man hoped to entice a girl into the woods by serenading her with his flute, and both men and women among the Ifugao of central Luzon, Philippines, used the lover's harp to generate ardor in a beloved.[24]

Perhaps the society most captivated by music is our own, however. From the "ghetto blaster" radios that teenagers carry through the streets to the loudspeakers that blare in almost every public place, music reigns wherever men and women congregate. And when you are invited to "his" or "her" house for dinner, you can be sure you will get more than pizza or a steak; you will get music too.

As might be expected, the melodies of human courtship are echoed in the songs of the animal community. Just step outdoors on a sultry summer night to hear the din. Frogs croak. Crickets chirp. Cats howl. Insects sing. Porcupines emit a piercing whine. Alligators bellow. Throughout the animal kingdom, the rutting calls of males—from the drumming air bladder of the haddock and muted rumble of the elephant to the "chip" of a tiny gecko lizard—serve as potent courting signs.

A few decades ago Otto Jespersen, the Danish philologist, even speculated that early human courting sounds stimulated the evolution of language. "Language," he said, "was born in the courting days of mankind; the first utterances of speech I fancy to myself like something between the nightly love-lyrics of puss upon the tiles and the melodious love-songs of the nightingale."[25] This sounds far-fetched. There were probably several reasons why early men and women needed advanced communication. But love songs, like national anthems, can certainly "stir the blood."

I would like to think that courtship starts when "he" or "she" makes a marvelous joke about an unlikable politician, an astute comment about the world economy, or a tantalizing remark about a recent play or sports event—something humorous, intelligent. But infatuation may begin with the slight tilt of a head, a gaze, a gentle touch, a tender syllable, a slab of roast beef in a fancy restaurant, or a whispered tune during a swaying dance. Then the body rushes forward, leaving the intellect to unravel this feeling of infatuation: "Why him?" "Why her?"

~2~

Infatuation

Why Him? Why Her?

*The meeting of two personalities is
like the contact of two chemical substances;
if there is any reaction,
both are transformed.*

—*Carl Jung*

"For should I see thee a little moment, / Straight is my voice hushed; / Yea, my tongue is broken, and through and through me, / 'Neath the flesh, impalpable fire runs tingling." So began a poem describing infatuation written by Sappho on the Greek island of Lesbos some twenty-five hundred years ago.[1]

Almost everybody knows what infatuation feels like. That euphoria. That torment. Those sleepless nights and restless days. Awash in ecstasy or apprehension, you daydream during class or business, forget your coat, drive past your turn, sit by the phone, or plan what you will say—obsessed, longing for the next encounter with "him" or "her." Then, when you meet again, his slightest gesture stops your pulse. Her laugh dizzies you. You take foolish risks, say stupid things, laugh too hard, reveal dark secrets, talk all night, walk at dawn, and often hug and kiss—oblivious to all the world as you tumble through a fever, breathless, etherized by bliss.

Despite thousands of poems, songs, books, operas, dramas, myths, and legends that have portrayed infatuation since before the time of Christ, despite the countless times a man or woman has deserted family and friends, committed suicide or homicide, or pined away because of love, few scientists have given this passion the study it deserves. Sigmund Freud dismissed infatuation as a blocked or delayed sex urge. Havelock Ellis called romantic attraction "sex-plus-friendship," an unconvincing description of this fever. And many people assume that infatuation is a mystical, intangible, inexplicable, even sacred experience that defies the laws of nature and the scrutiny of science. Hundreds of academics and philosophers mention infatuation in passing; few have tried to understand this animal attraction to another human being.

Falling in Love

One telling dissection of this madness, however, is found in *Love and Limerence,* by psychologist Dorothy Tennov.[2]

In the mid-1960s Tennov devised approximately two hundred statements about romantic love and asked four hundred men and women at and around the University of Bridgeport, in Connecticut, to respond with "true" or "false" reactions. Hundreds of additional individuals answered subsequent versions of her questionnaire. From their responses, as well as their diaries and other personal accounts, Tennov identified a constellation of characteristics common to this condition of "being in love," a state she calls limerence, which some psychiatrists call attraction and I will call infatuation.

The first dramatic aspect of this condition is its inception, the moment when another person begins to take on "special meaning." It could be an old friend seen in a new perspective or a complete stranger, but as one informant put it: "My whole world had been transformed. It had a new center and that center was Marilyn."

Infatuation then develops in a characteristic pattern, beginning with "intrusive thinking." Thoughts of the "love object," or the beloved, begin to invade your mind. A certain thing he said rings in your ear; you see her smile, recall a comment, a special moment, an innuendo—and relish it. You wonder what your love would think of the book you are reading, the movie you just saw, or the problem you are facing at the office. And every tiny segment of the time the two of you have spent together acquires weight and becomes material for review.

At first these intrusive reveries occur irregularly. Some informants reported that thoughts of their beloved invaded their consciousness less than 5 percent of their waking hours. But many said that, as the obsession grew, they spent from 85 to almost 100 percent of their days and nights in sustained mental attentiveness, doting on this single individual. Moreover, they began to focus on the most trivial aspects of the adored one and aggrandize them in a process Tennov calls crystallization.

Crystallization is distinct from idealization in that the infatuated person does indeed perceive the weaknesses of his or her idol. In fact, all of Tennov's limerent subjects could list the faults of their beloved. But they simply cast these flaws aside or convinced themselves that these defects were unique and charming. And they unremittingly doted on the positive parts of their sweetheart's physical features and personality.

Paramount in the daydreams of Tennov's infatuated informants were two overriding sensations: hope and uncertainty. If the cherished person gave the slightest positive response, the infatuated partner would replay these precious fragments in reverie for days. If he or she rebuffed one's overtures, uncertainty might turn to despair instead and the "limerent" would moon about listlessly, brooding until he or she had managed to explain away this setback and renew the quest. Interestingly, a key incendiary was adversity; this always intensified one's passion.

And underlying all of this angst and ecstasy was unmitigated fear. A twenty-eight-year-old truck driver summed up what most informants felt: "I'd be jumpy out of my head," he said. "It was like what you might call stage fright, like going up in front of an audience. My hand would be shaking when I rang the doorbell. When I called her on the phone I felt like I could hear the pulse in my temple louder than the ringing of the phone. . . ."

Most of Tennov's informants reported trembling, pallor, flushing, a general weakness, and overwhelming sensations of awkwardness, stammering, even loss of their most basic faculties and skills. Stendhal, the nineteenth-century French novelist, described this feeling perfectly. Recalling the afternoons he went strolling with his sweetheart, he wrote, "Whenever I gave my arm to Leonore, I always felt I was about to fall, and I had to think how to walk."[3]

Shyness, fear of rejection, anticipation, and longing for reciprocity were other central sensations of infatuation. Above all, there was the feeling of helplessness, the sense that this passion was irrational, involuntary, unplanned, uncontrollable. As a business executive in his early fifties wrote to Tennov, about an office affair, "I am advancing toward the thesis that this attraction for Emily is a kind of biological, instinct-like action that is not under voluntary or logical control. . . . It directs me. I try desperately to argue with it, to limit its influence, to channel it (into sex, for example), to deny it, to enjoy it, and, yes, dammit, to make her respond! Even though I know that Emily and I have absolutely no chance of making a life together, the thought of her is an obsession."

Infatuation, it seems, is a panoply of intense emotions, rollercoastering from high to low, hinged to the pendulum of a single being whose whims command you, to the detriment of everything around you—including work, family, and friends. And this involuntary mosaic of sensations is only partially related to sex. Ninety-five percent of Tennov's female informants and 91 percent of her male subjects rejected the statement "The best thing about love is sex."

Why do we fall in love with Ray instead of Bill, Sue instead of Ceciley? Why him? Why her? "The heart has its reasons which reason knows nothing of," contended philosopher Blaise Pascal. Scholars can, however, provide some "reasonable" explanations for this hurricane of emotion.

Odor Lures

Infatuation could be triggered, in part, by one of our most primitive traits—our sense of smell. Every person smells slightly different; we all have a personal "odor print" as distinctive as our voice, our hands, our intellect. As newborn infants we can recognize our mother by her smell, and as we grow up we come to detect over ten thousand different odors.[4] So if nature be our guide, we are probably susceptible to odor lures.

Many creatures use odors to seduce, as was made abundantly clear to the French naturalist Jean Henri Fabre almost a century ago. Fabre had found a cocoon of the beautiful emperor moth. He brought it into his country home and left it in his study overnight. The next morning a female emerged, sparkling from metamorphosis. Fabre put her in a cage. To his astonishment forty male emperor moths flapped through his open window that evening to woo the virgin; over the next few nights more than 150 males appeared. As Fabre finally established, this female moth had exuded an invisible secretion from her distended abdomen—a "pheromone," the smell of which had attracted suitors from over a mile across the country-side.[5]

Since the time of Fabre's experiments, the odor lures of over 250 insect species, and of many other animals, have been isolated. Some of these smells—such as castoreum, from the scent glands of Russian and Canadian beavers; musk, the red, jellylike pheromone of the East Asian musk deer; and civet, a honeylike secretion from the Ethiopian civet cat—have been worn by people as diverse as the ancient Greeks, Hindus, and Chinese to intoxicate a sweetheart.

But the human body may produce some of the most powerful olfactory aphrodisiacs of all. Both men and women have "apocrine" glands in their armpits, around their nipples, and in the groin that become active at puberty. These scent boxes differ from "eccrine" glands, which cover much of the body and produce an odorless liquid, because their exudate, in combination with bacteria on the skin, produce the acrid, gamy smell of perspiration.

Baudelaire thought one's soul resided in this erotic sweat. The nineteenth-century French novelist Joris Karl Huysmans, used to follow women through the fields, smelling them. He wrote that the scent of a woman's underarms "easily uncaged the animal in man." Napoleon agreed. He reportedly sent a letter to his sweetheart, Josephine, saying, "I will be arriving in Paris tomorrow evening. Don't wash."[6]

Today in parts of Greece and the Balkans, some men carry their handkerchiefs in their armpits during festivals and offer these odoriferous tokens to the women they invite to dance; they swear by the results. In fact, sweat is used around the world as an ingredient in love potions. In Shakespeare's day, a woman held a peeled apple under her arm until the fruit became saturated with her scent; then she presented this "love apple" to her lover to inhale. A contemporary recipe concocted by some Caribbean immigrants to the United States reads, "Prepare a hamburger patty. Steep it in your own sweat. Cook. Serve to the person desired."[7]

But could a man's smell actually *trigger* infatuation in a woman? This is extremely hard to test. In 1986 Winnifred Cutler, George Preti, and their colleagues at the Monell Chemical Senses Center, in Philadelphia, found an intriguing relationship between women, men, and odor.[8] They designed an experiment in which male volunteers wore pads in their armpits several days a week. "Male essence" was then extracted from these pads, mixed with alcohol, frozen, stored, and then thawed and dabbed on the upper lip of women who came to the clinic three times a week. The women reported they smelled nothing except alcohol.

The results were startling. Some of the women entered the test with irregular menstrual cycles, periods that were either longer or shorter than the average 29.5 days. After twelve to fourteen weeks of treatment, however, these women's monthly menstrual cycles became more normal. Male essence seems to stimulate normal cycling, an important aspect of fertility potential.

This possible link between male essence and female reproductive health may provide a clue to attraction. Women perceive odors better than men do. They are a hundred times more sensitive to Exaltolide, a compound much like men's sexual musk;[9] they can smell a mild sweat from about three feet away; and at midcycle, during ovulation, women can smell men's musk even more strongly. Perhaps ovulating women become more susceptible to infatuation when they can smell male essence and are unconsciously drawn toward it to maintain normal menstrual cycling.

Key to Cutler and Preti's data, however, is the finding that women are affected by male essence only when they are exposed through direct contact with their bodies. Whether male pheromones can attract a woman from a distance is unknown.

There is some evidence, though, that women's body smells can have a long-distance effect on men. Over a decade ago researchers reported that female roommates in college dorms and women who work or live in close proximity have synchronized menstrual cycles.[10] These data are speculative. But in other animals, estrus synchrony is caused by odor missiles, pheromones.

Could a "female essence" cause this synchrony in women too? To find out, Preti, Cutler, and their colleagues exposed ten women with normal cycles to the underarm sweat of other women.[11] They used the same technique: every few days these subjects received a dab of women's perspiration under their nostrils. Within three months the subjects' menstrual cycles began to coincide with the cycles of the sweat donors. If women do indeed exude smells potent enough to affect other women, perhaps these odors can actually intoxicate a man across a crowded room.

His smell or her smell could spark strong physical and psychological reactions. Between your eyes, within your skull, at the base of your brain, some five million olfactory neurons dangle from the roof of each nasal cavity, swaying in the air currents you inhale. These nerve cells transmit messages to the part of the brain that controls your sense of smell. But they also link up with the limbic system, a group of primitive structures in the middle of your brain that govern fear, rage, hate, ecstasy, and lust. Because of this brain wiring, smells have the potential to create intense erotic feelings.

A woman's or a man's smell can release a host of memories too. The limbic system contains the seat of long-term memory; thus you can remember odors years after smelling them, whereas many visual and auditory perceptions fade in days or weeks. A poignant literary evocation of this odor memory occurs in Kipling's poem "Lichtenberg," where he wrote that the smell of rain-soaked acacia trees meant home to him. No doubt you can remember the perfume of a

Christmas tree, the family dog, even a former lover—and all the feelings these evoke. So the right human smell at the right moment could touch off vivid pleasant memories and possibly ignite that first, stunning moment of romantic adoration.

But Americans, the Japanese, and many other people find body odors offensive; for most of them the smell of perspiration is more likely to repel than to attract. Some scientists think the Japanese are unduly disturbed by body odors because of their long tradition of arranged marriages; men and women were forced into close contact with partners they found unappealing.[12] Why Americans are phobic about natural body smells, I do not know. Perhaps our advertisers have swayed us in order to sell their deodorizing products.

But we certainly like commercially made aromas on a mate. We buy fragrant shampoos, scented soaps, after-shave lotions, and perfumes at exorbitant prices. Then smells of food, fresh air, tobacco, and smells of the office and the home all mix with our natural smells to make an odor soup. A silent label. And people respond. In a recent survey by the Fragrance Foundation, both men and women rated scent as an important aspect of sex appeal—giving odor an 8.4 rating on a scale of 10.[13] Like emperor moths, human beings find smells sexually exciting.

But cultural opinions about perspiration clearly vary. Climate, types of clothing, access to daily bathing, concepts of cleanliness, upbringing, and many other cultural variables condition one's appetite for odors. Moreover, the link between human pheromones and the euphoric, despairing state we call infatuation remains unknown.

This much I propose, however: when you meet someone new whom you find attractive, you probably "like the smell of him," and this helps predispose you to romance. Then, once infatuation flowers, the scent of your sweetheart becomes an aphrodisiac, a continuing stimulant to the love affair.

Love Maps

A more important mechanism by which human beings become captivated by "him" or "her" may be what sexologist John Money calls your love map.[14] Long before you fixate on Ray as opposed to Bill,

Sue instead of Ceciley, you have developed a mental map, a template replete with brain circuitry that determines what arouses you sexually, what drives you to fall in love with one person rather than another.

Children develop these love maps, Money thinks, between ages five and eight (or even earlier) in response to family, friends, experiences, and chance associations. For example, as a child you get used to the turmoil or tranquillity in your house, the way your mother listens, scolds, and pats you and how your father jokes or walks or smells. Certain temperamental features of your friends and relatives strike you as appealing; others you associate with disturbing incidents. And gradually these memories begin to take on a pattern in your mind, a subliminal template for what turns you off, what turns you on.

As you grow up, this unconscious map takes shape and a composite proto-image of the ideal sweetheart gradually emerges. Then in teenage, when sexual feelings flood the brain, these love maps solidify, becoming "quite specific as to details of the physiognomy, build, race and color of the ideal lover, not to mention temperament, manners and so on."[15] You have a mental picture of your perfect mate, the settings you find enticing, and the kinds of conversations and erotic activities that excite you.[16]

So, long before your true love walks past you in a classroom, at a shopping mall, or in the office, you have already constructed some basic elements of your ideal sweetheart. Then, when you actually see someone who fits within these parameters, you fall in love with him or her and project onto this "love blot" your unique love map. The recipient generally deviates considerably from your actual ideal. But you brush aside these inconsistencies to dote on your own construction. Hence Chaucer's famous words "Love is blynd."

These love maps vary from one individual to the next. Some people get turned on by a business suit or a doctor's uniform, by big breasts, small feet, or a vivacious laugh. Her voice, the way he smiles, her connections, his patience, her spontaneity, his sense of humor, her interests, his aspirations, her coordination, his charisma—myriad obvious as well as tiny, subliminal elements work together to make one person more attractive than the next. We can all list a few specific things we find appealing; deep in our unconscious psyche are many more.

American tastes in romantic partners show some definite patterns, however. In a test done in the 1970s, 1,031 Caucasian college students at the University of Wyoming rated what they found sexually appealing.[17] Their answers confirmed what you might expect. Men tended to prefer blondes, blue eyes, and lighter skin color, while women liked darker men. But there were some surprises. Few men liked very large breasts or the slender, boyish female figure, and almost none of the women were attracted to an extremely muscular physique. In fact, both sexes preferred the average. Too short, too tall, too slight, too "built," too pale or dark—the extremes were weeded out.

Averageness still wins. In a more recent study, psychologists selected thirty-two faces of American Caucasian women and, using computers, averaged all of their features. Then they showed these composite images to college peers. Of ninety-four photographs of real female faces, only four were rated more appealing than these fabrications.[18]

As you would guess, the world does not share the sexual ideals of Caucasian students from Wyoming. When Europeans first emigrated to Africa, their blond hair and white skin reminded some Africans of albinos, regarded as hideous. The traditional Nama of southern Africa particularly like dangling vulvar lips, so mothers conscientiously massage the genitals of their infant daughters to make them hang enticingly by teenage. Women in Tonga traditionally diet to stay slim, while Siriono women of Bolivia eat continually to stay fat.

In fact, there is seemingly no end to the varieties of human body embellishments designed to trigger infatuation: stretched necks, molded heads, filed teeth, pierced noses, scarred breasts, scorched or "tanned" skin, and high-heeled shoes in which women can hardly walk, not to mention the two-foot orange gourd penis sheathes of New Guinea tribesmen and the purple-dyed beards of distinguished Elizabethan gentlemen. Beauty truly is in the eyes of the beholder.

But everywhere people find particular aspects of those around them sexually appealing.

Despite wildly dissimilar standards of beauty and sex appeal, however, there are a few widely shared opinions about what incites romantic passion. Men and women around the world are attracted to those with good complexions. Everywhere people are drawn to partners whom they regard as clean. And men in most places generally prefer plump, wide-hipped women to slim ones.[19] Looks count.

So does money. From a study of thirty-seven peoples in thirty-three countries, the psychologist David Buss uncovered a distinct male/female difference in sexual preferences.[20] From rural Zulus to urban Brazilians, men are attracted to young, good-looking, spunky women, while women are drawn to men with goods, property, or money. Americans are no exception. Teenage girls are impressed by boys with flashy cars, and older women like men with houses, land, boats, or other expensive accoutrements. Hence the gentle, poetic carpenter will probably not attract the women an insensitive rich banker will collect.

These male/female appetites are probably innate. It is to a male's genetic advantage to fall in love with a woman who will produce viable offspring. Youth, clear skin, bright eyes, vibrant hair, white teeth, a supple body, and a vivacious personality indicate good health, vitality important to his genetic future. To women, belongings indicate power, prestige, success, and the ability to provide. For good reason: it is to a woman's biological advantage to become captivated by a man who can help support her young. As Montaigne, the sixteenth-century French essayist, summed it up, "We do not marry for ourselves, whatever we say; we marry just as much or more for our posterity."

The Chase

But let there be mystery. A degree of unfamiliarity is essential to infatuation; people almost never become captivated by someone they know well—as a classic study on an Israeli kibbutz clearly illustrates.[21] Here infants were placed in peer groups during the day while their parents worked. Before the age of ten these children often engaged in sexual play, but as they moved into adolescence boys and girls became inhibited and tense with one another. Then, in teenage, they developed strong brother–sister bonds. Almost none married within their peer group, however. A study of 2,769 kibbutzim marriages found that only 13 occurred between peers and that in each of them one mate had left the communal group before the age of six.

Apparently during a critical period in childhood, most individuals lose forever all sexual desire for those they see regularly. Mystery is critical to romantic love.

Barriers also seem to provoke this madness. The chase. If a person is difficult "to get" it piques one's interest. In fact, this element of conquest is often central to infatuation, hence what has become known as the Romeo and Juliet effect: if real impediments exist, such as the family feud between Shakespeare's Montagues and Capulets, these obstructions are likely to intensify one's passion. No wonder people fall for an individual who is married, a foreigner, or someone separated from them by an obstacle that appears almost insurmountable. Yet generally there must also be some slight possibility of fulfillment before one's first stirrings of infatuation escalate into an obsession.

Timing also plays an important role in infatuation.[22] When individuals are looking for adventure, craving to leave home, lonely, displaced in a foreign country, passing into a new stage in life, or financially and psychologically ready to share themselves or start a family, they become susceptible. From her questionnaires and interviews with over eight hundred Americans, Tennov reported that infatuation occurred only after one had become ready to shower attention on a love object.

Last, as a rule we are drawn to people like ourselves. Likes tend to marry likes—individuals of the same ethnic group, with similar physical traits and levels of education, what anthropologists call positive assortive mating.

Infatuation generally first takes place shortly after puberty. But it can happen at any stage in life. Children experience puppy love;

some octogenarians fall crazily in love. Once an individual becomes receptive, though, he or she is in danger of falling in love with the next reasonably acceptable person who comes along.

Love at First Sight

It is this constellation of factors appearing *all at once* —including timing, barriers, mystery, similarities, a matched love map, even the right smells—that make you susceptible to falling in love. Then, when that potential love object cocks his or her head, smiles or gazes at you, you get that rush. It can happen gradually or in a second— hence the phenomenon of love at first sight.

And this powerful, sometimes instantaneous attraction is not unique to Westerners.

Andreas Capellanus, a cleric at the court of Eleanor of Aquitaine in twelfth-century France, wrote of infatuation, "Love is a certain inborn suffering derived from the sight of and excessive meditation upon the beauty of the opposite sex, which causes each one to wish above all things the embraces of the other."[23] Since then some Westerners have come to believe that romantic love is an invention of the troubadours—those knights, poets, and romantics of eleventh- to thirteenth-century France who waxed eloquent on the vicissitudes of amour.

I find this preposterous. Romantic love is far more widespread. Vatsya, the author of the *Kama Sutra,* the classic work on love in Sanskrit literature, lived in India sometime between the first and sixth century A.D., and he clearly described romantic love between men and women. He even provided detailed instructions on how couples might court, embrace, kiss, fondle, and copulate. Despite the Confucian emphasis on filial piety that has long saturated Chinese mores, written tales dating back to the seventh century A.D. reveal the agony of men and women torn between obedience to their elders and romantic passion for a loved one.[24] In traditional Japan, star-crossed lovers sometimes chose double suicide, known as *shin ju,* when they found themselves betrothed to different partners.

The eastern Cherokee believed that if a young man sings to a girl at midnight, "she will dream of him, become lonesome for him and, when they next meet, be drawn irresistibly to him." Yukaghir girls of northeast Siberia wrote "love letters" on birch bark. In Bali, men believed a woman would "fall in love" if her suitor fed her a certain kind of leaf incised with the image of a god who sported a very large penis.

Even peoples who deny having concepts of "love" or "being in love" act otherwise. Mangaians of Polynesia are casual in their sexual affairs, but occasionally a desperate young man who is not permitted to marry his girlfriend kills himself. The Bem-Bem of the New Guinea highlands do not admit that they feel this passion either, but a girl sometimes refuses to marry the man whom her father has chosen for her and runs away with a "true love" instead. The Tiv of Africa, who have no formal concept of romance, call this passion "madness."[25]

Love stories, myths, legends, poems, songs, instruction manuals, love potions, love charms, lovers' quarrels, trysts, elopements, and suicides are part of life in traditional societies around the world. In fact, in a survey of 168 cultures, anthropologists William Jankoviak, and Edward Fischer were able to find direct evidence for the existence of romantic love in 87 percent of these vastly different peoples.[26]

This madness, this limerence, this attraction, this infatuation, this ecstasy so regularly ignored by scientists, must be a universal human trait.

It is entirely possible that infatuation is not unique to people either. What first made me suspect this was an anthropological account of a home-raised American gorilla named Toto. Toto regularly came into heat for about three days in the middle of her monthly menstrual cycle; apparently she also became infatuated with human males. One month it was the gardener, the next the chauffeur or the butler, at whom she gazed with "unmistakable lovesick eyes."[27]

Consorting lions show great tenderness for each other during the female's period of heat. Giraffes gently caress each other before they mate. Baboons, chimpanzees, and other higher primates show distinct preferences for one individual rather than the next, friendships that endure even when the female is not sexually receptive. And a pair of elephants will spend hours side by side during the female's period of receptivity, often stroking each other with their trunks. Many animals pat, nuzzle, coo, and gaze at one another affectionately as they court.

The most curious story of possible infatuation in another species, however, was reported in 1988. Newspapers carried the story of a moose that seemed to fall in love with a cow in Vermont.[28] The stricken herbivore trailed his idol for seventy-six days before he gave up his amorous "come hither" gesturing. That despair, that euphoria of infatuation, may strike more than just humankind.

Love at first sight. Could this human ability to adore another within moments of meeting come out of nature? I think it does. In fact, love at first sight may have a critical adaptive function among animals. During the mating season a female squirrel, for example, needs to breed. It is not to her advantage to copulate with a porcupine. But if she sees a healthy squirrel, she should waste no time. She should size him up. And if he looks suitable, she should grab her chance to copulate. Perhaps love at first sight is no more than an inborn tendency in many creatures that evolved to spur the mating process. Then among our human ancestors what had been animal attraction evolved into the human sensation of infatuation at a glance.

But how has nature actually created the bodily feeling of infatuation? What is this thing called love?

The Chemistry of Love

People probably began to discuss attraction more than a million years ago as they lay on riverbanks in Africa to rest and watch the sky. More-recent thinkers have come up with astute observations about this fever. W. H. Auden likened sexual craving to "an intolerable neural itch." H. L. Mencken described it differently, saying, "To be in love is merely to be in a state of perceptual anaesthesia." Both sensed that something physical was happening in the brain, anticipating what could be an astonishing discovery about the chemistry of love.

This violent emotional disturbance that we call infatuation (or attraction) may begin with a small molecule called phenylethylamine, or PEA. Known as the excitant amine, PEA is a substance in the brain that causes feelings of elation, exhilaration, and euphoria. But to understand exactly how PEA might contribute to attraction, you need to know a few things about the inside of your head.

The human brain is about the size of a grapefruit, weighing approximately three pounds, with an average volume of about 1,400 cubic centimeters. It is about three times larger than those of our closest relatives, chimpanzees and gorillas, whose average brain volumes are approximately 400 and 500 cubic centimeters respectively.

In the 1970s neuroscientist Paul MacLean postulated that the brain is divided into three general sections. Actually, it is a good deal more complex than this, but MacLean's perspective is still useful as an overview. The most primitive section surrounds the final bulb at the end of the spinal cord. This area, which deserves its reputation as the "reptilian brain," governs instinctual behaviors such as aggression, territoriality, ritual, and the establishment of social hierarchies. We probably use this area of the brain in courtship when we "instinctively" strut, preen, and flirt.

Above and surrounding the reptilian brain is a group of structures in the middle of the head known collectively as the limbic system. As was mentioned earlier, these structures govern the basic emotions — fear, rage, joy, sadness, disgust, love, and hate. So when you are overcome with happiness, paralyzed with fright, infuriated, revolted, or despondent, it is portions of the limbic system that are producing electrical and chemical disturbances. The storm of infatuation almost certainly has its physical origin here.

Overlaying the limbic system (and separated by a large layer of white matter that communicates between brain parts) is the cortex, a gray, convoluted rind of spongy matter that lies directly below the skull. The cortex processes basic functions like sight, hearing, speech, and mathematical and musical abilities. Most important, the cortex integrates your emotions with your thoughts. It is this section of the brain that *thinks* about "him" or "her."

Here, then, is how PEA (and probably other neurochemicals, such as norepinephrine and dopamine) may play a role. Within and connecting the three basic parts of the brain are neurons, or nerve cells; there are at least one hundred billion of them. Impulses travel through one neuron and jump across a gap—a synapse—to the next nerve cell. This way they gambol along the neuronal highways of the mind.

PEA lies at the end of some nerve cells and helps the impulse jump from one neuron to the next. Equally important, PEA is a natural amphetamine; it revs up the brain. So psychiatrist Michael Liebowitz of the New York State Psychiatric Institute speculates that we feel infatuation when neurons in the limbic system, our emotional core, become saturated or sensitized by PEA and/or other brain chemicals—and stimulate the brain.[29]

No wonder lovers can stay awake all night talking and caressing. No wonder they become so absentminded, so giddy, so optimistic, so gregarious, so full of life. Naturally occurring amphetamines have pooled in the emotional centers of their brains; they are high on natural "speed."

Romance Junkies

Liebowitz and his colleague Donald Klein arrived at this conclusion while treating patients they called attraction junkies. These people crave a relationship. In their haste they pick an unsuitable partner. Soon they are rejected, and their exhilaration turns to despair—until they renew their quest. As this cycle of miserable love affairs proceeds, the romance junkie swings from feeling brokenhearted and desperately depressed to feeling elated over each inappropriate, ill-fated romantic fling.

Both psychiatrists suspected that these lovesick people suffered from a tangle in their romantic wiring—specifically a craving for PEA. So in some highly experimental work they gave these attraction junkies MAO inhibitors. These antidepressant drugs block the action of a special enzyme in the brain—monoamine oxidase, or MAO, a class of substances that break down PEA and other neurotransmitters (norepinephrine, dopamine, and serotonin). Thus MAO inhibitors actually boost levels of PEA and these other natural amphetamines, heightening the infatuation high.

To everyone's astonishment, within weeks of receiving MAO inhibitors, one perpetually lovesick man began to choose his partners more carefully, even starting to live comfortably without a mate. Apparently he no longer craved the PEA high he used to get from his exciting yet disastrous love affairs. This patient had been in therapy for years, sessions that had helped him understand himself. "But it appears," says Liebowitz, "that until the MAO inhibitor was administered, he was largely unsuccessful in applying what he had learned, because of his overriding emotional response."

Psychiatrist Hector Sabelli independently arrived at the same conclusion about PEA. In a study of thirty-three people who were happily attached to a "significant other" and who reported to Sabelli that they were feeling great, *all* were found to have high levels of the PEA metabolite in their urine too. PEA levels were low in a man and woman who were going through a divorce—probably, he says, because both spouses were suffering from a low-grade depression as they parted.[30]

PEA seems to have a powerful effect on nonhuman creatures as well as people. When mice are injected with PEA, they jump and squeal, a display of mouse exhilaration known in laboratory jargon as "popcorn behavior." Rhesus monkeys injected with PEA-like chemicals make pleasure calls and smack their lips, a courting gesture, and baboons press levers in their cages more than 160 times in a three-hour period to obtain supplements that maintained a PEA high.

Auden and Mencken probably described romantic attraction astutely. The feeling of infatuation may result from a deluge of PEA and/or other natural stimulants that saturate the brain, transforming the senses, altering reality.

But infatuation is more than exhilaration. It is part of love, a deep, "mystical" devotion to another human being. Is this complex sensation due solely to natural stimulants in the brain?

Not at all. In fact, PEA may give us no more than a generalized sense of awakeness, alertness, excitement and an elevated mood, as Sabelli suggests. Sabelli measured the amount of PEA released in the urine of parachute jumpers before and after a jump. During free-fall, PEA levels soared. A divorcing couple also experienced a PEA high during court proceedings.[31] It appears, then, that PEA gives us no more than a shot of exhilaration and apprehension—a chemical high that accompanies a range of experiences, including infatuation.

Cupid's Second Arrow: Culture

Liebowitz's and Sabelli's work on the chemistry of love has caused a great deal of controversy, not only among colleagues who, like them, recognize that this research is still speculative, but also among those embroiled in the old nature/nurture controversy—that perennial debate about how much of our behavior derives from genes, from nature and heredity, how much of human conduct stems from childhood experiences, from culture, from what we learn.

So here I should stress a critical concept. The brain and body produce dozens (if not hundreds) of different chemicals that affect behavior. Adrenaline, for example, is secreted by the adrenal glands when one gets angry, frightened, or euphoric; it makes the heart pump faster, quickens breathing, and prepares the body for action in several other ways. But it is not adrenaline that triggers rage, fear, or joy; it is stimuli from the environment.

For example, a colleague at the office says something snide about your work. You are insulted—a largely learned response. Your body secretes adrenaline. You feel this fuel. Then your culturally conditioned mind *converts* this natural energy into fury, as opposed to fear or joy. And you shoot a caustic comment at your peer.

In the same way, culture plays a major role in love. You begin in childhood to like and dislike the smells in your environment. You learn to respond to certain kinds of humor. You get used to the peace or hysteria in your home. And you begin to build your love map from your experiences. Then, in teenage, you join the military, go away to college, or become otherwise displaced. These and many other *cultural* events determine *whom* you love, *when* you love, *where* you love. But after you find that special person, it is probably PEA and/

or other natural neurochemicals in the brain that direct *how* you feel *as* you love. As usual, culture and biology go hand in hand.

There seems to be some variation in this experience from one individual to the next, however. Some of those who report they have never felt romantic love suffer from hypopituitarism, a rare disease in which the pituitary malfunctions in infancy, causing hormonal problems—as well as "love blindness." These men and women lead normal lives; some marry for companionship; but that rapture, that heartache are mythology to them.[32]

Tennov also found variation among the over eight hundred Americans she polled about romance in the 1960s and 1970s. A few men and women claimed that they had never felt infatuation, whereas others fell in love quite frequently. But Tennov reports that the vast majority of both genders experienced the ecstasy of romantic love— and they felt it "in roughly equal proportions." Sexologists John Money and Anke Ehrhardt confirm this; like Tennov, they found no gender differences in the experience of infatuation.[33]

Scientists are far from understanding this obsession. But one fact is becoming undeniable: infatuation is a physical as well as a psychological phenomenon. And physical mechanisms evolve through evolution. The limbic system, the emotional core of the brain, is rudimentary in reptiles but well developed in all mammals. So I shall maintain in following chapters that our first ancestors inherited the primal emotion of animal attraction and then evolved the engulfing sensation of infatuation as they adapted to an entirely new world in the grasslands of Africa some four million years ago.

Alas, infatuation fades. As Emerson put it, "Love is strongest in pursuit, friendship in possession." At some point, that old black magic wanes. For teenagers a "crush" can last a week. Lovers who see each other irregularly, because of some barrier like an ocean or a wedding ring from another person, can sometimes sustain that smitten feeling for several years.

Yet there does seem to be a general length to this condition. Tennov measured the duration of romantic love, from the moment infatuation hit to when a "feeling of neutrality" for one's love object began. She concluded, "The most frequent interval, as well as the average, is between approximately 18 months and three years." John Money agrees, proposing that once you begin to see your sweetheart regularly the passion typically last two to three years.[34]

Liebowitz suspects that the end of infatuation is also grounded in brain physiology. He theorizes that the brain cannot eternally maintain the revved-up state of romantic bliss. Either the nerve endings become habituated to the brain's natural stimulants or levels of PEA (and/or other natural amphetamine-like substances) begin to drop. The brain can no longer tolerate the onslaught of these drugs. As he sums it up, "If you want a situation where you and your long-term partner can still get very excited about each other, you will have to work on it, because in some ways you are bucking a biological tide."[35]

Now an even more insidious emotion emerges—attachment. This is the warm, comfortable, secure feeling that so many couples report. And Liebowitz is convinced that, as infatuation wanes and attachment grows, a new chemical system is taking over—the opiates of the mind. These substances, the endorphins (short for "endogenous morphines"), are chemically similar to morphine, an opiate, a narcotic. Like PEA, the endorphins reside at the brain's nerve endings, travel between synapses from one nerve cell to the next, and pool in specific areas in the brain. Unlike PEA, they calm the mind, kill pain, and reduce anxiety.

Liebowitz theorizes that partners in the attachment stage of love trigger the production of endorphins in each other, giving each the sense of safety, stability, tranquillity. Now lovers can talk and eat and sleep in peace.[36]

No one has speculated about how long the stage of attachment lasts, either in the brain or in relationships. I suspect it varies with different human brains, with social circumstances, and with age. As you will see during the course of this book, the older you get, the easier it is to remain attached. But the sensation of infatuation has both a beginning and an end. As Stendhal brilliantly put it, "Love is like a fever that comes and goes quite independently of the will."

Why does love ebb and flow? The pulse of infatuation, like many of our courting gestures, may be part of nature's scheme—soft-wired in the brain by time, by evolution, and by ancient patterns of human bonding.

~ 3 ~

Of Human Bonding

Is Monogamy Natural?

Breathes there a man with hide so tough
Who says two sexes aren't enough?

—*Samuel Hoffenstein*

When Darwin used the term *survival of the fittest* he was not referring to your good looks or your bank account; he was counting your children. If you raise babies that have babies, you are what nature calls fit. You have passed your genes to the next generation and in terms of survival you have won. So the sexes are locked in a mating dance, endlessly adjusting their moves to complement those of each other. Only in tandem can either men or women reproduce and pass on the beat of human life.

This mating dance—our basic human "reproductive strategy"—began long, long ago when the world was young and our primordial ancestors evolved into two sexes.

Why Sex?

Different species replicate differently. A few, like a variety of whiptail lizards, have done away with sex entirely. These little reptiles roam the semiarid chaparral of the American Southwest. During the breeding season, each develops eight to ten unfertilized ova, eggs that will hatch as perfect replicas of themselves. This type of asexual reproduction—parthenogenesis, or virgin birth—has its practical side. Whiptails do not expend their time or energy courting one another. They do not mix their genes with those of other whiptails, individuals that may have inferior genetic makeups. They don't have to haul about heavy antlers like male elk to fight other courters, or outlandish tail feathers like male peacocks to woo females. They don't even attract predators as they court or copulate. And they produce offspring that carry 100 percent of their DNA.

Is love between the sexes necessary? Not for desert-grassland whiptails, some dandelions, blackberries, quaking aspen trees, or the asexual wild grasses. For these species, even mating has been dispensed with.[1]

Despite the enormous Darwinian advantages of asexuality, however, our ancestors and many other creatures went the way of sexual reproduction—for at least two reasons. Individuals who mate create one vital asset in their offspring: variety. A collie and a poodle may produce a puppy that looks nothing like either of its parents. This can have bad consequences; sometimes mixture produces a poor match. But recombination creates new genetic "personalities." Some will die. But some will live and overcome nature's tireless effort to weed out poor strains.

Recently biologists proposed a more subtle explanation for why our primitive forebears evolved sexual reproduction: to confuse enemies.[2] This is known as the Red Queen hypothesis, after an incident in Lewis Carroll's book *Through the Looking Glass.*

The Red Queen takes Alice by the arm, and together they run madly, hand in hand. But when they stop, they are exactly where they started. The Queen explains this bizarre situation to Alice, saying, "Now here, you see, it takes all the running you can do, to keep in the same place." Translated into evolutionary thinking, this means that creatures that change regularly remain biologically less susceptible to the bacteria, viruses, and other parasites that kill them. Thus sexual reproduction evolved to elude one's germs.[3]

But why *two* sexes, males and females? Why didn't our primeval progenitors choose a reproductive strategy in which any individual could exchange its genetic material with that of any other?

Bacteria do this. Organisms simply come together and exchange DNA. A can mate with B; B can mate with C; C can mate with A; everybody can mate with everybody else; bacteria have no sexual distinctions.[4] Unlike bacteria, however, the remote ancestors of human beings (and many other creatures) developed into two distinct types: females with big, sluggish eggs composed of DNA and rich, surrounding nutriments and males with little, agile sperm stripped bare of all but genes.

No one knows how two separate sexes evolved in the primordial goo. One suggestion is that our first sexual ancestors somewhat resembled bacteria but were larger, multicellular life forms that produced sex cells (gametes) containing half their DNA. Like bacteria, each individual produced gametes that could combine with any other gamete. But some organisms disseminated big gametes surrounded by a lot of nutritious cytoplasm. Others sprayed forth smaller sex cells with less fodder. Still others propelled tiny gametes with almost no added food aboard.

All of these sexual creatures cast their sex cells into the ocean currents. When two small gametes united, however, they lacked enough nutriments to survive. When two big sex cells joined, they were too ungainly to live on. But when a lithe, little, unencumbered gamete, a proto-sperm, united with a big, nutrient-laden gamete, a proto-egg, the new organism lived through its precarious beginning. And with time two separate sexes evolved, one carrying eggs, the other transporting sperm.[5]

There are problems with this theory, as well as alternative hypotheses.[6] And, regrettably, there are no living organisms that portray the lifeways of our first sexual ancestors. But somehow, billions of years ago, individuals of two complementary strains developed. Then two separate sexes emerged. And their continually varying offspring lived and multiplied across the eons of our restless, changing past.

Sexual Paths Our Ancestors Overlooked

It is a wonder our rude antecedents did not opt for the sex life of strawberries—creatures that, like the little whiptail lizard, can reproduce asexually but also engage in sexual mating. When strawberries feel secure, the patch is unexploited, and the environment is unchanging, they clone. Why bother with sex? Only when space runs out, forcing strawberries to disperse into uncharted lands, do they put forth flowers and mate. When the pioneer berries settle in, however, they start to clone again.

Earthworms have another variation of sexuality. These creatures are both male and female at the same time; they can impregnate themselves. But most hermaphroditic plants and animals go to great lengths to avoid self-fertilization, a process that has the deficits of both sexuality and asexuality.

Perhaps the most eccentric form of reproduction, by human standards, exists in species in which individuals are able to transform themselves from one sex into the other. Among these are fish that live along the Great Barrier Reef of Australia. Known as cleaner fish, or *Labroides dimidiatus,* these reef combers live in groups of one male and five or six females. If the single male dies or disappears, the most dominant female begins to metamorphose into a male. Within a few days "she" is "he."

If men and women were able to clone themselves, if we could be both sexes simultaneously, or if we could totally transform ourselves within hours from one sex into the other, we probably would not have evolved our courting gaze, our flirting brow, or the brain physiology for infatuation and attachment. But the ancestors of human beings, like the vast majority of other living species, did not elect the sex lives of cloning strawberries, hermaphroditic earthworms or transsexual fish. Instead, we became men and women, subspecies that must mix our genes or slip into oblivion.

Copulation is not the only way that you and I ensure our genetic futures. A second means by which sexual organisms propagate their

DNA is a process known as kin selection.[7] This is derived from a reality of nature: every individual shares his or her genetic makeup with blood relatives. From the mother the child receives half its genes; from the father, the other half. If a child has full brothers or sisters, it shares half its genes with each of them. One-eighth of its genes it shares with cousins, and so forth. So if a man or woman spends a lifetime nurturing genetic relatives, he or she is actually helping his or her own DNA; when kin survive, you survive—hence the concept of "inclusive fitness."[8] No wonder people around the world tend to favor their genetic kin.

Our surest way to posterity, however, is through mating. In fact, all of our human rituals concerning courtship and mating, marriage and divorce, can be regarded as scripts by which men and women seduce each other in order to replicate themselves—what biologists call reproductive strategies. What are these mating games?

Well, men have two choices, as do women, and the elegance of each is that it is easily distinguished by counting heads. A man can mate with a single woman at a time, monogyny (from the Greek *mono*, "one," and *gyny*, "female), or he can have several mates simultaneously, polygyny (many women). Women have two similar options: monandry (one man) or polyandry (many men). These terms are commonly used to describe human marriage types. Thus the dictionary defines *monogyny* as "the state or custom of having only one wife at a time," *monandry* as "one husband," *polygyny* as "many wives," and *polyandry* as "many husbands." *Monogamy* means "one spouse"; *polygamy* connotes "many spouses" without designating gender.[9]

Hence monogamy does not imply fidelity.

This is important to remember: the word *monogamy* is regularly misused. The *Oxford English Dictionary* defines monogamy as "the condition, rule or custom of being married to only one person at a time." This does not suggest that partners are sexually faithful to one another. Zoologists James Wittenberger and Ronald Tilson use the term *monogamy* to refer to "a prolonged association and essentially exclusive mating relationship between one male and one female."[10]

But fidelity is not central to this scientific definition either. They add, "By 'essentially exclusive' we imply that occasional covert matings outside the pair bond, (i.e. 'cheating') do not negate the existence of monogamy."

So *monogamy* and *fidelity* are not synonymous. What is more, adultery often goes hand in hand with monogamy, as well as with the other reproductive strategies mentioned here.[11]

Nature's Peyton Place

Male red-winged blackbirds, for example, oversee large territories of marsh during the breeding season; several females join a single male on his patch of real estate and copulate with only him—monandry. Or so the story goes. Recently scientists vasectomized some of these males prior to the breeding season.[12] Females then joined these neutered males, copulated with them, and nested in their home ranges—nothing unusual.

Many of these females laid fertile clutches, though. Clearly these monandrous females had not been sexually faithful to their partners. To be positive of this, scientists took blood samples from the infant nestlings of thirty-one female red-winged blackbirds. Almost half of all nests contained one or more chicks whose father was not the landlord. Most of these females had copulated with "floaters" or with a male that lived next door.[13]

Adultery is common in other species too. Ornithologists have observed these extrapair copulations, or "sneakers," in over one hundred species of monogamous birds. The little South American monkeys, female marmosets and tamarins, as well as many other monogamous female mammals once thought to be paragons of virtue, also "cheat." The marshes, the meadows, the forests across the earth may be nature's Peyton Place.

And if you have missed the combination of monogamy and cheating in red-winged black birds or marmosets, surely you have noticed philandering in people. All married men and women in the United States are, by definition, monogamous; bigamy is against the law. According to some recent estimates, over 50 percent of all married Americans are adulterous as well.[14] No one knows how accurate these figures are. But no one would deny that adultery occurs in every culture around the world.

So here's the point. Men in some cultures have only one wife, while some men in other societies have a harem; some women marry only one man at a time, while others have several husbands simultaneously. But marriage is only part of our human reproductive strategy; extramarital sex is often a secondary, complementary component of our *mixed* mating tactics. However, before I explore the amorphous tangle of human adultery, I would like to examine the human mating patterns that are quite visible—our marriage systems.[15]

Perhaps the most remarkable thing the sexes have in common is that they bother to marry at all. Marriage is a cultural universal; it predominates in every society in the world. Over 90 percent of all American men and women marry; modern census records go back to the mid-1800s.[16] From church ledgers, court records, mortuary lists, and marriage files of ninety-seven industrial and agricultural societies, the Statistical Office of the United Nations has culled data on weddings since the 1940s. Between 1972 and 1981 an average of 93.1 percent of the women and 91.8 percent of the men married by age forty-nine.[17]

Marriage is also the norm where record keepers have not arrived. Among the Cashinahua Indians of Brazil, marriage is a casual affair. When a teenage girl becomes eager to marry and gets her father's permission, she asks her husband-to-be to visit her in her hammock after the family is asleep. He must be gone by daybreak. Gradually he moves his possessions into the family home. But the marriage is not taken seriously until the girl becomes pregnant or the liaison has lasted at least a year. In contrast, Hindu parents in India sometimes pick a husband for their daughter before the child can walk. There are several separate wedding rites. And long after the marriage has been consummated, the families of the bride and groom continue to exchange property according to terms negotiated years before.

Marriage customs vary. But from the steppes of Asia to the coral atolls of the western Pacific, the vast majority of men and women take a spouse. In fact, in all traditional societies marriage marks a critical step into adulthood; spinsters and bachelors are rare.

What are the marriage strategies of men and women? Although I will maintain that monogamy, or pair-bonding, is the hallmark of the human animal, there is no question that a minority of men and women follow other sexual scripts. Men are the more variable of the genders, so let's begin with them.

Harem Building

"Hogamus, higamus, men are polygamous." So the ditty goes. Only 16 percent of the 853 cultures on record actually prescribe monogyny, in which a man is permitted only one wife at a time.[18] Western cultures are among them. We are in the minority, however. A whopping 84 percent of all human societies permit a man to take more than one wife at once—polygyny.

Although anthropologists have used a lot of ink and paper to describe cultural reasons for the widespread permissibility of harem building, it can be explained by a simple principle of nature: polygyny has tremendous genetic payoffs for men.[19]

The most successful harem builder on record was Moulay Ismail the Bloodthirsty, an emperor of Morocco. *The Guinness Book of World Records* reports that Ismail sired 888 children with his many wives. But even Ismail may have been surpassed. Some "hardworking" Chinese emperors copulated with over a thousand women, all carefully rotated through the royal bedroom when they were most likely to conceive. These privileged heads of state are not the only men to experience harem life, however. Polygyny is exceedingly common in some West African societies, where about 25 percent of all older men have two or three wives at once.

The most colorful example of harem building, by Western standards, is the traditional Tiwi, who live on Melville Island, about twenty-five miles off the northern coast of Australia.

In this gerontocracy, custom dictated that all women be married—even those not yet conceived. So after her first menstruation, a pubescent girl emerged from temporary isolation in the bush to greet her father and her future *son*-in-law. As soon as she saw these men, she lay in the grass and pretended to be asleep. Carefully her father placed a wooden spear between her legs; then he handed this ceremonial weapon to his companion, who stroked it, hugged it, and called it wife. With this simple ceremony, her father's friend—a man in his thirties—had just married all of the *unborn* daughters this teenage girl would someday bear.

Because men were betrothed to babies not yet conceived, boys had to wait until their mid-forties to make love to their pubescent wives. Young men had sex, of course; sweethearts sneaked into the bush together all the time. But young men craved the prestige and power that marriage brought. So they learned to wheel and deal, bartering promises, food, and labor for wealth and potential wives in later life. Then, as they accumulated spouses and begot children, men gained control of their daughters' unborn daughters—whom they proceeded to marry off to their friends in exchange for even more potential wives.[20] By his seventieth birthday, a very rich and clever Tiwi gentleman might have collected as many as ten brides, although most had far fewer.

This traditional Tiwi marriage system worked before the coming of the Europeans. Because of the great age difference between spouses, men and women married several times. Women liked choosing new young husbands as they got older. Men and older women savored the wits and bargaining it took to manipulate marriage negotiations. And the Tiwi said that everybody enjoyed the sexual variety.

Women in most societies try to prevent their husbands from taking a junior spouse, although they are less reluctant to accept a younger sister as a co-wife. Nor do women want to be a junior wife. Apart from the chronic jealousy and battles for attention, women married to the same man tend to war with one another over food and the other resources their mutual husband provides. There comes a point, however, when a woman becomes willing to join a harem—a Rubicon known as the polygyny threshold.[21]

This occurred among the Blackfoot Indians of the northern plains of North America at the end of the nineteenth century. By this time warfare had become chronic and casualties were enormous, so eligible Blackfoot men were in short supply. Women needed husbands. At the same time, men needed extra wives. The horses and guns they had acquired from the Europeans enabled these Indians to kill many more buffalo than they had been able to kill on foot with bows and arrows. Successful hunters needed extra hands to tan these hides— the backbone of their trading power. This tipped the balance; unwed girls preferred being the second wife of a rich man to being the only wife of a poor one or a woman with no spouse at all.[22]

Polygyny also occurs in the United States. Although harem building is illegal here, some Mormon men take several wives for religious reasons. Their forefathers in the Church of Jesus Christ of Latter-day Saints, founded in 1831 by Joseph Smith, originally held that men should take more than one wife. And although the Mormon church officially turned away from polygyny in 1890, some devout fundamentalist Mormons still practice plural marriages. Not surprisingly, many of these polygynous Mormon men are also rich.[23]

If polygyny were permitted in New York, Chicago, or Los Angeles, an Episcopalian man with $200 million could probably also attract several women willing to share his love—and his cash.[24]

So men seek polygyny to spread their genes, while women join harems to acquire resources and ensure the survival of their young. But it is important to remember that these are not conscious motivations. If you ask a man why he wants a second bride, he might say he is attracted to her wit, her business acumen, her vivacious spirit, or splendid thighs. If you ask a women why she is willing to "share" a man, she might tell you that she loves the way he looks or laughs or takes her to fancy vacation spots.

But no matter what reasons people offer, polygyny enables men to have more children; under the right conditions women also reap reproductive benefits. So long ago ancestral men who sought polygyny and ancestral women who acquiesced to harem life disproportionately survived, selecting for this unconscious motivation. No wonder harems crop up where they can.

Man: A Monogamous Primate

Because of the genetic advantages of polygyny for men and because so many societies permit polygyny, many anthropologists think that harem building is a badge of the human animal. I cannot agree. Certainly it is a secondary *opportunistic* reproductive strategy. But in the vast majority of societies where polygyny is permitted, only about 5 to 10 percent of men actually have several wives simultaneously.[25] Although polygyny is widely discussed, it is much less practiced.

In fact, after surveying 250 cultures, anthropologist George Peter Murdock summarized the controversy: "An impartial observer employing the criterion of numerical preponderance, consequently, would be compelled to characterize nearly every known human society as monogamous, despite the preference for and frequency of polygyny in the overwhelming majority."[26] Around the world men tend to marry one woman at a time.

"Higamus, hogamus, women monogamous." Indeed, women also tend to take a single spouse—monandry. All women in so-called monogamous societies have only one husband at a time; they never have two spouses simultaneously. In so-called polygynous societies, a woman also marries only one man at a time, despite the fact that she may have co-wives. Because women in 99.5 percent of cultures around the world marry only one man at once, it is fair to conclude that monandry, one spouse, is the overwhelmingly predominant marriage pattern for the human female.

This is not to suggest that women never have a harem of men. Polyandry is rare; only 0.5 percent of all societies permit a woman to take several husbands simultaneously.[27] But it does occur under peculiar circumstances—such as when the women are very rich.

The Tlingit Indians of southern Alaska were wealthy before the Europeans arrived. They lived, as they do today, along the coast of one of the most abundant fishing grounds in the world, the Alaskan archipelago. During the summer months Tlingit men fished for salmon and trapped myriad animals in the woods along the shore. Women joined their husbands at summer fishing and hunting camps, collected berries and wild plants, and converted the catch into dried fish, rich oils, smoked meats, pelts, and valuable trade items of wood and shell. Then, in the autumn, men and women went on trading expeditions along the coast.

But commerce among the Tlingit was fundamentally different from that of Europeans. Women were the traders. Women set the prices, women did the bargaining, women finalized transactions, and women pocketed the gains. Women were often high ranking.[28] And it was not uncommon for a wealthy woman to have two husbands.

Polyandry also occurs in the Himalayas, for a different ecological reason. Well-to-do Tibetan families in the highlands of Limi, Nepal, are determined to keep their estates together; if they divide their landholdings among their heirs, the precious property will lose its value. Besides, parents need several sons to work the soil, herd the cattle, yak, and goats, and work for overlords. So if a couple bear several sons, they coax these boys to share a wife. From the woman's perspective this is polyandry.

Not surprisingly, these co-husbands have problems with one another. Brothers are often of different ages, and a wife of twenty-two may find her fifteen-year-old husband immature and her twenty-seven-year-old spouse sexually exciting. Younger brothers endure the sexual favoritism in order to remain on the family land, however, surrounded by the jewels, the rugs, the horses—the good life. But resentments fester.

Polyandry is rare in people as well as in other creatures, for a good biological reason.[29] Female birds and mammals can bear only a limited number of offspring during their lives. Gestation takes time. The young often require additional care before weaning. And females have distinct intervals between successive births. Women, for example, cannot bear more than about twenty-five children during a lifetime. The record is held by a Russian woman who had sixty-nine babies, mostly multiple births, during the course of twenty-seven pregnancies. But this is phenomenal. Most women in gathering-hunting cultures bear no more than about five infants.[30] Polyandry may help a woman's young survive, but it does not help a woman bear more than a limited number of infants.

For men, polyandry can spell genetic suicide. Male mammals do not go through pregnancy; nor do they lactate. So like the ancient Chinese emperors, all men can have thousands of offspring—if they can get a parade of cooperative partners and withstand sexual exhaustion. Hence if a man joins the harem of a single woman, much of his sperm is wasted.

Horde Living

Even rarer than polyandry is "group marriage," polygynandry, from the Greek meaning "many females males." This sexual tactic deserves mention not because of its frequency but because it reveals the single most important point about human bonding.

You can count on the fingers of one hand the number of peoples that practice group marriage. Among them are the Pahari, a tribe in northern India. There wives are so expensive that two brothers sometimes have to pool their money to pay the "bride price" to a girl's father. She marries both at once. Then, if the brothers become prosperous, they purchase a second bride. Apparently both wives make love to both husbands.[31]

Group wedlock also occurs in the United States in sex communes that crop up decade after decade.[32] But the classic example is the Oneida community—and what went on at this colony illustrates the most essential point about our human mating game.

This avant-garde colony was started in the 1830s by a religious zealot, John Humphrey Noyes, a daring and sexually energetic man who wished to create a Christian, communist utopia.[33] In 1847 his community settled in Oneida, New York, where it functioned until 1881. In its heyday over five hundred women, men, and children worked the communal lands and manufactured the steel traps they sold to the outside world. Everyone lived in one building, Mansion House, which still stands. Each adult had his or her own room. But everything else was shared, including the children they brought into the commune, their clothes, and their sex partners.

Noyes ruled. Romantic love for a particular person was considered selfish, shameful. Men were forbidden to ejaculate unless their partners had passed menopause. No children were to be born. And everybody was supposed to copulate with everybody else.

In 1868 Noyes lifted the ban on reproducing, and, by special permission, several women conceived. Noyes and his son sired twelve of the sixty-two children born within the next few years. But there was growing friction among community members. The younger men were expected to have sex with the older women, while Noyes had first claim to the pubescent girls. In 1879 the men revolted and accused Noyes of raping several young women. He fled. Within months the community disbanded.

Most interesting about the Oneida sexual experiment is this: despite his dictatorial regulations Noyes was never able to keep men and women from falling in love and forming clandestine pair-bonds with one another. Attraction between people was more powerful than his decrees. In fact, no Western experiment in group marriage has managed to thrive for more than a few years. As Margaret Mead put it, "No matter how many communes anybody invents, the family always creeps back."[34] The human animal seems to be psychologically built to form a pair-bond with a single mate.

Is monogamy natural?

Yes.

There certainly are exceptions. Given the opportunity, men often opt for multiple spouses to further their genetic lines. Polygyny is also natural. Women join harems when the resources they can garner outweigh the disadvantages. Polyandry is natural. But co-wives fight. Co-husbands argue too. Both men and women have to be cajoled by riches to share a spouse. Whereas gorillas, horses, and animals of many other species *always* form harems, among human beings polygyny and polyandry seem to be optional opportunistic exceptions; monogamy is the rule.[35] Human beings almost never have to be cajoled into pairing. Instead, we do this naturally. We flirt. We feel infatuation. We fall in love. We marry. And the vast majority of us marry only one person at a time.

Pair-bonding is a trademark of the human animal.

Arranged Love

This is not to suggest that all wives and husbands are infatuated with each other when they wed. In most traditional societies the first marriage of a son or daughter is arranged.[36] Where marriage has been a family's means of making alliances—for example, among many traditional peoples who farmed in Europe and North Africa, as well as in preindustrial India, China, and Japan—a young couple might not even meet until their wedding night. But in the vast majority of cultures, the views of both the boy and girl are sought before wedding plans proceed.

Modern Egyptians provide a good example. Parents of potential spouses design a meeting between the youths; if the two like each other, parents begin to plan the marriage. Even in New York City, traditional Chinese, Korean, Russian-Jewish, West Indian, and Arab parents often introduce their sons or daughters to appropriate partners and encourage them to wed.

Interestingly, many of these people fall in love. This is well documented in India. Hindu children are taught that marital love is the essence of life. So men and women often enter married life enthusiastically, *expecting* a romance to blossom. Indeed romance often does. As the Hindus explain it, "First we marry, then we fall in love."[37] I am not surprised. Since love can be triggered by a single glance in a single moment, no wonder some of these arranged courtships rapidly turn into romantic attachments.

So where are we? The basic human reproductive strategy is monogamy, one spouse, although human beings sometimes live in harems. But you can't kill romantic love. Even where men and women live with several spouses simultaneously, individuals generally have one partner that they prefer. In free sex communes men and women tend to pair up. Even where marriages are strictly arranged and romantic attachments are prohibited, love blossoms—as the novel *The Family,* by Pa Chin, powerfully illustrates.

Chin wrote about life in a traditional Chinese household in the 1930s. Teetering between the ancient Chinese concept of filial piety and modern values of individualism, the young sons of a tyrannical old man struggle to make life meaningful. The eldest accepts his fate and his arranged marriage. But daily he pines for his beloved, a sweetheart who dies of unrequited love for him. The family's chambermaid hurls herself into a lake and drowns; she is of the wrong station to marry the son she loves and wants to avoid an arranged marriage with a hideous old man. The youngest son steals out of the family compound by moonlight to seek fulfillment in one of the freer cities of Westernizing China. All the while, the patriarch dines with his concubine, a woman he fell in love with years before.

For hundreds of years Chinese tradition tried to curb infatuation. Fate, resignation, and obedience were drummed into the young. And the most painful of all the world's fashions—the thousand-year-old practice of foot-binding—kept a young wife at her loom, preventing her from fleeing her husband's house. Today, however, the Chinese have begun to shed their custom of arranged marriages. More and more are buying pulpy romance novels, playing sentimental tunes, dating, divorcing partners they never loved, and choosing spouses for themselves. They call their new convention "free love."

Taboos, myths, rituals, myriad cultural inventions coax the young around the world into arranged marriages. Yet where these marriages can be dissolved, as in New Guinea, on atolls in the Pacific, in much of Africa and Amazonia, people regularly divorce and remarry mates they choose themselves. To court, to fall in love, to form a pair-bond is human nature.

Why are some of us sexually unfaithful to our vows?

～ 4 ～

Why Adultery?
The Nature of Philandering

That we can call these delicate creatures ours,
And not their appetites. I had rather be a toad,
And live upon the vapor of a dungeon,
Than keep a corner in the thing I love
For others' uses.

— *William Shakespeare,* Othello

Along the southern Adriatic coast, the flat Italian beaches are broken by rocky hills that descend into the sea. Here, behind the boulders, in secluded caverns with shallow pools and sandy shoals, young Italian men seduce foreign women they pick up in the resort hotels, on the beaches, and in the bars and discos. Here the boys lose their virginity in their late teens, and here they hone their sexual skills, count their conquests, and build their reputations as dexterous, passionate Italian lovers, personas they will cultivate throughout their lives.

Because local Italian girls are too supervised to be enticed and because prostitution is not practiced in these villages, young men are dependent on the seasonal tourist trade for their sexual education until they wed. But by middle age, these men enter a new network of sexual liaisons, an elaborate quasi-institutionalized system of ex-

tramarital affairs with local village women. With time each philand-
erer learns to exercise discretion and follow strict rules that everybody understands.

As psychologist Lewis Diana reports, adultery is the rule rather
than the exception in these towns that dot the central and southern
Adriatic coast; almost every man has a lover he visits regularly during
weekdays, either late in the morning or in the early evening while
husbands are still at work in the vineyards, on fishing boats, in their
retail shops, or off on their own clandestine business.

Generally middle- and upper-class men have long affairs with married women of the same or lower social standing. Sometimes younger
male servants visit the wives of landowners, while prestigious men
occasionally have trysts with their maids or cooks. But the most
enduring relationships are those between men and women who are
married to others; many of these affairs last for several years or even
life.

The only dalliances that are taboo are those between older, unattached women and young, unmarried men—largely because young
men boast. Gossip is intolerable. In these villages, family is still the
warp and weft of social life, and whispering threatens to expose the
network of extramarital relationships, seriously disrupting community cohesion and destroying family life. So although infidelity is
commonplace among adults—and known to most because of the
lack of privacy—a code of absolute silence prevails. Family life must
not be undermined.

One breach of this collective complicity occurred when a retired
Italian businessman who had lived in America since childhood made
a comment in a men's club about a woman he hoped to lure into a
sexual rendezvous. All listeners immediately fell silent. Then, one by
one, each man rose and walked out. As Diana reports, "The man had
pulled a monumental blunder. No married man ever speaks of his
interest in other women. The taboo is stringent and unbreakable.
Life is difficult enough not to jeopardize one of its rare diversions."[1]

An ocean away in Amazonia extramarital affairs are equally cov-
eted—but much more complex. Among the Kuikuru, a group of

about 160 people who live in a single village along the Xingu River in the jungles of Brazil, men and women often marry shortly after puberty. But sometimes, within months of matrimony, both spouses begin to take lovers known as *ajois*. [2]

Ajois get their friends to arrange their assignations; then they stroll out of the communal compound at the planned moment under the pretense of fetching water, bathing, fishing, or going to tend the garden. Instead, sweethearts rendezvous and sneak off to a distant clearing in the forest, where they talk, exchange small gifts, and copulate. Even the oldest Kuikuru man and woman in the village regularly slip away for an afternoon rendezvous, says anthropologist Robert Carneiro. Most villagers have between four and twelve extra lovers at a time.

Unlike the men of coastal Italy, however, the Kuikuru enjoy discussing these affairs. Even small children can rattle off the lattice of *ajois* relationships, much as American youngsters recite their ABCs. Only husband and wife refrain from speaking of their outside sexual adventures with one another, largely because once faced with the facts, a spouse might feel obliged to confront the offending party publicly, a disruption and embarrassment that all wish to avoid. If a woman flaunts her friendship with a paramour, however, or spends so much time outside the village that she neglects her daily chores, a husband sometimes does get irritated. Then a public argument erupts. But the Kuikuru consider sexual freedom normal; retribution for adultery is rare.

Dozens of ethnographic studies, not to mention countless works of history and fiction, testify to the prevalence of extramarital sexual activities among men and women around the world. [3] Although we flirt, fall in love, and marry, human beings also tend to be sexually unfaithful to a spouse. So this chapter explores this second aspect of our human reproductive strategy—how clandestine relationships vary; why adultery evolved.

The Many Faces of Adultery

The Turu of Tanzania enjoy sexual license during the puberty ceremony of their teenage boys. On the first day's festivities, extramarital lovers dance to imitate intercourse and sing songs extolling the penis, vagina, and copulation. If these dances are not "hot," or full of sexual passion, as the Turu say, the celebration will be a failure. That evening sweethearts consummate what they have suggested all day.[4] Closer to home, the festival of Mardi Gras has an air of sexual license too.

Wife lending, known as wife hospitality, is customary among several Inuit (Eskimo) peoples. This form of adultery stems from their concept of kinship. If a husband is eager to cement his ties with a hunting companion, he may offer the sexual services of his wife—but only with her permission. If all agree, she copulates with this business partner for several days or even weeks. Women also offer sex to visitors and strangers. But Inuit women see these extramarital couplings as precious offerings of everlasting kinship, not as social indiscretions.[5]

Perhaps the most curious custom prescribing overt adultery comes from our Western heritage. In several European societies, a feudal lord had the right to deflower the bride of a vassal on his wedding night—a custom known as the *jus primae noctis,* or "right of the first night." Some historians question whether this rite was widely exercised; but there seems to be some evidence that medieval Scottish nobles did indeed bed their subjects' brides.[6]

Which raises the question: What constitutes adultery? Definitions vary. The Lozi of Africa do not associate adultery with intercourse. The Lozi say that if a man accompanies a married woman he is not related to as she walks along a path, or if he gives her a beer or some snuff, he has committed adultery. This sounds farfetched. But Americans do not always associate adultery with intercourse either. If an American businessman finds himself in a foreign city buying dinner for an attractive colleague and then performing every sexual act with her except copulation, he might think that he has been adulterous—despite the lack of coitus. In fact, in a poll taken by *People* magazine in 1986, some 74 percent of the 750 respondents believed that one does not actually need to engage in intercourse to be unfaithful.[7]

Among the Kofyar of Nigeria, people define adultery quite differently. A woman who is dissatisfied with her husband but does not wish to divorce can take a legitimate extra lover who lives openly with her in her husband's homestead. Kofyar men are permitted the same privilege. And no one regards these extramarital relationships as adultery.

The *Oxford English Dictionary* defines *adultery* as sexual intercourse by a married person with someone other than one's spouse. So, by Western standards, the Italian man, the Eskimo woman, and the Kofyar wife who have engaged extra lovers are committing adultery, while the Lozi husband and the married American who bought a woman a drink, perhaps even reached orgasm with her—but did not have coitus—have not philandered. Cultural mores do indeed affect one's definition of and attitude toward adultery.

This is nowhere more evident than in all agricultural societies where people use the plow (rather than the hoe) to grow crops— cultures such as the traditional Japanese, Chinese, Hindu, and pre-industrial European. In these patriarchal societies *adultery* was not a term even regularly applied to men; it was considered largely a female vice.

The sexual double standard for adultery arose in farming cultures in tandem with the belief that the male was the bearer of the family "seed." It was his duty to reproduce and pass on his lineage. But only in India were men supposed to be faithful to their brides. Throughout much of Asia, husbands were encouraged to have concubines.[8] In China, where a man could have only a single legal wife, concubines were often taken into the family compound and given private apartments, luxuries, and attention. Moreover, these women were treated with much more respect than is a mistress in the West today—largely because concubines served an important purpose, to bear sons. And because their children supplied the blood of the patrilineage, all infants born out of wedlock in China were considered legitimate.

A traditional Chinese or Japanese man could be branded as adulterous only if he slept with the wife of another man. This was taboo. Illicit sex with a married woman was a violation against the woman's husband and his entire ancestry. In China these lawbreakers were burned to death. If a man seduced the wife of his guru in India, he might be made to sit on an iron plate that was glowing hot, then chop off his own penis. A Japanese man's only honorable course was suicide. In traditional Asian agricultural societies, only geishas, prostitutes, slaves, and concubines were fair game. Sex with them was simply not considered adultery.

A woman's sexual rights in traditional India, China, and Japan were an entirely different matter. A woman's worth was measured in two ways: her ability to increase her husband's property and prestige with the dowry she brought into the marriage and her womb's capacity to nurture her husband's seed. Because a woman's responsibility in life was to produce descendants for her mate, she had to be chaste at marriage and sexually faithful to her husband all her life—paternity had to be secure so as not to jeopardize her husband's family line. As a result, a respectable girl was often married off by age fourteen, before she succumbed to clandestine suitors. Then she was tethered to her husband's home under lifelong surveillance by his kin.

And extramarital sex was strictly forbidden to women. An unfaithful wife was not fit to live. A Hindu man could kill an adulterous spouse. In China and Japan a guilty woman was expected to kill herself instead. In these patriarchial societies, a promiscuous wife threatened a man's land, his wealth, his name, his status. Both his ancestors and his descendants were at risk.

This same double standard for adultery was first recorded among the forebears of Western civilization in several law codes written in Semitic dialects between 1800 and 1100 B.C. in towns in ancient Mesopotamia.[9] Surviving portions dealt with the legal position and rights and duties of women.

Like those of other agrarian communities, these early peoples of the Tigris-Euphrates valley felt that a woman had to "maintain her virtue." A wife who was adulterous could be executed or have her nose chopped off. Meanwhile, a husband had license to fornicate with prostitutes whenever he chose; philandering was a transgression only if he coupled with another man's wife or took the virginity of a peer's eligible daughter. Only for these crimes could he receive a stiff fine, castration, or death.

As in America today, however, more than one sexual code operated simultaneously. Some ancients engaged in fertility celebrations in which extramarital coitus was expected.[10] For them sex had an aura of sanctity; the sex act brought fertility and power. But for the most part, stricter codes prevailed in the cradle of Western civilization. Only women, however, were expected to be faithful to a spouse. Among most historical agricultural Asian peoples, male adultery was essentially a trespass against another's property. Moreover, as in other ancient agrarian societies, adultery was not considered sinful, an offense against God.

This would change.

"Thou Shalt Not Commit Adultery."

Adultery first became allied with sin in Western history, according to historian Vern Bullough, among the ancient Hebrews. Prior to the Babylonian exile, earliest Judaism had a simple code of sexual conduct; few sexual practices were equated with immorality. But in the postexile period, from roughly 516 B.C. until the Romans destroyed Jerusalem in A.D. 70, Jewish sexual mores became increasingly identified with God. By Mosaic law a woman had to be a virgin on her wedding night, then remain permanently faithful to her husband's bed. But prostitutes, concubines, widows, and maidservants were permitted to men. Only intercourse with a married woman was banned.[11] God had spoken: "Thou shalt not commit adultery."

In the following, talmudic period, during the first few centuries of the Christian era, Hebrew attitudes toward sex became more explicit.

God, it was said, decreed that husband and wife engage in the marital act on the eve of the Sabbath. Lists were drawn up prescribing the minimal sexual obligations of different social classes. Gentlemen of leisure were to copulate with their wives nightly; laborers who resided in the same city where they worked should engage in intercourse two times a week; businessmen who traveled to other cities should indulge once a week; camel drivers were obliged to have marital sex every thirty days. And scholars should perform their marital duties on Friday night.[12] Sex within marriage became blessed, celebrated, holy.

"Awake, O north wind, and come, O south wind! Blow upon my

garden, let its fragrance be wafted abroad. Let my beloved come to his garden, and eat its choicest fruits." This was but a part of the Song of Solomon, the extravagant and joyous ode to love between husband and wife that the Jews included in the Hebrew Bible in about A.D. 100. A wife's hair, her teeth, her lips, her cheeks, her neck, her breasts were all cause for celebration before the Lord.[13] The Jews likened the adoration between husband and wife to the love between the peoples of Israel and the Lord. But homosexuality, bestiality, transvestitism, masturbation, and adultery by a wife or by a man with a married woman were condemned by God.

This Hebraic attitude toward adultery would greatly influence Western mores, as would some curious customs of the ancient Greeks.

Often called the first people in history to devote themselves to play, the classical Greeks reveled in their games. As Greek gods indulged their concupiscence, so would Greek mortals. By the fifth century B.C. sexual frolic was among the favorite pastimes—for men. Greek men considered themselves superior to women. Well-bred girls were married off in their early teens to men twice their age, then treated more like wards than wives, cloistered in the house to bear sons. A husband's only heinous sexual misdeed was coitus with another man's wife, a transgression for which he could be put to death.

But these life-threatening liaisons seem not to have occurred with any frequency. Instead, most married gentlemen in classical Athens and Sparta amused themselves with a host of legitimate extramarital pursuits. Concubines looked after their daily needs. Educated courtesans known as hetaerae entertained them outside the home. And some men, particularly among the upper classes, partook regularly of homosexual rendezvous with teenage boys.

Early Christians would react violently to these appetites, but they would cherish other Greek ideals. Although the Greeks generally celebrated sex, some of them also harbored a deep misgiving that sex was contaminating, defiling, impure.[14] Heavenly celibacy. As early as 600 B.C. cultists had even begun to espouse asceticism and celibacy, concepts that would be adopted by fringe groups within the Hebraic tradition, then seep from generation to generation to influence early Christian leaders and eventually saturate the mores of Western men and women.[15]

Asceticism and celibacy remained alive—yet peripheral to daily life—in classical Rome. The ancient Romans were well known for their libertinism.[16] By 100 B.C. many Romans apparently regarded adultery the way some Americans feel about cheating on taxes— justified.

But the Romans also had their stoic side. Many liked to hark back to the good old days when Rome, they maintained, was a village of high moral integrity and everybody displayed *gravitas*, a sense of dignity and responsibility. An undercurrent of morality, continence, and abstinence was common in the Roman character.[17] And despite the sexual excesses of emperors and ordinary citizens—women as well as men—during Rome's glory days, some philosophers and teachers in these centuries continued to nurture and spread the little-known Greek philosophy of self-denial of all carnal pleasures.

This strain of Greco-Roman asceticism, commingled with the Hebrew concept that certain forms of sexual activity, including adultery, were sinful in the eyes of God, appealed to early Christian leaders.

Interpretations of Jesus' teachings on the subject of sexual conduct vary widely. Perhaps Jesus held sex within marriage in high esteem. But Mark 10:11 has Jesus speak as follows on adultery: "Whoever divorces his wife and marries another, commits adultery against her; and if she divorces her husband and marries another, she commits adultery." Even divorce and remarriage were seen as licentious actions.

Then in the centuries after Jesus, some influential leaders of the Christian faith became more and more hostile to sex of any kind. Although some suggest that Paul may have been a sex-affirming Jew of the Hebraic tradition, he certainly had a fondness for celibacy too. As he wrote in 1 Corinthians 7:8–9, "To the unmarried and the widows I say that it is well for them to remain single as I do. But if they cannot exercise self-control, they should marry. For it is better to marry than to be aflame with passion."[18]

Sex begone. Celibacy was not officially imposed on all Christian clergy until the eleventh century. But as the generations passed in early Christendom, sexual abstinence was becoming increasingly allied with God, adultery with sin—for both men and women.

Saint Augustine, who lived from A.D. 354 to 430, would spread these teachings across the Christian world. As a young man, Augustine was eager to convert to Christianity, but he could not overcome his lust for his mistress and his devotion to their son. As he wrote in his *Confessions,* the classic book of Christian mysticism and the story of his conversion, he prayed regularly to God, saying, "Give me chastity and continency, but do not give it yet."[19]

At the behest of his strong-willed mother, Monica, Augustine eventually cast out his concubine in order to take a legal wife of the correct social standing. But this wedding never came to pass. During the two years he waited to marry, he took a temporary mistress. And this led him to a watershed. Suffering a stricken conscience, he abandoned his marriage plans, converted to Christianity, and adopted a life of continence instead. It was not much later that Augustine came to see coitus as vile, lust as shameful, all acts surrounding intercourse as unnatural.[20] Celibacy he called the highest good. Intercourse between husband and wife should be for procreation only. And adultery, by men as well as women, was the devil incarnate.

This attitude that adultery is a moral transgression *for both sexes* has dominated Western mores ever since.

Unfaithfully Yours in America

This moral code has not deterred Western men and women—or people in any other society—from cheating on their spouses. Americans are no exception. Despite our attitude that philandering is immoral, regardless of our sense of guilt when we engage in trysts, in spite of the risks to family, friends, and livelihood that adultery inevitably entails, we indulge in extramarital affairs with avid regularly. As George Burns once summed it up, "Happiness is having a large, loving, caring, close-knit family in another city."[21]

How many Americans are adulterous we will never know. In the 1920s psychiatrist Gilbert Hamilton, a pioneer in sex research, reported that 28 of 100 men and 24 of 100 women interviewed had strayed.[22] This was the talk of American dinner tables for more than a decade.

The famous Kinsey reports in the late forties and early fifties stated that a little over a third of husbands in a sample of 6,427 men were unfaithful. Because so many of these subjects were reluctant to discuss their escapades, however, Kinsey surmised that his figures were low, that probably about half of all American men were unfaithful to their wives at some point during marriage. Twenty-six percent of the 6,972 married, divorced, and widowed American women sampled, Kinsey reported, had engaged in extramarital coitus by age forty. Forty-one percent of the female adulterers had copulated with a single partner; 40 percent had made love with two to five; 19 percent had engaged more than five paramours.[23]

Almost two decades later these figures apparently had not changed significantly—despite enormous changes in American attitudes toward sex during the sixties and seventies, the pinnacle of the "sexual revolution." A survey commissioned by *Playboy* magazine and conducted by Morton Hunt in the seventies reported that 41 percent of the 691 men and about 25 percent of the 740 married white middle-class women in the sample had philandered.

Two new trends stood out, however: both sexes started their trysts earlier than in former decades, and the double standard had eroded. Whereas only 9 percent of the wives under age twenty-five in the 1950s had taken a paramour, about 25 percent of young wives in the 1970s had done so. Hunt concluded, "Woman will go outside marriage for sex as often as will man, if she and her society think that she has as much right to do so as he."[24] A poll taken by *Redbook* confirmed Hunt's data for the 1970s. Of about 100,000 women surveyed, 29 percent of those who were married had engaged in an extramarital affair—but they were cheating sooner after wedding.[25] "Why wait?" seemed to have become the motto.

Have these figures for the 1970s gone up?

Maybe—and maybe not. A survey of 106,000 readers of *Cosmopolitan* magazine in the early 1980s indicated that 54 percent of the married women had participated in at least one affair,[26] and a poll of 7,239 men reported that 72 percent of those married over two years had been adulterous.[27] These figures for both men and women were then independently verified by other researchers.[28] As the June 1, 1987, issue of *Marriage and Divorce Today* reported, "Seventy percent of all Americans engage in an affair sometime during their marital life."[29] And adultery continues to start earlier. In a recent poll of 12,000 married individuals, about 25 percent of the men and women under twenty-five had cheated on a spouse.[30]

But who knows whether any of these figures are accurate?

Men tend to brag about sex, whereas women more regularly conceal their escapades. Perhaps married women in former decades admitted to fewer of their love affairs, whereas those of the 1980s are more honest. Maybe middle-class women today have more "opportunities," because they work outside the home. Perhaps men feel freer to philander as women become more financially independent. Undoubtedly pollsters do not reach a random sample of Americans either. And these researchers may be asking different questions or polling audiences more likely to have committed infidelities or more willing to admit their dalliances in a poll.

"Who's been sleeping in my bed?" asks Papa Bear in one of our folktales. No one knows the extent of adulterous sex in America now or in yesteryear. After all, unlike Hawthorne's Hester Prynne, adulterers do not display their trysts by wearing the letter *A*. And although adultery laws still exist in twenty-five states, our current laws concerning "no fault" divorce have shifted the emphasis of marriage to an economic partnership; sexual transgressions rarely reach the courts or census takers. So scientists who think they know the truth about American philanderers are naive.

But of one thing I am sure: despite our cultural taboo against infidelity, Americans are adulterous. Our societal mores, our religious teachings, our friends and relatives, urge us to invest all of our sexual energy on one person, a husband or a wife. But in practice a sizable percentage of both men and women actually spread their time, their vigor, and their love among multiple partners as they sneak into other bedrooms.[31]

And we are hardly extraordinary. I recently read forty-two ethnographies about different peoples past and present and found that adultery occurred in every one. Some of these peoples lived in tenements; others in row houses or thatched huts. Some raised rice; some raised money. Some were rich, some poor. Some espoused Christianity; others worshiped gods embodied in the sun, the wind, the rocks, and trees. Regardless of their traditions of marriage, despite their customs of divorce, irrespective of any of their cultural mores about sex, they all exhibited adulterous behavior—even where adultery was punished with death.

These forty-two peoples are not alone in their taste for cheating. As Kinsey concluded, "The preoccupation of the world's biography and fiction, through all ages and in all human cultures, with the non-marital sexual activities of married females and males, is evidence of the universality of human desires in these matters."[32] Adultery is a major reason for divorce and family violence in America and many other places. There exists no culture in which adultery is unknown, no cultural device or code that extinguishes philandering.

"Friendship is constant in all other things, save the office and affairs of love," Shakespeare wrote. Our human tendency toward extramarital liaisons seems to be the triumph of nature over culture. Like the stereotypic flirt, the smile, the brain physiology for infatuation, and our drive to bond with a single mate, philandering seems to be part of our ancient reproductive game.

Why Adultery?

Public whipping, branding, beating, ostracism, mutilation of genitals, chopping off of nose and ears, slashing feet, chopping at one's hips and thighs, divorce, desertion, death by stoning, burning, drowning, choking, shooting, stabbing—such cruelties are meted out by people around the world for philandering. Given these punishments, it is astonishing that human beings engage in extramarital affairs at all. Yet we do.

Why? From a Darwinian perspective, it is easy to explain why men are—by nature—interested in sexual variety. If a man has two children by one woman, he has, genetically speaking, "reproduced" himself. But if he also engages in dalliances with more women and, by chance, sires two more young, he doubles his contribution to the next generation. So, as the biological explanation goes, those men who tend to seek variety also tend to have more children. These young survive and pass to subsequent generations whatever it is in the male genetic makeup that seeks "fresh features," as Byron said of men's need for sexual novelty.[33]

But why are women adulterous? A woman cannot bear another child every time she sneaks into bed with another lover; she can get pregnant only at certain times of her menstrual cycle. Moreover, a woman takes nine months to bear the child, and then it is often several more months or years before she can conceive again. Unlike a man, a woman cannot breed every time she copulates. In fact, anthropologist Donald Symons has argued that, because the number of children a woman can bear is limited, women are biologically less motivated to seek fresh features.

Are women really less interested in sexual variety? This puzzle has several angles. So I shall take the role of devil's advocate and explore the possibility that women are just as interested in sexual variety and just as adulterous as men—albeit for different reasons. Let's begin with Symons, who has an intriguing argument for men's greater drive for sexual novelty.

Symons bases his premise that men are more interested in sexual variety than women are not only on the above genetic logic but also on the sexual habits of American homosexuals. These individuals, he believes, provide the "acid test" for gender differences in sexuality because homosexual behavior is not "masked by the compromises heterosexual relations entail and by moral injunctions."[34]

Accepting this as gospel, Symons then cites several studies in the 1960s and 1970s of gay Americans and concludes that gay men are inclined to one-night stands, to easy, anonymous, unencumbered sex, to coitus with several different, uncommitted partners, and to collecting harems and extra lovers, whereas gay women tend to seek longer relationships instead, as well as more commitment, fewer lovers, familiar partners, and sex with feeling rather than sex for sex itself.

Symons then proposes that these differences in male and female "sexual psychologies" stem from mankind's long hunting-gathering past: over countless millennia, males who liked sexual variety impregnated more females, produced more young, and bulked up their genetic lineages; hence for ancestral males philandering was adaptive.

But an ancestral woman's primary goal was to find a single protector who would ensure the survival of her children. A woman who sought sexual variety ran the risk of a jealous mate who might desert her. Moreover, female sexual escapades took time away from gathering vegetables and caring for her children. So those females who coupled with a variety of partners disproportionately died out or bred less often—passing on to modern women the propensity for fidelity.

With his Darwinian logic, his homosexual sample, and his evolutionary scenario, Symons concludes that men are, *by nature,* more interested in sexual variety than women are.

Man the natural playboy, woman the doting spouse—Americans already believed it. Because of our agrarian background and sexual double standard it became acceptable to view men as would-be Don Juans and women as the more virtuous of the genders. So when Symons presented an evolutionary explanation for men's philandering nature, many scholars bought it like a better chocolate bar. The idea that men crave sexual novelty more than women do now saturates academic books and academic minds.

Which Gender Philanders More?

I am not convinced that homosexual behavior illustrates essential truths about male and female sexual natures however. Most experts believe that about 5 percent of all American men and fewer American women are gay.[35] Homosexual behavior does not constitute the norm in the United States or anywhere else on earth. Moreover, I cannot agree with Symons that homosexual behavior constitutes the "undiluted" nature of either sex; instead, homosexuals are probably equally affected by their environment. In the 1970s, when his sample was collected, fast, loose sex was "in" for men. Lesbians, on the other hand, may well have been constrained by the cultural belief that women should curtail their sexual escapades.

Equally important, sexuality varies with age and other factors.

Kinsey and his colleagues found that young men of the blue-collar class indulged in a great deal of infidelity in their early twenties and then diminished their sexual pursuits by their forties whereas white-collar, college-educated men tended to philander less in their twenties, then increase their dalliances to almost once a week by age fifty. Women, on the other hand, reached the peak of their adultery in their middle thirties and early forties.[36] If, for example, Symons's homosexual men and women were largely *young* and blue-collar workers, it would not be surprising that he found men sought more sexual variety than women.

Simple math raises another problem. After all, every time a heterosexual man is "sleeping around," he is copulating with a woman. And since the vast majority of adults in almost all of the world's societies are married, logic upholds the proposition that when a married man is sneaking into the bushes in Amazonia, behind a rock in the Australian outback, or into a hut in Africa or Asia, he is most likely copulating with a married woman.

In modern urban cultures our rotating pool of singles warps this simple mathematical correlation. Moreover, some 8 to 15 percent of all American men's dalliances occur with prostitutes.[37] But its fair to say that the vast majority of the world's heterosexual trysts involve married men *and married women*. And it's hard to believe that all the married women across the planet who have copulated with paramours throughout all of human history were coerced into philandering.

In fact, there are at least four reasons why adultery could have been biologically adaptive for our female forebears.

The most obvious of these was elegantly put by Nisa, a !Kung woman who lives in the Kalahari Desert in southern Africa today. When anthropologist Marjorie Shostak met Nisa in 1970, Nisa was living in a hunting-gathering band along with her fifth husband. Nisa had engaged a lot of lovers too. When Shostak asked Nisa why she had taken on so many paramours, Nisa replied, "There are many kinds of work a woman has to do, and she should have lovers wherever she goes. If she goes somewhere to visit and is alone, then someone there will give her beads, someone else will give her meat, and someone else will give her other food. When she returns to her village, she will have been well taken care of."[38]

Nisa summed up in a few sentences a fine adaptive explanation for female interest in sexual variety—supplementary subsistence. Extra goods and services would have provided our adulterous female forebears with more shelter and extra food, perquisites that gave them more protection and better health, ultimately enabling their young to survive disproportionately.

Second, adultery probably served ancestral females as an insurance policy. If a "husband" died or deserted home, she had another male she might be able to enlist to help with parental chores.

Third, if an ancestral woman was "married" to a poor hunter with bad eyesight and a fearful or unsupportive temperament, she stood to upgrade her genetic line by having children with another man— Mr. Good Gene.

Fourth, if a woman had offspring with an array of fathers, each child would be somewhat different, increasing the likelihood that some from among them would survive unpredictable fluctuations in the environment.

As long as prehistoric females were secretive about their extramarital affairs, they could garner extra resources, life insurance, better genes, and more varied DNA for their biological futures. Hence those who sneaked into the bushes with secret lovers lived on—unconsciously passing on through the centuries whatever it is in the female spirit that motivates modern women to philander.

Thus female philandering was probably adaptive in the past. So adaptive, in fact, that it has left its mark on female physiology. At orgasm the blood vessels of a man's genitals eject the blood back into the body cavity, the penis goes limp, and sex is over. The man must start from the beginning to achieve orgasm again. For a woman, however, sex may have just begun. Unlike her mate's, a woman's genitals have not expelled all the blood. If she knows how, she can climax again soon and again and again if she wants to. Sometimes orgasms occur in such rapid succession that one is indistinguishable from the next, a phenomenon known as continual orgasm.

This high sex drive of the human female, in conjunction with data on other primates, has led anthropologist Sarah Hrdy to a novel hypothesis about the primitive beginnings of human female adultery.[39]

Hrdy points out that female apes and monkeys engage in a great deal of nonreproductive coitus. During estrus, for example, a female chimp will copulate with every male in the vicinity except her sons. This ancillary sexuality in chimps and many other female primates is not necessary to conceive a child. Hrdy therefore proposes that the female chimp's pursuit of sexual variety has two Darwinian purposes: to befriend males who may try to kill a female's coming newborn and to confuse paternity so that each male in the community will act paternally toward her forthcoming child.

Hrdy then applies this reasoning to women, attributing the high female sex drive to an ancient evolutionary tactic to copulate with multiple partners, thereby obtaining supplementary paternal investment and insurance against infanticide from each. This is a good idea. Perhaps our primitive female ancestors living in the trees pursued sex with a variety of males to keep friends. Then, when our forebears were driven onto the grasslands of Africa some four million years ago and pair-bonding evolved to raise the young, females turned from open promiscuity to clandestine copulations, reaping the benefits of resources and better or more varied genes as well.

Much of the world would not agree with Donald Symons or the American belief that men are the Don Juans whereas women are the shy, retiring recipients of sex.

The custom of the veil evolved in Moslem societies partly because Islamic people firmly believe that women are highly seductive. Clitoridectomy, the excising of the clitoris (and often some of the surrounding genital tissues), is done in several African cultures to curb the high female libido. Talmudic writers in the early Christian era stipulated that it was a husband's duty to copulate with his wife regularly precisely because they thought women had a higher sex drive than men. The Cayapa Indians of western Ecuador think women are lechers. Even the Spanish men who strut, preen, and philander in the small towns of Andalusia are convinced that women are dangerous, potent, and promiscuous—hence the practice of the chaperone.

In fact, had you asked Clellan Ford and Frank Beach, sex researchers of the 1950s, which sex was more interested in sexual variety, they would have replied, "In those societies which have no double standard in sexual matters and in which a variety of liaisons are permitted, the women avail themselves as eagerly of their opportunity as do the men."[40] Kinsey agreed, saying, "Even in those cultures which most rigorously attempt to control the female's extramarital coitus, it is perfectly clear that such activity does occur, and in many instances it occurs with considerable regularity."[41]

All these data certainly lead one to suspect that women avail themselves of illicit lovers with relish, perhaps even as avidly as men.

So the picture on the adultery puzzle is taking shape: men's biological need to spread their genes and the noticeable number of highly sexually active male homosexuals support the proposition that men are by nature more interested in sexual variety than women are. On the other hand, every time a heterosexual man is philandering, he is philandering with a woman. Moreover, women's biological drive to acquire resources, to obtain an insurance policy, and to secure better or more varied DNA, the potentially intense and long female sexual response, and the high incidence of female adultery in societies where there is no sexual double standard all suggest that women seek sexual variety regularly, perhaps as regularly as men.

There is a last line of evidence to toss into your thinking cap: that offered by prostitution.

The Oldest Profession

In agrarian societies with a strict double standard, women long embarked on one of two quite different sexual careers, becoming either cloistered housewives or courtesans, concubines, or prostitutes. In these cultures, therefore, some women had only a single partner, while others copulated with a lot of men. These "ladies of the night" were not unique to farming peoples either.[42]

Among the Mehinaku of Amazonia, the most sexually active person in the jungle village was a woman—who received fish, meat, or trinkets in payment for her trysts with a variety of partners.[43] Some traditional Navajo women chose not to marry; instead, they lived alone and entertained a variety of male visitors for a fee.[44] Women in many other American Indian tribes traditionally accompanied men on their hunting expeditions, returning home with meat in exchange for satisfying *several* of these hunters' sexual needs.[45]

An unmarried Canela girl of central Brazil who wished to earn food or services selected a would-be lover and asked her brother to arrange a date. Many of these trysts became long-term business relationships.[46] Madams flourished among the traditional Sierra Tarascans of Mexico. These older women had a string of girls they could summon at a moment's notice.[47] Nupe women of sub-Saharan Africa came to the marketplace at night dressed in their finery and jewels; here they sold kola nuts; but buyers could also purchase the woman for the night.[48]

You may wish to argue that these women (and women in many other cultures) all engaged in prostitution for purely economic reasons. But many women say they like the sexual variety.

And the women who pursue this vocation are not alone. The animal kingdom is rife with loose females. As you recall from chapter 1, female chimpanzees, other mammals, and many female birds, bugs, and reptiles solicit males and copulate in return for food. Among Australian bush crickets and other insects, the male's offering is called the nuptial gift. Prostitution deserves its venerable title "the oldest profession in the world."

A Modest Proposal

So back to the refrain: Who seeks more sexual variety, men or women?

My own modest proposal is that during our long evolutionary history most males pursued trysts to spread their genes, while females evolved two *alternative* strategies to acquire resources: some women elected to be relatively faithful to a single man in order to reap a lot of benefits from him; others engaged in clandestine sex with many men to acquire resources from each. This scenario roughly coincides with the common beliefs: man, the natural playboy; woman, the madonna or the whore.

It is an old axiom in science that what you are looking for, you tend to find. And this may well have become the case in the scientific examination of adultery. In a recent study by Donald Symons and Bruce Ellis, for example, 415 college students were asked whether they would have sex with an anonymous student of the opposite sex. In this imaginary scenario, participants were told that all risk of pregnancy, discovery, and disease was absent. The results were those you would expect. Males were consistently more likely to say yes, leading these researchers once again to conclude that men are more interested in sexual variety than women are.[49]

But here's the glitch. This study takes into consideration the primary genetic motive for male philandering (to fertilize young women). But it does not take into account the primary motive for female philandering—the acquisition of resources.

What if Symons and Ellis had asked these same men a different question: "Would you be willing to have a one-night stand with a woman from the nearby senior citizens' home?" I doubt these men would have expressed such craving for sexual variety. And what if Symons and Ellis had asked these same young women a different question too: "Would you be willing to have a one-night stand with Robert Redford if he gives you a brand new Porsche?" Evolutionary logic holds that women sleep around for goods and services. And until scientists take into account the underlying genetic motivations of each gender, as well as the age and social status of their informants, we will never know which sex is more interested in sexual variety.

Whatever you chose to make of all these data and ideas, there is no evidence whatsoever that women are sexually shy or that they shun clandestine sexual adventures. Instead, both men and women seem to exhibit a mixed reproductive strategy: monogamy *and* adultery are our fare.

The "Perfect" Love

We may never know who philanders more. But we do know why men and women *say* they are adulterous.

When polls ask men and women *why* they engage in extramarital affairs, adulterers regularly say, "for lust," "for love," or "I don't know." Psychologists would add that some philanderers want to get caught in order to patch up a marriage. Others use their dalliances to improve their marriage by satisfying some of their needs outside the home. Still others use their escapades as an excuse to leave a spouse. Some seek attention. Some are searching for autonomy. Some want independence. Some want to feel special, desired, more masculine or feminine, more attractive or better understood. Some want more communication, more intimacy, or just more sex. Others crave drama, excitement, or danger. A few seek revenge. Some want to find the "perfect" love. And some want to prove to themselves they are still young, the so-called last-chance affair.[50]

Carol Botwin tells us that some men can't be faithful because they are arrested in the "baby phase"; these people need another parent when they are traveling or when their partner is unavailable. Other sexually unfaithful men and women grew up in households where parents were never intimate, so as adults these people create shallow marriages and pursue noncommittal relationships. Some men put their wives on a pedestal but like to sleep with women from "the gutter." Some women and men are narcissistic; they need multiple lovers to show off their glitzy facade. A few like a triangle, a tug-of-war. Others get high on secrecy. Some want to solve a sex problem.[51]

Many other sociological and psychological factors are associated with adultery as well. Full-time work for the woman, one's level of education, one's decade of birth, frequency of attendance in church, one's degree of financial independence, one's premarital sexual career, one's parents' values and occupations, the chronic illness of a spouse, the frigidity of the wife, or constant travel by one's mate all affect one's susceptibility to adultery.

But as a Darwinist, I prefer the simple explanation of the man who says he seeks variety and that of Nisa, who reports, "One man gives you only one kind of food to eat. But when you have lovers, one brings you something and another brings you something else. One comes at night with meat, another with money, another with beads."[52] These answers have an evolutionary honesty. For although the woman who climbs into bed with a colleague is certainly not thinking of her genetic future as she draws down the bedcovers, and the last thing a husband wants is to impregnate the co-worker he seduces after the Christmas party, it is the millennia of sneaking off with lovers—and the genetic payoffs these dalliances accrued—that have produced the propensity for adultery around the world today.

"Thou shalt commit adultery." Because of a printer's error in the 1805 edition of the Bible, this commandment suddenly dictated philandering. It soon became known as the wicked Bible.[53] But the human animal seems cursed with a contradiction of the spirit. We search for true love, find him or her, and settle in. Then, when the spell begins to fade, the mind begins to wander. As Oscar Wilde summed up our plight, "There are two great tragedies in life, losing the one you love and winning the one you love."

Alas, winning often leads to another part of our reproductive strategy, our human tendency to divorce.

~5~

Blueprint for Divorce
The Four-Year Itch

She was a worthy womman al hir lyve,
Housbondes at chirche dore she hadde fyve.

—*Geoffrey Chaucer*, the Wife of Bath

"Oh eyes be strong, you cherish people and then they're gone." Safia, a middle-aged Bedouin woman of Egypt's Western Desert, held back her tears as she recited this sad poem to anthropologist Lila Abu-Lughod.[1] A year earlier her spouse of almost twenty years had come to her while she was baking and said, "You're divorced." At the time Safia had acted aloof, nonchalant. She still feigned indifference, saying to the anthropologist, "I didn't care when he divorced me. I never liked him." But Safia was concealing her despair. Only in a little poem could she reveal her vulnerability, longing, or attachment.

Although their songs and stories express passion between women and men, the Bedouins think romantic love is shameful. Individuals in their society are supposed to marry according to their family's bidding. One should feel deep love only for parents, brothers, sisters, and children—not for a spouse. So the Bedouins are horrified by public displays of affection between husband and wife. And although they believe spouses can fall deeply in love, honorable people must maintain *hasham*—sexual modesty and propriety. Unveiled passions appear only in short verse.[2]

Today these nomads have settled down to herd sheep, tend fig and olive groves, smuggle, or pursue other business ventures, but they carry with them an ancient love of love.

Before the railroad, before the Toyota truck, their ancestors traversed the deserts of North Africa, moving caravans of dates and other goods from oases in the sand to markets in the Nile valley. With them they brought their Arabian tribal mores—a love for independence, honor, courage, gallantry, and hospitality, a penchant for vendettas, and, above all, a taste for women, wine, and song.[3] Safia's short poem, like all modern Bedouin verse on the despair of love or the exhilaration of romance, is today's remembrance of desert song masters long deceased.

"I divorce thee; I divorce thee; I divorce thee." These words, too, come from pre-Islamic times. In those days women were honored and respected. They were also prized goods. Girls were wards of the family; after marriage, women became the property of a spouse and could be dismissed if unsatisfactory. As al-Ghazali, the outstanding eleventh-century intellectual and author, described divorce in ancient Arabian society, it was easy to obtain.[4] One merely had to pronounce a statement of divorce three times.

In the sixth century A.D. the Prophet Muhammad built on this tribal custom. Unlike early Christian fathers who venerated celibacy, Muhammad believed that coitus was one of the great joys of life and that marriage guarded men and women from the irreligious world of promiscuity. So he insisted that his followers wed. As he declared, "I fast and I eat, I keep vigil and I sleep, and I am married. And whoever is not willing to follow my Sunna (tradition) does not belong to me."[5] There would be no celibacy in Islam.

To this day Muhammad's influence has produced what scientists call a sex-positive Islamic culture, a society that venerates man/woman love, sex, and marriage. Western society, on the other hand, is sometimes called sex negative because our historical reli-

gious precepts extolled the virtues of celibacy and monasticism instead.

Muhammad sealed other traditions. Although he saw women as subordinate to men, a belief inherited from pre-Islamic peoples, he introduced a host of social, moral, and legal codes to protect women, as
well as a list of explicit rights and duties of each spouse. Among these
guidelines: a man should have no more than four wives, and he must
circulate among them on consecutive nights. Above all, a husband
must provide for each without favoritism.

A wife had responsibilities, too, particularly to bear and raise children, to cook, and to obey her husband. In Islam, marriage rested on
a legal contract. And unlike Christian matrimony, which became a
sacrament and hence indissoluble, the Muslim wedding pledge
could be broken. The Prophet's bidding was from God.

Today these traditional divorce procedures still exist in much of
the Islamic world, although in some places divorce has become
harder to obtain. The most acceptable means of divorce is still Tala-
qus-Sunna, in conformity with the dictates of the Prophet. This
form of *talaq*, or divorce, can be done in either of two slightly varied,
approved ways. One of them, *talaq ahsan*, consists of a single pro-
nouncement, "I divorce thee; I divorce thee; I divorce thee," made
while the wife is not menstruating, along with sexual abstinence for
three months. The divorce is revoked if the husband withdraws his
words or if the couple resume intercourse during this three-month
waiting period.

Islamic law gives a host of other stipulations about divorce—
when it is appropriate for a wife to leave a husband and how either
spouse can negotiate their separation with grace—for Muhammad
savored harmony between men and women, be they together or
apart. As the Koran enjoined, "Then, when they have reached their
term, take them back in kindness or part from them in kindness."[6]

Still, Safia felt sorrow when her husband went away.

Parting

We all have our share of troubles. But probably one of the hardest things we do is leave a spouse. Is there any way to do this well?

I doubt it. But people have devised many formal ways to end a marriage. In some societies special courts or councils negotiate divorces. Sometimes the village headman hears divorce cases. Most often divorce is considered a private matter to be handled by the parties and their families.[7] This can be as easy as moving a hammock from one fireplace to the next, or it can disrupt an entire community—as recently occurred in India.

In 1988 the *New York Times* reported the divorce case of a young Hindu girl, Ganga, who fled her husband of five years after he had severely beaten her.[8] The next day over five hundred people met in a field near the village to hear the couple and their kin answer questions posed by respected elders of their caste. But when Ganga accused her husband's father and uncle of trying to assault her sexually, an argument erupted. Insults soon led to combat with long sticks, and in no time several men lay in the field—clubbed and bleeding. The ruckus stopped only when word spread that the police were coming. Divorce proceedings no doubt continued with bitter words behind mud walls.

Whether done in anger or dispassion, with full state regalia, or with a minimum of fuss, divorce is indisputably a part of the human condition. Almost everywhere in the world people permit divorce. The ancient Incas did not. The Roman Catholic church refuses to acknowledge it. A few other ethnic groups and societies do not allow marital dissolution.[9] And in some cultures divorces are difficult to obtain.[10]

But from the tundras of Siberia to the jungles of Amazonia, people accept divorce as regrettable—although sometimes necessary. They have specific social or legal procedures for divorce. And they do divorce. Moreover, unlike many Westerners, traditional peoples do not make divorce a moral issue. The Mongols of Siberia sum up a common worldwide attitude, "If two individuals cannot get along harmoniously together, they had better live apart."[11]

Why Do People Divorce? Bitter quarrels, insensitive remarks, lack of humor, watching too much television, inability to listen, drunkenness, sexual rejection—the reasons men or women give for why they leave a marriage are as varied as their motives for having wedded in the first place. But there are some common circumstances under which people around the globe choose to abandon a relationship.

Overt adultery heads the list. In a study of 160 societies, anthropologist Laura Betzig established that blatant philandering, particularly by the wife, is the most commonly offered rationale for seeking to dissolve a marriage. Sterility and barrenness come next. Cruelty, particularly by the husband, ranks third among worldwide reasons for divorce. Then come an array of charges about a spouse's personality and conduct. Bad temper, jealousy, talkativeness, nagging, disrespect, laziness by the wife, nonsupport by the husband, sexual neglect, quarrelsomeness, absence, and running off with a lover are among the many explanations.[12]

I am not surprised that adultery and infertility are paramount. Darwin theorized that people marry primarily to breed. Unquestionably, many people wed to gain an economically valuable spouse or to accumulate children to support them as they age; still others marry to cement political ties with relatives, friends, or enemies. But as Betzig has neatly proven, Darwin was correct: since the main reasons given for divorce are closely linked to sex and reproduction, it follows that people wed primarily to reproduce.[13]

It should also follow that most divorced persons of reproductive age remarry. And indeed they do.[14] Despite dashed dreams, with full memory of the vicious quarrels, regardless of the inevitable realization that marriage can be irritating, dull, and painful, the vast majority of people who divorce take another spouse. In America 75 percent of the women and 80 percent of the men who separate wed again.[15] And because marriage defines one as an adult in most traditional societies, divorced people around the world find another partner.

We seem to have an eternal optimism about our next mate.

Money Talks

Samuel Johnson defined remarriage as the triumph of hope over experience. Americans joke about the "seven-year itch." Anthropologists know this human habit as "serial monogamy." Call it what you will, the human penchant to divorce and remarry is worldwide. And it displays several other striking patterns.

First of all, divorce is common in societies where women and men *both* own land, animals, currency, information, and/or other valued goods or resources and where *both* have the right to distribute or exchange their personal riches beyond the immediate family circle. If you own a bank in New York City, if you possess the rights to the only local water hole in the Kalahari Desert of southern Africa, or if you take your grain to market in Nigeria and come home with wealth that you can keep, invest, sell, barter, or give away, you are rich. Where men and women are not dependent on each other to survive, bad marriages can end—and often do.

A telling example of the power of economic autonomy is offered by the !Kung Bushmen of the Kalahari Desert. Among these people, men and women often marry more than once.[16] And it is no coincidence, I think, that !Kung women are economically and socially powerful as well.

Although the !Kung are rapidly adopting Western values and twentieth-century technology, their high divorce rate is not a new development. When anthropologists recorded their lifeways in the 1960s, these people lived in small groups of some ten to thirty individuals during the rainy season. Then, as the weather turned and the blistering October sun sucked up the surface water, they assembled in larger communities around permanent water holes. But even when the !Kung were scattered across the bush, men and women traveled regularly between communities, connecting a fluid network of several hundred kin.

!Kung women commuted to work. Not every morning. But every two to three days when staples waned, a wife needed to go collecting. Carrying her nursing infant in her shawl and leaving her older youngsters in the "day care" of friends and relatives, she joined a group of women and marched off through the chaparral.

Each foraging expedition was novel. Sometimes a woman re-turned with baobab fruit, wild onions, tsama melons, and sweet mongongo nuts. On other days she gathered sour plums, tsin beans, leafy greens, and water roots. Honey, caterpillars, tortoises, and birds' eggs were groceries too. And regularly a woman returned with valuable information. From the animal tracks she discovered as she walked, she could tell which beasts had passed by, when, how many were in the herd, and where the group was headed.

!Kung men went hunting two to three days a week, in quest of dove or sand grouse, a springhare, a porcupine, an antelope, even a giraffe. Sometimes a husband came home with just enough meat to feed his wife and children; sometimes a group of men felled a beast large enough to divide with hunting companions, relatives, and friends. Meat was a delicacy. And good hunters were honored. But men brought home meat only one day in four.

Consequently women provided 60 to 80 percent of dinner almost every night. Women also shared the rights to water sites in the desert—a situation not unlike owning the local bank. During repro-ductive years women held high status as child bearers. Older women often became shamans and leaders in community affairs as well.

So !Kung women were powerful.

And when a husband and wife found themselves in a desperate marriage, either one or the other generally packed up a few belong-ings and departed for another camp. Why? Because they could. !Kung spouses often argued for months before breaking up. Cruel words and bitter tears spilled onto the desert sand. Neighbors invari-ably got involved. But eventually most unhappy relationships ended. Of the 331 marriages !Kung women reported to sociologist Nancy Howell in the 1970s, 134 ended in divorce.[17] Then men and women wed again. Some !Kung women had as many as five consecutive spouses.

This correlation between economic independence and divorce is seen in a host of cultures.[18] Among the Yoruba of West Africa, for example, women traditionally controlled the complex marketing system. They grew the crops, then took their produce to a weekly market—a market run entirely by women. As a result Yoruba women brought home not only staples but also money and luxuries, independent wealth. Up to 46 percent of all Yoruba marriages ended in divorce.[19]

The Hadza live on the grasslands around Olduvai Gorge, Tanzania. Although the gorge area is dry and rocky, it abounds with roots, berries, and small game, and during the rainy season spouses regularly leave camp separately in the morning to forage for themselves. Then in the dry season, bands assemble around permanent water holes, men hunt large game, and all dance, gamble, gossip, and share the meat. But Hadza men and women are not dependent on one another to provide the evening meal. And their marriages reflect this independent spirit. In the 1960s their divorce rates were roughly five times higher than those in the United States.[20]

Personal economic autonomy spells freedom to depart. And for me the most vivid illustration of this correlation are the Navajo of the American Southwest—undoubtedly because I lived with them for several months in 1968.

Take Route 66 west out of Gallup, New Mexico, drive some forty-five minutes, swing north on a broad dirt road through the chaparral, the dust, and the smell of sage, go past the Pine Springs trading post, beyond the abandoned hogan (a seven-sided log house), and curve right past the big pine tree and up the hill of wildflowers. There's our wooden house—with a potbellied stove for heat, a gas range for cooking fried bread, coffee, and mutton soup, two big brass beds, a kitchen table, and three kerosene lamps we used to sit around at night and talk. A usually jolly home, with a front door looking east, two big tanks of precious water nestled in a nearby grove of pines, and an orange canyon ribboning through our vast front yard.

My Navajo "mother" orchestrated daily life. She collected Indian paintbrush and other wildflowers, carded and dyed wool, and wove Navajo blankets to support a family of five. She also owned the land around her. The Navajo are matrilineal; children trace their descent through their mother's lineage, so women own a great deal of property. Women are also medical diagnosticians, who play a vital role in Navajo ritual life.[21] They analyze the sick, identify spiritual and

physical illnesses, and prescribe the appropriate Navajo curing ceremony. So women enjoy a lot of prestige; they participate in all community affairs—and about one out of three divorces.[22]

"One shouldn't marry only to be unhappy the remainder of one's
days," the Micmac of eastern Canada say.[23] Much of the world
agrees. Where women and men *can* leave each other, unhappy people often do. Then usually they wed again.

Divorce rates are much lower where spouses are dependent on each
other to make ends meet. The most notable correlation between
economic dependence and low divorce rates is seen in preindustrial
Europe and in all other societies that use the plow for agriculture—
such as India and China.[24] Some people trace this low divorce rate
among historical Christian Europeans to religious causes—for understandable reasons. Jesus forbade divorce.[25] And as I have mentioned, by the eleventh century A.D. Christian marriage had become
a sacrament; divorce was impossible for Christians.

But culture often complements nature's laws, and the low divorce
rates seen in preindustrial European societies were also due to an
inescapable ecological reality: farming couples needed each other to
survive.[26] A woman living on a farm depended on her husband to
move the rocks, fell the trees, and plow the land. Her husband
needed her to sow, weed, pick, prepare, and store the vegetables.
Together they worked the land. More important, whoever elected to
leave the marriage left empty-handed. Neither spouse could dig up
half the wheat and relocate. Farming women and men were tied to
the soil, to each other, and to an elaborate network of stationary kin.
Under these ecological circumstances, divorce was not a practical
alternative.

No wonder divorce was rare throughout preindustrial Europe,
across the breadbasket of the Caucasus, and among many agrarian
peoples stretching to the Pacific Rim.

The Industrial Revolution changed this economic relationship between men and women and helped stimulate modern patterns of
divorce (see chapter 16).

The United States is a good example. When factories appeared beyond the barns of agricultural America, women and men began to leave the farm for work. And what did they bring home but money—movable, divisible property. During much of the 1800s most women still ran the house. But in the early decades of the twentieth century American middle-class women began to join the labor force in greater numbers, giving them economic autonomy.

Not coincidentally, the American divorce rate, which started to rise with the advent of the Industrial Revolution, continued its slow but steady climb. For an unhappy husband will leave a wife who brings home a paycheck long before he will desert the woman who weeds his garden. And a woman with a salary is often less tolerant of marital despair than one dependent on her spouse to provide the evening meal. Many observers identify women's employment outside the home—and control over their own money—as a prime factor in this rising frequency of divorce.[27]

A rise of divorce rates in tandem with female economic autonomy has been seen before in Western history. When the Romans won several foreign wars in the centuries preceding Christ, trade monopolies brought unprecedented wealth to Rome. An urban upper class emerged. Rich Roman patricians were now less eager to let massive dowries pass into the hands of sons-in-law. So with a series of new marriage regulations in the first century B.C., upper-class women came to control more of their fortunes—and their futures. And as a class of increasingly financially independent women rose in ancient Rome, divorce became epidemic.[28]

Ties That Bind

"All you need is love," the Beatles sang. Not so. Many other cultural factors besides economic autonomy contribute to the stability or instability of a marriage.

Traditionally divorce rates were higher in the United States among partners who came from different socioeconomic, ethnic, and religious backgrounds.[29] This may be changing, though. In a study of 459 women in Detroit, sociologist Martin Whyte discovered that these factors had little effect on the fate of a relationship. Instead, similar personality traits, shared habits, parallel interests, common values, joint leisure activities, and mutual friends were the best predictors of marital stability. Interestingly, Whyte also concluded, "It helps if you marry at a mature age, if you are very much in love, if you are white and come from a close and loving home."[30] People without these attributes are at greater risk.

Psychologists report that inflexible people make unstable marriages.[31] Therapists say that where the ties holding a couple together outweigh the forces pulling them apart, individuals tend to stay together.[32] How spouses adjust to one another, how they bargain, how they fight, and how they listen and persuade make a difference too; where there is little compromise, marriages are more likely to dissolve.[33] Demographers have shown that when there is an excess of men or a dearth of women, wives become scarce commodities and people are less likely to separate.[34] American couples who bear a boy have a statistically better chance of remaining married,[35] as do spouses with preschool children.[36] And couples that marry very young tend to divorce.[37]

Anthropologists have added a cross-cultural perspective to our understanding of divorce.[38] Divorce is common in matrilineal cultures like that of the Navajo, probably because a wife has resources, her children are members of her clan, and her husband has more responsibilities for his sister's offspring than for his own; hence spouses are companions, not vital economic partners. Where a husband must pay a "bride price" to the family of his intended for the privilege of marrying her, divorce rates are often lower because at divorce these goods must be returned. Endogamy, marrying within one's own community, is associated with more-permanent relationships because common relatives, friends, and obligations tend to bind the pair into a common network.[39]

Polygyny has a curious effect on divorce. When a man has several wives, these women tend to fight for the attention and resources of their single husband. Jealousies lead to showdowns and divorce. More important, a man with several women can spare the services of one, while a man with only a single wife will think hard before he deserts the only woman who cooks for him. As a matter of fact, divorce rates have *declined* in Muslim societies since contact with Western mores;[40] our tradition of monogamy is stabilizing Islamic family life.

"There is no society in the world where people have stayed married without enormous community pressure to do so," Margaret Mead once said.[41] She was right. Divorce rates are just as high in many traditional societies as in the United States.[42]

This seems curious. After all the smiles and gazes, the dizzying sensations of adoration, the shared secrets and private jokes, the lovely times in bed, the days and nights with family and friends, the children they have borne, the property they have collected, the colorful experiences they have amassed through all the hours, months, and years they laughed and loved and struggled as a team, why do men and women leave rich relationships behind?

Perhaps this restlessness is driven by currents buried in our human psyche, profound reproductive forces that evolved across eons of daily mating throughout our shadowed past.

The Four-Year Itch

Hoping to get some insight into the nature of divorce, I turned to the demographic yearbooks of the United Nations. These volumes were begun in 1947 when census takers in countries as culturally diverse as Finland, Russia, Egypt, South Africa, Venezuela, and the United States started to ask their inhabitants about divorce. In these data, collected every decade by the Statistical Office of the United Nations on dozens of societies, I culled the answers to three questions: How many years were you married when you divorced? How old were you when you divorced? How many children did you have at the time of your divorce?

Three remarkable patterns emerged.

And they ring of evolutionary forces.

Most striking, divorce generally occurs early in marriage—peaking in or around the fourth year after wedding—followed by a gradual decline in divorce as more years of marriage go by (See appendix A).[43] Actually I was disappointed to discover this; I had expected to find a divorce peak during and around the seventh year of marriage.[44] Not to be. Finland offered a typical example. In 1950 the number of Finnish divorces peaked during the fourth year of marriage; it gradually declined after this four-year peak. In 1966 Finnish divorces occurred most often during the third year of marriage. Divorces once again clustered around a four-year pinnacle in 1974, 1981, and 1987 (see appendix, figure 1, A–E).

When I put these four Finnish divorce peaks ("modes," to statisticians) and the divorce peaks for all years available for all the other sixty-one cultures on a master chart (appendix, figure 2), it became evident that among these diverse peoples divorces tended to peak during *and around* the fourth year of marriage. There was no seven-year itch; a four-year itch emerged instead.

There certainly were variations off this four-year divorce peak. In Egypt and other Muslim countries, for example, divorces occurred most frequently during the first few months of marriage—nowhere near the four-year mark (appendix, figure 3).

These variations were not surprising, though. In these cultures the groom's family is expected to return their new daughter-in-law to her parents if she is not fitting into her new home—something in-laws do rapidly when they do it.[45] Moreover, the Koran exempts a Muslim husband from paying half of the wedding fee if he dissolves the union before consummating it.[46] Thus social pressure and economic incentive both spur unhappily married Egyptians and other Muslim people to divorce early. Last, these statistics include "revocable divorces," provisional decrees that require few financial reparations. Revocable divorces make the process of separation quick and easy and the duration of marriage short.[47]

The American divorce peak hovers somewhat below the common four-year peak, and it is interesting to speculate on this variation too. In some years, such as 1977, divorces peaked around the fourth year of marriage.[48] But in 1960, 1970, 1979, 1981, 1983, and 1986 the divorces peaked earlier—between the second and third year after wedding (appendix, figure 4).[49] Why?

I know that this American divorce peak has nothing to do with the rising divorce *rate* in America. The divorce rate doubled between 1960 and 1980, yet couples divorced in or around the second year of marriage throughout this time. I know that it cannot be explained by the growing number of couples who live together either. The numbers of men and women who took up residence without marrying almost tripled in the 1970s—but the American divorce peak did not budge.[50]

Purely as a guess, I would say that this American divorce peak may have something to do with American attitudes toward marriage itself. We tend not to marry for economic, political, or family reasons. Instead, as anthropologist Paul Bohannan once said, "Americans marry to enhance their inner, largely secret selves."[51]

I find this remark fascinating—and correct. We marry for love *and to accentuate, balance out, or mask parts of our private selves.* This is why you sometimes see a reserved accountant married to a blond bombshell or a scientist married to a poet. Perhaps it is no coincidence that the American divorce peak corresponds perfectly with the normal duration of infatuation—two to three years. If partners are not satisfied with the match, they bail out soon after the infatuation high wears off.

So there are exceptions to the four-year itch.

These data have other problems.[52]

In some societies, partners court for months; in others they marry quickly. The time involved in preparing for the wedding, the months or years a person will endure an awful marriage, the ease or difficulty of obtaining a divorce, and the length of time needed to get the divorce decree also vary from one culture to the next. In actuality, then, human relationships begin before they are legally recorded and founder before they become legally defunct.

There is no way to measure all the variables that skew these data collected by the United Nations. But here is a focal point of this book: given the vast number of cultural factors and individual variations involved in marriage and divorce, one would expect even fairly significant patterns to disappear; it is remarkable that *any* pattern appears at all. Yet, despite the varying traditions for marrying, the myriad worldwide opinions about divorce, and the diverse procedures for parting, men and women desert each other in a roughly common pattern.

Some of these people are bankers; others garden, herd cattle, fish, or trade to make a living. Some have a college education; some neither read nor write. Among these hundreds of millions of men and women from sixty-two different cultures, individuals speak different languages, ply different trades, wear different clothes, carry different currencies, intone different prayers, fear different devils, and harbor different hopes and different dreams. Nevertheless, their divorces regularly cluster around a four-year peak.

And this cross-cultural divorce pattern is unrelated to divorce rate. It occurs in societies where the divorce rate is high and in cultures where divorce is rare.[53] It even remains constant in the same society over time—despite a soaring incidence of divorce. What a curiosity. *Marriage has a cross-cultural pattern of decay.*

This pattern of human bonding is even embedded in Western mythology. During the twelfth century traveling European minstrels called together lords and ladies, knights and commoners, to hear the fatal epic saga of Tristan and Iseult—the first modern Western romance. "My lords," a bard began, "if you would hear a high tale of love and of death, here is that of Tristan and Queen Iseult; how to their full joy, but to their sorrow also, they loved each other, and how at last, they died of that love together upon one day; she by him and he by her."[54]

As the French writer Denis de Rougemont has said of this myth about adultery, it is "a kind of archetype of our most complex feelings of unrest." His observation is even more astute than he may know. The tale begins when a young knight and a beautiful queen share an elixir known to induce love for *about three years.*

Is there an inherent weak point in human pair-bonds? Perhaps. There are others.

Divorce Is for the Young

Between 1946 and 1964 some 76 million Americans were born. Hail the "baby boom," a mass production following World War II. Today these people range from their late twenties to their mid-forties. And because they see divorce among their peers, they assume that marital dissolution is most prevalent in middle age. It is not. Divorces peak among the young.

In America divorce *risk* peaks between ages 20 and 24 for both women and men. This is slightly low by world standards. In the twenty-four societies for which data are available in the United Nations yearbooks, divorce risk is highest in age category 25–29 for men, while divorce risk peaks about equally in age groups 20–24 and 25–29 for women. Divorce then becomes less and less frequent in older age groups. And by middle age divorce becomes uncommon. Eighty-one percent of all divorces occur before age 45 among women; 74 percent of all divorces happen before age 45 among men.[55]

This seems strange. You would think that partners would become bored or sated with one another as they age, or that they would abandon their marriage after their children have left home for work or college. Not so. Instead, men and women divorce with impressive regularity when they are in their twenties—during the height of their reproductive and parenting years.

We leave one another with children too.

A third pattern to emerge from the United Nations data regards "divorce with dependent children." Among the hundreds of millions of people recorded in forty-five societies between 1950 and 1989, 39 percent of all divorces occurred among couples with no dependent children, 26 percent among those with one dependent child, 19 percent among couples with two "issue," 7 percent among those with three children, 3 percent among couples with four young, and couples with five or more dependent young rarely split.[56] Hence it appears that the more children a couple bear, the less likely they are to divorce.

This third pattern is less conclusively demonstrated by the UN data than the first two.[57] Yet it is strongly suggested and it makes genetic sense. From a Darwinian perspective, couples with no children should break up; both individuals will mate again and probably go on to bear young—ensuring their genetic futures. As couples bear more children they become less economically able to abandon their growing family. And it is genetically logical that they remain together to raise their flock.

But we can say this "for sure": one-quarter of all divorces involve one dependent child; almost 20 percent occur among couples with two offspring. A lot of people divorce after they have had a child or two.

I am often asked, "Which sex more often leaves the other?"

We will never know. Laws and customs often dictate which spouse begins divorce proceedings. But which individual actually initiates the emotional, physical, and legal separation is not measurable. After all the arguing and tears are over, sometimes even the parties involved are not sure who left whom. But one thing is certain: the vast majority of people wed again.

American women "typically" remarry about four years after divorcing, whereas men "typically" wed three years after breaking a former tie.[58] The average period of time between divorce and remarriage is three years.[59] And the median number of years between divorce and remarriage ranges from three to four and a half years, depending on one's age.[60] Moreover, 80 percent of all divorced American men and 75 percent of all divorced American women take another spouse.[61]

In 1979 the peak age category for remarriage among American men was 30–34; the peak age category for remarriage among American women was 25–29. The percentage of men and women in other cultures who remarry is not calculated by United Nations census takers. But among ninety-eight cultures surveyed between 1971 and 1982, the peak age for remarriage among men was 30–34 while the peak age for remarriage among women was 25–29—the same as in the United States.[62]

Planned Obsolescence of the Pair-bond?

Perhaps. Marriage clearly shows several general patterns of decay. Divorce counts peak among couples married about four years. Divorce risk is greatest among spouses in their twenties—people at the height of their reproductive years. A great many divorces occur among partners with one or two children. Divorced persons remarry while they are young. And the longer a couple remain together, the older the partners get, and probably the more offspring they produce, the less likely spouses are to leave each other.[63]

This is not to say that everybody fits this mold. George Bush, for example, does not. But Shakespeare did. He left his wife, Anne, in Stratford to pursue his career in London some three to four years after wedding.[64] Etched in Shakespeare's marriage and in all these other divorces recorded from around the world is a blueprint, a primitive design. *The human animal seems built to court, to fall in love, and to marry one person at a time; then, at the height of our reproductive years, often with a single child, we divorce; then, a few years later, we remarry once again.*

Why did this script evolve? The explanation for these patterns of human bonding is the core of coming chapters in this book.

Along the headwaters of the Amazon, on coral atolls in the Pacific, in the Arctic wastes, in the Australian outback, and in other remote parts of the world, men and women leave each other too. Few scientists or census takers have asked these out-of-the-way peoples how long their marriages lasted, how old they were when they divorced, or how many children were involved. But the scant data should be reviewed.

Among the traditional jungle-living Yanomamo of Venezuela, nearly 100 percent of all infants live with their natural mother; the majority also have their natural father living with them. But the co-residence of the biological parents declines sharply after the child reached the age of five—not just because a parent dies but because spouses divorce.[65] Among the Fort Jameson Ngoni of southern Africa divorces peak between the fourth and fifth year of marriage too.[66] These data are consistent with the four-year itch.

Also consistent with the United Nation data are all the marriages that break up among the young. On the Truk Islands of Micronesia, and among several gardening-hunting peoples of New Guinea, Africa, the Pacific, and the Amazon, marriages are exceedingly brittle among couples in their teens and twenties.[67]

People around the world will tell you that a marriage strengthens when a child is born.[68] For example, in rural Japan a marriage is often not even noted by village record keepers until a child is produced.[69] Andaman Islanders of India do not consider a marriage fully consummated until spouses become parents.[70] And the Tiv of Nigeria call a union a "trial marriage" until an infant cements the pair.[71]

But we shouldn't assume that the birth of a child necessarily produces *lifelong* marriage.[72] I suspect the Aweikoma of eastern Brazil best illustrate trends in traditional societies. Here typically "a couple with several children stays together til death. . . . But separations before many children are born are legion."[73] This is exactly the pattern that emerges from the United Nations data.

There are exceptions, of course. Among the Kanuri Muslims of Nigeria divorces peak prior to the first full year of marriage. Anthropologist Ronald Cohen thinks this early divorce peak occurs because "young girls tend not to stay with first husbands whom they are forced to marry by parents."[74] Interestingly, the !Kung Bushmen also divorce within months of wedding, and they also have arranged first marriages.[75]

Even this is consistent with the United Nations sample, although it is the exception, not the rule. As you recall, Egypt and other Muslim countries all exhibit a divorce peak before the first full year of marriage. And these countries have high incidences of arranged first marriages. An arranged marriage may provoke one to bail out fast, accelerating the four-year itch.

All sorts of cultural mores skew patterns of human bonding; the economic autonomy of women, urbanism, secularism, and arranged marriages make up but a fraction. Despite these influences, human mating has some general rules: women and men from western Siberia to the southern tip of South America marry. Many leave each other. Many depart around the fourth year after wedding. Many leave when they are young. Many divorce with a single child. And many remarry once again.

Year upon decade upon century we replay these ancient scripts— strutting, preening, flirting, courting, dazzling, then capturing one another. Then nesting. Then breeding. Then philandering. Then abandoning the fold. Soon drunk on hope, we court anew. Eternal optimist, the human animal seems restless during reproductive years, then settles in as he or she matures.

Why? The answer lies, I think, in the vagaries of our past, "when wild in woods the noble savage ran."

～ 6 ～

"When Wild in Woods the Noble Savage Ran"

Life among Our Ancestors in the Trees

I am as free as Nature first made man
Ere the base laws of servitude began
When wild in woods the noble savage ran.

—*John Dryden*, The Conquest of Granada

Mahogany trees, tropical evergreens, laurels, wild pear trees, litchi fruit trees, mango trees, rubber trees, myrrh trees, ebony trees—trees, trees, and more trees stretched from Kenya's sandy shores to the Atlantic Ocean.[1] Twenty million years ago equatorial Africa was a curtain of impenetrable green. Glades, pools, swamps, and streams, even more open woodlands and grassy plains occasionally interrupted these forests. But fossilized seeds, fruits, and nuts dug up at Rusinga Island in Lake Victoria, and nearby sites suggest that East Africa was largely windless woods.[2]

Butterflies danced in the dim light that filtered through the sky of leaves. Flying squirrels glided from bow to bow and bats hung in darkened crevices. Ancient relatives of rhinos, elephants, hippos, warthogs, okapi, tusked deer, and other forest creatures fed among the ferns. And golden moles, elephant shrews, hamsters, hedgehogs, mice, gerbils, and many other small creatures gathered insect larvae, earthworms, herbs, or berries on the damp forest floor. The temperature was slightly higher than it is today, and almost every afternoon rain poured onto the steamy jungles, feeding the lakes and streams with fresh water, pelting the upper stories of the thick forest canopy.

Ancient relatives of ours roamed among these trees.

They have an array of scientific names, but they are known collectively as the hominoids—the ancestors of apes and humans. Hundreds of their fossil teeth and bones have been found in East Africa (as well as in Eurasia), dating from between twenty-three and fourteen million years ago. Each had a mixture of ape-like and monkey-like features, although some looked more like monkeys while others had more characteristics of apes.[3]

The bones of one species found on Rusinga Island suggest that this creature was about the size of a modern house cat, whereas others were as big as modern chimps. None resembled human beings. But from among these kin both our ancestors and the living great apes would one day emerge.

How the hominoids spent their days and nights is difficult to say. Perhaps some ran along the tops of tree limbs the way many monkeys do, leaping from branch to branch and climbing to follow adjacent highways above the ground. Some may have hung below the tree limbs and swung beneath them instead.

This distinction is actually important to human evolution, for these are quite different ways to move around. When the precursors of apes and humans abandoned life atop the stronger central limbs to hang below smaller branches, they evolved the basic structures of our human frame. To begin with, our ancestors lost their tails. These graceful appendages served their predecessors as the balancing pole serves the acrobat—a righting device perfectly designed to provide added stability as they scurried along the top of sturdy boughs. But as the forebears of the apes and man began to hang below the branches, tails became baggage that nature could discard.

Other streamlining features were adopted for swinging below the branches, too, particularly adjustments of the shoulder, arm, and torso. Gently pick up the family kitten by its forelimbs and watch its head dangle behind its paws; the cat cannot see between its limbs.

Then find a jungle gym in a playground and hang by your arms. Notice how your shoulders do not collapse before your face; you can see between your elbows as you suspend. The human collarbone, the position of our shoulder blades across our backs, our broad breast-bone, or sternum, our wide, shallow ribcage, and our reduced lumbar vertebrae all evolved for hanging the body from above rather than supporting it from underneath.

Equally distinctive, humans and all the apes can rotate their wrists 180 degrees. Hence you and I can swing across a jungle gym palm up or palm away. Our ancestors acquired all of these anatomical features of the arms and upper body in order to dangle from tree limbs, swing below these delicate boughs, and feed on fruit and flowers long ago.

Exactly when this occurred has been debated for decades. One suggestion is that these ancestors began to diverge from primitive monkeys and hang below the branches as early as thirty million years ago[4] but remained generalized ape-like and monkey-like creatures until some sixteen million years ago.[5] So we do not know how the hominoids propelled themselves twenty million years ago.

But they lived among the leaves. And from the dozens of jaws and teeth they left behind it is obvious that these creatures spent much of their days collecting fruit.[6] With their projecting snouts, shearing fangs, and bucked front teeth, these hominoids plucked, stripped, husked, and shelled their daily fare. They must have drunk from tulip-shaped bromeliads, from other plants, and from crannies that cupped water from the daily rains. And certainly they chattered with their companions, jockeyed for rank and food, and tucked into the crotches of sturdy limbs to sleep.

Jungle Love

No doubt the hominoids "made love" too. Perhaps they even felt mild infatuation as they sniffed and stroked and groomed one another prior to copulation. But it is unlikely that sex was daily fare for these early relatives of ours. Why? Because all female primates— except women—have a period of heat, or estrus. Female monkeys of some species come into heat seasonally; other monkeys and all the apes have a monthly menstrual cycle, much like that of women. But in the middle of each rotation, which can last from about twenty-eight days to more than forty-five, they come into heat for a period of one to about twenty days, depending on the species and the individual.

Baboons illustrate a common primate pattern of sexuality, and their sex lives say several things about coitus among our hominoid relatives twenty million years ago.

With the beginning of estrus a female baboon's odor changes, and the "sex skin" around her genitals swells, announcing her fertility like a flag. She begins to "present," tipping her buttocks, looking over her shoulder, crouching, and backing toward males to invite copulation. When her period of heat wanes, however, a female baboon regularly refuses coitus—until next month. Females do not normally copulate when they are pregnant. And after parturition they do not resume estrus or regular sexual activity until they have weaned their young—a period of about five to twenty-one months. Hence female baboons are available for sex only about one twenty-fifth of their adult lives.[7]

Our ancestors may have been no more sexually active.

The sex lives of several apes confirm this. Female "common" chimps have a period of heat that lasts some ten to fourteen days; female gorillas come into heat for one to four days; and orangutans display estrus about five to six days of their monthly menstrual cycles.[8] Among these wild relatives of ours, the vast majority of copulations occur during this period of heat.[9] At pregnancy these apes cease cycling and stop regular sexual activity. And estrus does not resume until a mother has weaned her young—a period of postpartum sexual quiescence that lasts three to four years among common chimps and gorillas, much longer among orangutans.[10] Only pygmy chimps copulate more regularly. But because these creatures exhibit an unusual pattern of sexuality, they probably do not qualify as a useful model for life as it was some twenty million years ago.[11]

Indeed, our ancestors in the trees were probably like ordinary primates—and sex was periodic. Some females were sexier than others, just as some apes and women are today. Some had longer periods of heat; some were more popular with the males. But coupling was most likely confined to the time of estrus. Placid days may have become orgiastic as females came into heat and males struggled among the branches for the privilege of coitus. But females must have resumed sexual quiescence during pregnancy, then abstained until they weaned their young. They probably had sex no more than a few intermittent weeks every few years.

Even ordinary primates make exceptions, however, and that leads me to offer a few more speculations about sex among our furry forebears. Because social upheaval stimulates females of many species to copulate at times other than midcycle estrus, it is likely that a new leader, a new member in the group, or some special food item like meat provoked some females to copulate when they were not in heat.[12] Females probably used sex to get delicacies and make friends.

Females probably occasionally stole a little sex while pregnant or nursing too. Rhesus monkeys, as well as common chimps and gorillas, sometimes copulate during the first few months of pregnancy[13] or before they have weaned an infant.[14] So it is reasonable to suggest that our ancestors also did so. Sometimes they may have masturbated, as gorillas do.[15] Since homosexuality is known among female gorillas, chimps, and many other species, our female forebears must have mounted or rubbed against one another for stimulation.[16] Last, because male apes sometimes force females into coitus when they are not receptive, female hominoids were no doubt occasionally raped.[17]

We can say nothing more about the sexuality or mating system of these early creatures except that profound changes in the weather would push some of them imperceptibly toward humanity—and our worldwide penchant to flirt, to fall in love, to marry, to be unfaithful, to divorce, and to pair again.

It all began with churning molten currents of the inner earth.

Commotion in the Ocean

Twenty million years ago Africa and Arabia formed a single island continent that lay slightly south of its position today.[18] To the north lay a sea, the Tethys Ocean, that stretched from the Atlantic in the west to the Pacific in the east, connecting the waters of the world. At the time, this sluice was the earth's radiator. Hot bottom waters from the Tethys swept around the globe, heating tides and winds that bathed the world's beaches with warm waves and its forests with warm rain.[19]

This furnace would disappear. Pulled by fiery currents beneath the land, the African-Arabian plate of the earth's crust began to shift to the north some seventeen or more million years ago and slammed into what we now call the Middle East to make the Zagros, the Taurus, and the Caucasus mountain ranges. Soon an immense land corridor stretched from Africa into Eurasia, connecting the vast forests of the ancient world.[20]

Now the Tethys was squeezed in half. From its western portion, what would become the Mediterranean Sea, warm salty water still spilled into the Atlantic Ocean. But the eastern Tethys, what later evolved into the Indian Ocean, no longer received tropical currents. The Atlantic and the Indo-Pacific oceans were disconnected: warm tides no longer swept around the globe, warming the jungles of the ancient world.[21] Since the dawn of the Cenozoic era, when the mammals replaced the dinosaurs over sixty-five million years ago, world temperatures had begun to drop. Now they plunged again. In Antarctica ice caps formed on mountaintops. Along the equator the land began to dry.

The earth was cooling down.

Further climatic upheavals struck East Africa. Earlier jostling of the earth's crust had left two yawning gashes, parallel rifts that stretched five thousand kilometers from today's northern Ethiopia south through Malawi. But as the African-Arabian continent drifted north, these rifts began to spread apart. Between them the ground sank, forming the East African landscape we know today, a series of low valleys nestled between mountainous highlands on either side.[22]

Clouds from equatorial Africa now dumped warm moisture before they rose over the western shoulder of the Western Rift, while trade winds from the Indian Ocean dumped their rain before rising over the Eastern Rift. The Rift Valley region of East Africa came into "rain shadow." Where mists had veiled the morning sun, now days were clear and parched.

Seasons soon marked the ceaseless round of births and deaths. Monsoons still swept off the Indian Ocean between October and April seventeen million years ago, but by May many of the tropical plants were dormant. Fig trees, acacia trees, and mango and wild pear trees no longer bore their fruit or flowers all year long; tender buds, new leaves, and shoots burgeoned only in the rainy season.[23] Hot rains that had soaked East Africa every afternoon were becoming a thing of the past.

Even worse, volcanoes began to spray forth molten rock. Some had begun to spout as early as twenty million years ago. But by sixteen million years ago, Tinderet, Yelele, Napak, Moroto, Kadam, Elgon, and Kisingeri threw off streams of lava and clouds of ash on the animals and plants below.[24]

With the cooling of the earth, the effects of rain shadow, and the active volcanoes in the region, the tropical forests of East Africa began to shrink—as woods were thinning around the world.

Replacing all these trees were two new ecological niches: the woodlands and the savannahs.[25] Along lakes and riverbanks, trees still packed together. But where the ground rose and streams turned into rivulets, the woodlands appeared. Here single-story trees stretched out, barely touching one another with their boughs. And where water was even scarcer, herbs and grasses that had struggled to survive below a dome of branches began to spread into miles and miles of wooded and savannah plains.[26] By fourteen million years ago the lush, protective world of the hominoids was coming to an end.

Havoc reigned.

So did opportunity.

Around this time many forest animals died out. The tiny ancient relatives of the horse and other creatures migrated into Africa from the dwindling forests of Eurasia. And many other species emerged from forest glades to congregate in larger groups and evolve into novel species on the veldt. Among these immigrants to the grasslands were the forerunners of the modern rhino and giraffe, the ostrich, myriad kinds of antelopes, and other browsing and grazing herbivores that swarm the Serengeti Plains today. Evolving with them were their predators, lions, cheetahs, and other carnivores, as well as jackals and hyenas—the garbage collectors of the ancient world.[27]

Turmoil in the ocean, the new land bridge to the north, seasonality, the thinning forest canopy, and the expanding woodlands and grassy plains would enormously affect the hominoids. By fifteen million years ago our precursors had experienced an "adaptive radiation." Due undoubtedly to the new highway out of Africa, some trickled into France, Spain, and Hungary and on to Asia before most vanished from the fossil record some eleven million years ago. Several strains flourished, then disappeared—dead ends.

Most interesting of these explorers was a group known collectively as the ramamorphs (including *Ramapithecus* and *Sivapithecus*), some of which have long been hailed the missing link. These "nutcrackers" appeared in East Africa about fourteen million years ago, then radiated through the Middle East to India and China. The thick enamel on their molar teeth suggests they roamed the woods eating nuts and fruits with tough rinds, although they probably also forayed into more-open countryside.[28] They appear to have died out some eight million years ago.

Who were the ramamorphs? Today some anthropologists think these animals were ancient relatives of the orangutans, crumpled-looking, red-haired apes that still live in the shrinking jungles of Southeast Asia.[29] Others maintain that from within this general stock, our humanlike forebears (as well as all the living apes) would emerge.[30] This argument isn't resolved. At its core remains the basic question: What was the missing link—that breed of hominoid to descend from the fast-disappearing trees of Africa and begin the march toward humankind? We still don't know.

By six million years ago grasses reigned across East Africa; conditions were ripe for the emergence of humankind. Bits and pieces of humanlike fossil bones have been found, but not enough to fill a shoe box. And virtually no fossils of primitive apes have been uncovered from this time block. So scientists have no extensive evidence of that arboreal ancestor who would emerge on the plains to build the world of sex we struggle with today.

One essential clue has materialized, however. From biochemical similarities of blood proteins and other molecules, scientists have established that the ancestors of the orangutan split off from this basic ramamorph stock somewhere around ten million years ago. Consequently we are most closely related to the African apes, goril-

las, and chimpanzees. Our hominid forebears probably diverged
from the ancestors of these creatures as recently as four or five million years ago.[31]

~ Friends you pick, relatives you are stuck with. So this genetic link
to the African apes is important to the story of human love; nature
plays with what she's got—upon the adaptations of one creature she
selects new designs. So although the African apes have certainly
evolved over past millennia, their close biological ties to humankind
make them excellent models for reconstructing life as it may have
been just before our ancestors were forced from the vanishing forests
of East Africa, just before human patterns of marriage, adultery, and
divorce evolved.

Gorilla Tactics

Gorillas live in harems. Today these shy, beguiling creatures still
roam the dormant Virunga volcanoes of Zaire, Uganda, and
Rwanda. Until her murder in the jungle in 1985, anthropologist
Dian Fossey studied thirty-five of these gorilla bands, recording their
daily lives for some eighteen years.

Each gorilla harem is led by a single adult silverback male (so-
called because of the saddle of silvery hair that spreads across his
back) and at least two "wives." Often a black-backed (subadult) or a
younger fully adult male occupies a lesser position at the flank of a
gorilla band, accompanied by his younger wives. So the leader, the
younger males, their wives, and a gaggle of sundry young wander
together among the moss-laden hagenia trees, foraging for thistle
and wild celery in the mist and underbrush, deep in the heart of
Africa.

Female gorillas begin to copulate by age nine to eleven. As her
monthly one- to four-day estrous period starts, a female begins to
court the group's highest-ranking male that is not her father or full
sibling.[32] She tips her buttocks toward him, looks into his brown
eyes, and backs assertively toward him, rubbing her genitals rhythmi-
cally against him or sitting on his lap to copulate face-to-face. All the
while she makes soft, high, fluttering calls.[33]

If no eligible "husband" is available, however, she leaves her natal band to join another group where a suitable male resides. And if no partner is present there either, she joins a solitary bachelor and travels independently with him. If her mate cannot entice a second female to join them within a few months, however, a female will desert her lover and travel with a harem. Female gorillas do not tolerate monogamy; they seek harem life.

Young males are also mobile. If a black-backed male reaches puberty in a band where one or more young adult females reside, he often remains in his natal group to breed with them. But if no females have reached puberty or if all are full siblings, he either transfers to another group or wanders as a solitary bachelor in order to attract young females for a harem of his own. This mobility inhibits incest. In fact, on only one occasion did Fossey witness incest: a silverback mated with his daughter. Curiously, months after she gave birth, the infant was killed by family members. Evidence of bone splinters in their feces indicates that the baby was partially eaten too.[34]

Once a harem is established, the husband and his co-wives settle down; normally they mate for life—sunbathing when the sun breaks through, moving in their rhythmic round of work and play. Occasionally a female leaves her spouse to join a different mate—serial monandry.[35] But this is rare. Mates are not necessarily sexually faithful to their partners, though. An estrous female mates only with her husband, who interrupts her sexual overtures to other males. Once pregnant, however, a female often begins to copulate with lower-ranking males—directly under her husband's nose. And unless sex becomes too vigorous, her spouse does not interrupt these rendezvous. Gorillas philander and tolerate adultery.

Did our arboreal ancestors living six million years ago travel in harems as gorillas do? Did males and females mate for life, then copulate occasionally with other members of the band? Perhaps.

There are major differences between human sexual tastes and the reproductive habits of gorillas, however. Gorillas always copulate in public, whereas a hallmark of human coupling is privacy. More important, male gorillas *always* form harems. Not so men. As you know, the vast majority of human males have only a single wife at once. Female gorillas and human females have even less in common.

Although women do join harems, they usually bicker with their co-wives. Women are not temperamentally built for harem life.

What most distinguishes human beings from gorillas, though, is the length of our "relationships." Gorillas almost always mate for life. People, on the other hand, tend to switch partners—sometimes several times. For us, long marriages take work.

The Primal Horde

Darwin, Freud, Engels, and many other thinkers have postulated that our earliest ancestors lived in a "primal horde"—that men and women copulated with whom they liked, when they liked.[36] As Lucretius, the Roman philosopher, wrote in the first century A.D., "The human beings that lived in those days in the fields were a tougher sort of people, as the tough earth had made them. . . . They lived for many revolutions of the sun, roaming far and wide in the manner of wild beasts. And Venus joined the bodies of lovers in the forest; for they were brought together by mutual desire, or by the frenzied force and violent lust of the man, or by a bribe of acorns, pears, or arbute-berries."[37]

Lucretius may have been correct. Our closest relatives, common chimpanzees and pygmy chimpanzees, live in hordes, and sexual bribery is commonplace—particularly among pygmy chimps, the smaller of the two species. Moreover, we are as genetically similar to these chimpanzees as the domesticated dog is to the wolf. So we can surmise a lot about our past from examining their lives.

Today pygmy chimps (*Pan paniscus*), commonly called bonobos, remain in a few swampy jungles that hug the Zaire (Congo) River. Here they display feats of acrobatics, arm swinging, leaping, diving, and walking on two limbs like tightrope artists often a hundred feet above the ground. They spend most of their time moving on the forest floor, however, strolling through the woods on all four limbs, looking for juicy fruits, seeds, shoots, leaves, honey, worms, and caterpillars, digging holes to excavate mushrooms, or stealing sugarcane and pineapples from farmers.[38]

They eat meat too. On two occasions anthropologists saw males stalk flying squirrels—unsuccessfully. In two other instances males silently caught and killed a small forest antelope, a duiker, and shared its meat. And the local villagers say bonobos dig in the mud beside streams to collect fish and scatter termite mounds to eat the milling residents.[39] Perhaps our ancestors hunted animals and collected other proteins to supplement their diet of fruit and nuts.

Anthropologists are just beginning to learn about bonobo social life. From what they can make out, these creatures travel in mixed groups of males, females, and young. Some parties are small; two to eight individuals often travel in a relatively stable band. Yet fifteen to thirty, even a hundred individuals sometimes assemble to eat, relax, or sleep near one another. And individuals come and go between groups, depending on the food supply, connecting a cohesive community of several dozen animals. Here is a primal horde.

Sex is almost a daily pastime. Female bonobos have an extended monthly period of heat, stretching through almost three-quarters of their menstrual cycle. But sex, as mentioned earlier, is not confined to estrus. Females copulate during most of their menstrual cycles—a pattern of coitus more similar to women's than any other creature's.[40]

And females bribe their male friends with sex quite regularly. A female will walk up to a male who is eating sugarcane, sit beside him, beg palm up, as people do, and then look plaintively at the delicacy and back at him. He feels her gaze. When he gives her the treat, she tips her buttocks and copulates; then she ambles off with the cane in hand. A female is not beyond soliciting another female either, sauntering up to a comrade, climbing into her arms face-to-face, wrapping her legs around her waist, and rubbing her genitals on those of her partner before accepting sticks of cane. Male–male homosexuality, fellatio, also occurs.[41]

Bonobos engage in sex to ease tension, to stimulate sharing during meals, to reduce stress while traveling, and to reaffirm friendships during anxious reunions. "Make love, not war" is clearly a bonobo scheme.

Did our ancestors do the same?

Bonobos, in fact, display many of the sexual habits people exhibit on the streets, in the bars and restaurants, and behind apartment doors in New York, Paris, Moscow, and Hong Kong. Prior to coitus bonobos often stare deeply into each other's eyes. As I have mentioned, this copulatory gaze is a central component of human courtship too. And bonobos, like human beings, walk arm in arm, kiss each other's hands and feet, and embrace with long, deep, tongue-intruding French kisses.[42]

Darwin suspected kissing was natural to people. Although aware that this practice was unknown in several cultures, he thought the drive to caress a beloved was innate.

He was right. Over 90 percent of all peoples on record kiss. Until Western contact, kissing was reportedly unknown among the Somali, the Lepcha of Sikkim, and the Siriono of South America, whereas the Thonga of South Africa and a few other peoples traditionally found kissing disgusting.[43] But even in these societies lovers patted, licked, rubbed, sucked, nipped, or blew on each other's faces prior to copulation. The world's great kissers are the Hindus and Westerners; we have made the kiss an art. But bonobos—and a lot of other animals—share our fondness of the kiss.

Bonobos in the San Diego Zoo also copulate in the missionary position (face-to-face with the male on top) 70 percent of the time, although this may be because they have access to a flat dry surface.[44] In the African forest 40 of 106 observed copulations were face-to-face; the balance were in the rear-entry pose instead.[45] But pygmy chimpanzees like variety. A female will sit on a male's lap to copulate, couple face-to-face from on top of him, crouch while her partner stands, have intercourse while both are standing, or have coitus while hanging in a tree. Sometimes the two manipulate each other's genitals while mating. And they always gaze at each other as they "make love."

Our last tree-dwelling ancestors probably kissed and hugged prior to coitus too; maybe they even "made love" *en face* while looking deep into each other's eyes.[46]

Because bonobos appear to be the smartest of the apes, because they have many physical traits quite similar to people's, and because these chimps copulate with flair and frequency, some anthropologists conjecture that bonobos are much like the African hominoid prototype, our last common tree-dwelling ancestor.[47] Maybe pygmy chimps are living relics of our past. But they certainly manifest some fundamental differences in their sexual behavior. For one thing, bonobos do not form long-term pair-bonds the way humans do. Nor do they raise their young as husband and wife. Males do care for infant siblings,[48] but monogamy is no life for them. Promiscuity is their fare.

If pygmy chimpanzees are what remains of our primordial ancestors living in the trees, then human adultery is very old indeed.

Chimpanzee Days

Just as promiscuous are common chimpanzees, *Pan troglodytes,* named after Pan, the spirit of Mother Nature and a god to the ancient Greeks. Since 1960 Jane Goodall has been watching these creatures at the Gombe Stream Reserve, Tanzania, and she has observed some remarkable behaviors that help us visualize life as it may have been among our tree-dwelling ancestors six million years ago.

These chimps live in communities of fifteen to eighty individuals in ranges of five to twelve square kilometers along the eastern shore of Lake Tanganyika. "Home" varies from thick forests to more open woodlands to stretches of savannah grass with scattered trees. Because the food supply is dispersed and uneven, individuals are obliged to travel in small, temporary groups.

Males move along the ground in parties of about four or five. Two or more mothers with infants sometimes join one another for a few hours as a "nursery" party. And individuals often amble by themselves or with one or more friends in a small mixed-sex group. Parties are flexible; individuals come and go. But if members of one party find a particularly lush supply of figs, new buds, or some other delicacy, they hoot through the forest or drum on trees with their fists. Then all assemble for the meal.

Female common chimps have a midcycle estrus that often lasts ten to sixteen days, and their patterns of sexuality strike me as the best model for life as it was among our ancestors long ago.[49]

As a female comes into heat, the sex skin around her genitals balloons like a huge pink flower—a passport to male activities. She often joins an all-male party and proceeds to seduce all except her sons and brothers. As many as eight males may line up and wait their turn, in what is known as opportunistic mating. Males copulate within two minutes of one another; intromission, thrusting, and ejaculation normally take only ten to fifteen seconds.[50]

More dominant courtiers may attempt to monopolize an estrous female instead, what is called "possessive mating." A male will stare intently to get a female's attention, sit with his legs open to display an erect penis, flick it, rock from side to side, beckon her with outstretched arms, swagger in front of her, or follow a female doggedly.[51] One male slept on the ground in the rain all night waiting for a nesting estrous female to arise. When a male succeeds in attracting a female to his side, he sticks close to her and tries to prevent copulations with other males. Sometimes males even chase, charge, or attack other suitors. But confrontations of this sort take precious time—minutes the female sometimes uses to copulate with as many as three other admirers.

Female chimps are sexually aggressive. On one occasion Flo, the sexiest of the chimps at Gombe, copulated several dozen times during the course of a single day. Adolescent females are sometimes insatiable, even tweaking the flaccid penises of uninterested companions. Some females appear to masturbate as well. Moreover, female chimps can be picky. They prefer males who groom them and give them food—not necessarily the most dominant individuals in the male hierarchy.[52] Some courtiers they flatly refuse. With others they have long-standing friendships and copulate more regularly. And both sexes avoid coitus with close relatives, such as mother or siblings.[53]

Female chimps like sexual adventure. Adolescent females at Gombe often leave their natal group for the duration of estrus to join males in a neighboring community, a habit many continue as adults. Strange males see the enlarged, pink sex skin of an estrous female and inspect her vulva. Then they copulate rather than attack the stranger. Like some human teenagers, female common chimps regularly leave home to mate. Some return; others transfer permanently instead.

Were ancestral hominoid women sexually aggressive? Did they join all-male parties during estrus, copulate with these bachelors, masturbate at times, and make friends with specific males? Probably.

They may have made longer partnerships as well.

Making Dates

Sometimes an estrous female and a single male chimp vanish to copulate out of sight and earshot—what is known as going on safari.[54] These trysts are often initiated by the male. With hair and penis erect, he beckons, rocks from side to side, waves branches, and gazes intently at his potential paramour. When she moves toward him, he turns and walks away, hoping she will follow. These gestures become more intense until she does his bidding. Sometimes a male even attacks a female until she acquiesces.

Here, then, are traces of monogamy—complete with coitus in privacy. These clandestine consortships often last several days; a few last several weeks. And they have reproductive payoffs. At least half of the fourteen pregnancies recorded at Gombe occurred while a female was on safari.[55] Perhaps our ancestors in the trees occasionally made similar short-term pair-bonds, vanished into the leaves to copulate face-to-face, hugged, stroked, kissed each other's faces, hands, and bodies, lay in each other's arms, fed each other bits of fruit, and bore young from these "affairs."

But once again these chimps differ in a vital respect from human beings. When a female common chimp becomes noticeably pregnant, she begins to roam alone or joins a group of mothers and infants. And as she nears parturition, she settles in a small "home" range. Some females pick a spot in the center of a community; some make home at the periphery of the neighborhood. On this turf she bears her infant and raises it alone. Chimpanzees do not form pair-bonds to rear their young. To chimps, fathering is unknown.

Common chimps display many other social habits, however, that would germinate among our forebears, then flourish in humankind. Among them is war.

The males at Gombe guard the borders of their turf. Three or more adult males set off together. Sometimes they call loudly, perhaps to scare off outsiders, but usually they scout in silence. They stop to stand and peer over tall grass or climb trees to scan adjacent property. Some inspect discarded food, examine strange nests, or listen for intruding chimps as they steal along. When they encounter neighbors, they urinate or defecate out of nervousness and touch one another for reassurance; then they call aggressively and perform mock charges. Some wave branches. Some slap the ground. Some hurl or roll stones. Then both sides retreat.[56]

In 1974 a chimpanzee war erupted. In the early 1970s a splinter group of seven males and three females had begun to travel chiefly in the southern portion of the Kasakela community's real estate, and by 1972 these emigrants had established themselves as a separate community, known to observers as Kahama, after this river valley to the south. Intermittently Kasakela males met Kahama males at their new border and called, drummed on trees and dragged branches in unfriendly displays before mutually retreating.

In 1974, however, five Kasakela males penetrated deep into southern territory, surprised a Kahama male, and beat him up. As Goodall described the incident, one Kasakela male held the victim down while others bit him, kicked him, pummeled him with their fists, and jumped on him. Finally one male rose onto his hind legs, screamed above the melee, and hurled a rock at the enemy. It fell short. After ten more minutes of mayhem, the warriors abandoned the Kahama male with bleeding wounds and broken bones.[57]

Over the next three years five more Kahama males and one female met the same fate. By 1977, Kasakela males had exterminated most of their neighbors; the rest vanished. The Kasakela community soon extended its range south along the shores of Lake Tanganyika.[58]

Had our tree-dwelling ancestors begun to wage war on one another some six million years ago? It seems plausible.

They probably had begun to hunt for meat as well.[59] Chimpanzee hunters are always adults, almost always males. The victims are normally juvenile baboons, monkeys, bushbuck, or bushpigs. Sometimes a male simply seizes an unsuspecting monkey feeding nearby in a tree and tears it to shreds, "opportunistic hunting." But planned, cooperative group hunting expeditions are also common. The hunt is always silent. Only the direction of the hunter's gaze, his ruffled hair, his cocked head, the determination of his gait, or exchanged glances alert others that the chase is on. Then a group of males surround their victim together.

As soon as one chimp grabs the prey, a tug-of-war begins. Each hunter hollers and retreats with pieces, and minutes later all in ear-shot assemble to form "sharing clusters" around possessors of the spoils. Some chimps beg, palm up; others stare at the possessor or the meat; still others retrieve dropped morsels from the foliage below. Then everyone sits to eat, leisurely adding leaves to supplement the protein—the proverbial steak-and-salad dinner. Sometimes it takes a dozen chimps all day to consume a carcass weighing less than twenty pounds, an event not unlike an American Christmas dinner.

Chimps do fight over meat. Tempers sometimes flare, but interestingly rank does not guarantee a larger portion. In this one aspect of chimpanzee social life, subordinates do not defer to leaders. Instead, age has clout. So does sex appeal. And estrous females always receive extra pieces.[60]

Forethought, group hunting, cooperation, sharing—these hunting skills would be greatly improved by our ancestors, for one key element of human hunting is often missing among these chimps: the use of weapons. On only one occasion did a Gombe chimp use an implement to fell quarry. A group of males had surrounded four bushpigs, and the hunters were trying to extricate a piglet from their midst. Finally one aged male hurled a melon-sized rock, striking an adult pig. The bushpigs fled. Immediately the chimp hunters captured, disassembled, and devoured the youngster.[61]

Chimps use weapons more often when confronting one another, however.[62] They drop tree limbs on those beneath them, whip their enemies with saplings, rise onto their hind legs to brandish sticks, hurl rocks and branches, and drag logs or roll stones as they charge their adversaries. Perhaps when our tree-dwelling ancestors were not courting estrous females, they were making war, hunting, or attacking one another with sticks and stones. Most likely they also spent a good deal of time just trying to keep the peace.[63]

Male chimps use weapons regularly, but females make and use tools more often—particularly when they gather insects.[64] Female chimps "dip" for ants, opening a subterranean ant nest with their fingers and inserting a slender twig. As the ants stream up the pole, the hunter plunges the tiny, milling creatures into her mouth like peanuts—chewing frantically to devour the ants before they bite her tongue. Chimps also use rocks to open nuts and tough-skinned fruits. They fish in the tunnels of termite compounds with long grass stems, and they use leaves to wipe dirt from their bodies, sticks to pick their teeth, leaves to fan away flies, chewed leaves to sop water from a tree crotch, and sticks and stones to hurl at cats and snakes and hostile chimpanzees.[65]

Our ancestors must have used tools regularly.

Dentistry and doctoring probably also came from our tree-dwelling predecessors. At Gombe the budding chimp "dentist," Belle, used twigs to clean the teeth of a young male as he held his mouth wide open. On one occasion she made a successful extraction too—pulling out an infected tooth as her patient lay still, head back, mouth gaping.[66] At the Primate Research Center at Central Washington University a young male used a twig to clean a foot sore on one of his companions.[67] Chimps also pick away scabs when they groom one another.

Chimps do not desert their dying either. After a female chimp at Gombe was attacked by a group of males, her daughter sat beside her crushed body for hours, brushing off the flies until her mother passed away. But the juvenile did not leave a leaf, a branch, or stone to commemorate the death. Only elephants "bury" their companions, placing branches over the head and shoulders of their deceased.[68]

In addition, our tree-dwelling ancestors probably had a rich world of etiquette six million years ago. Chimps today give gifts of leaves and twigs to their chimp superiors. They bow to high-ranking companions. They keep "friends" and travel with these companions. They shake hands, stroke one another reassuringly, and pat each other's fannies the way football players do. They clench their teeth and draw back their lips into the "human" nervous social smile. They pout, sulk, and stage tantrums. And they groom each other regularly, picking grass and dirt from each other's hair much as we pick lint from someone else's sweater.

Noble Savages

Did our last tree-dwelling relatives live in communities like chimpanzees?[69] Did they gang up on one another, protect their boundaries, and war on neighbors, a consuming passion of humanity today? Did they think ahead, use sticks to dip for ants, cooperate to hunt for meat, and share the spoils? It seems reasonable.

Some may have been early doctors; others, warriors. They probably played practical jokes like dumping water or foliage on an unsuspecting comrade, because chimps love to be buffoons and play pranks on one another. Some of our forebears must have been serious, some inventive, some shy, some courageous, some sweet, some self-centered, some patient, some sneaky, some petty—as people and all the apes can be.

They must have had a sense of family too. Chimpanzees, gorillas, and all the higher primates associate regularly with mother, sisters, and brothers. And they probably gave gifts to friends, were scared of strangers, had tiffs with peers, bowed to superiors, kissed their lovers, walked arm in arm, and held hands and feet. They undoubtedly communicated their fondness, amusement, irritation, and many other emotions with facial expressions, giggles, pants, and hoots. And surely they spent a great deal of time sitting on the forest floor, patting, stroking, hugging, picking dirt and leaves from one another, playing with their infants, friends, and lovers.

Maybe they vanished into the forest with a consort for a few days or weeks of private sex. Perhaps some even felt adoration for this temporary mate or sadness when the safari ended. But most likely sex was a casual affair. Six million years ago children grew up under the tutelage of mother and her female friends. The "father," the "husband," the "wife," our human reproductive strategy of serial monogamy and clandestine adultery had not yet evolved.

But the stage was set; the players in the wings. Soon our ancestors would be forced out of Eden—into the woodlands and grasslands of the ancient world. Here they would develop a dual craving for devotion and philandering that would plague their descendants to this day.

~7~

Out of Eden

A Theory on the Origin of Monogamy and Desertion

The beast and bird their common charge attend,
The mothers nurse it, and the sires defend;
The young dismiss'd to wander earth or air,
There stops the Instinct, and there ends the care;
The link dissolves, each seeks a fresh embrace,
Another love succeeds, another race.
A longer care Man's helpless kind demands;
That longer care contracts more lasting bands.

—*Alexander Pope,* An Essay on Man

It was the beginning of the wet season in East Africa some 3.6 million years ago. For weeks the volcano Sadiman had periodically belched forth clouds of gray volcanic ash, daily spreading a blanket of dust on the plains below. Every afternoon showers moistened the ash; then during the cool evenings it hardened—engraving raindrops, acacia leaf prints, and the tracks of passing antelopes, giraffes, rhinos, elephants, pigs, guinea fowl, baboons, hares, insects, hyenas, a saber-toothed cat, and some ancient relatives of ours.[1]

Three primitive hominids,[2] among the earliest individuals ever found in the line toward modern people, had picked their way through the volcanic muck, leaving their footprints for posterity. The largest had walked across the ash, sinking about five centimeters with every step. Beside these prints were those of a smaller hominid, perhaps a female, who stood a little over four feet tall. And because a third pair of tracks were superimposed on those of the largest creature, we deduce that a somewhat smaller hominid had followed, stepping carefully in the footsteps of the leader. All three were heading north to a small gorge, perhaps to camp in the trees beside the stream, because the tracks proceed seventy-seven feet to the canyon's edge. Then abruptly they disappear.

In 1978 Mary Leakey, the well-known archaeologist and wife of Louis Leakey, the now deceased grand old man of African paleoanthropology, and her team discovered these footprints eroding out of an ancient geologic stratum.[3] Since the mid-1970s Leakey had been excavating a site called Laetoli, an area in northern Tanzania named by the local Masai tribesmen for a red lily that carpets the area today. Within weeks of the 1978 field season she found these signatures of our past. With minor variations, the footprints were just like those of modern men and women.

Whether these creatures strolled, strode, or picked their way, even whether they walked together or at different times, is not clear from the many analyses of these tracks. But that they lived and died near the gorge is beyond doubt. In other field seasons Leakey unearthed a host of other hominid fossils—mostly skull and jaw fragments and the isolated teeth of more than twenty-two individuals who wandered across these grasslands below Mount Sadiman between 3.5 and 3.8 million years ago.[4]

They were not alone. To the north, along what is today the Hadar River of the Afar region of Ethiopia, lived Lucy. Anthropologist Donald Johanson and teammates unearthed her in 1974. Named after the Beatles song "Lucy in the Sky with Diamonds," Lucy once stood some three and a half feet tall, weighed about sixty pounds, and dined along the edge of a shallow lake in what was then the rolling wooded countryside of Ethiopia. She suffered from arthritis and died in her early twenties, around three million years ago.[5]

Johanson's team recovered about 40 percent of Lucy's skeleton. And although her toes and fingers were curved and somewhat longer than ours, suggesting that Lucy spent time in the trees, the remains of her hip, knee, ankle, and foot confirm that she walked on two feet instead of four.[6] The following year Johanson unearthed what could have been Lucy's friends, the partial remains of at least thirteen more individuals who strode through the woods of Ethiopia so long ago. Now bits and pieces of perhaps fifteen more ancient hominids have been unearthed as well.

Exactly who these hominids at Laetoli and Hadar were, we do not know. Those who study hominid footprints are known as ichnologists, and they, as well as many other anthropologists, think a foot like Lucy's could also have left the prints at Laetoli. So they place all these individuals in the same early species, *Australopithecus afarensis*, a branch of hominids somewhere near the beginning of the human line.[7]

These creatures probably looked something like modern chimps, with brains that were slightly larger (but no more than a third the size of ours), heavy ridges at their brows, dark eyes and skin, thin lips, no chins, and protruding jaws with bucked front teeth and shearing fangs. Many details of their craniums, jaws, and skeletons were reminiscent of apes, but their bodies were remarkably human. And they walked erect. Humankind had emerged on earth.

Where had these "people" come from? How had their ancestors turned down the road toward humanity?

(overleaf) A moment in our human ancestry: The scene depicted on the following pages shows members of the species *Australopithecus afarensis*, the first of our humanlike forebears, who had begun to live in the woodlands and plains of East Africa by some four million years ago. These "people" had long (and somewhat curved) fingers and toes, short legs, long arms, small brains, projecting jaws, and other anatomical details that distinguish them from contemporary people. But they walked erect and had begun their march toward modern human life. Individuals such as these probably traveled in bands of twelve to twenty-five friends and relatives, formed pair-bonds shortly after puberty, shared food with a mate, remained paired for at least the infancy of a single child (about four years), and often parted when the child became old enough to join community activities. Then typically each formed a new pair-bond with a partner in a neighboring group and bore more young. In subsequent chapters I propose that modern human sexual anatomy and the human sexual emotions evolved in conjunction with the evolution of the reproductive strategy of serial monogamy and clandestine adultery. *Illustration by Michael Rothman.*

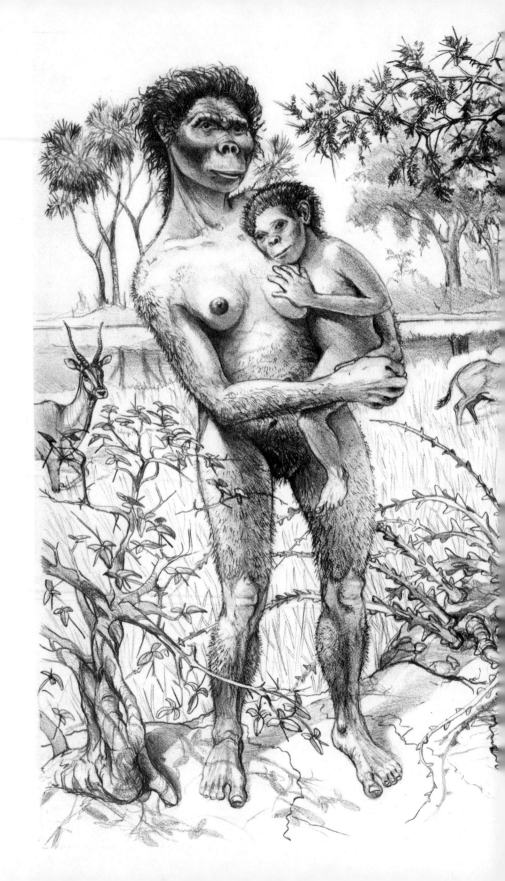

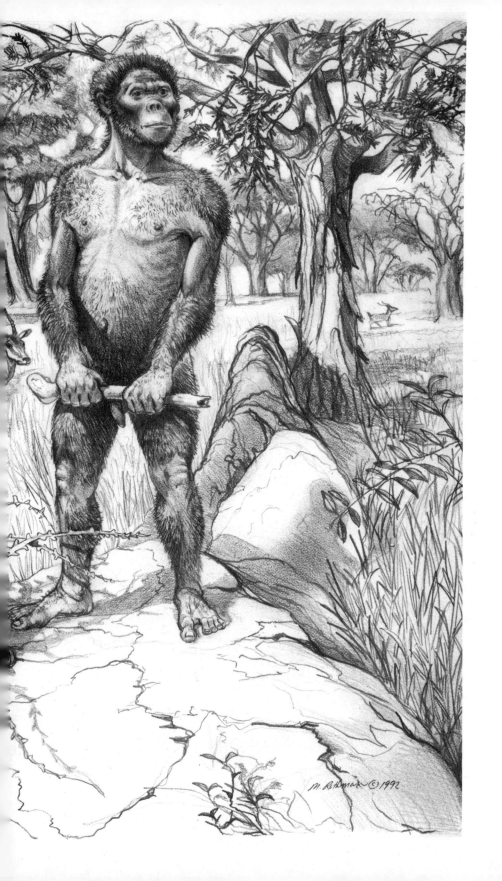

M. Rothman © 1992

The Crucible

"Two roads diverged in a wood, and I—I took the one less traveled by, and that has made all the difference." Robert Frost captured that moment in life that irrevocably changes everything that follows. Such a time occurred in human evolution, an era when our first ancestors stepped irreversibly away from their tree-dwelling relatives and began along the path toward modern human social life. Silent is the fossil record of this nativity. The "missing link" is lost in time and rock. Yet through the centuries theologians, philosophers, and scientists have woven, from threads of knowledge, theories of our genesis.

The following is another version. It stems from scientific data in a variety of disciplines, including what we know of the animals and plants that flourished across East Africa millennia ago, the lifeways of modern apes and monkeys, the mating habits of other monogamous species such as foxes and robins, the life-styles of modern hunting-gathering peoples, and human patterns of infatuation, attachment, and abandonment that I have presented in this book. Here, then, is an hypothesis for the origin of marriage, divorce, and remarriage.

The time was somewhere between four and six million years ago; let's make it four million—somewhat before Lucy's contemporaries left their bones and footprints below Mount Sadiman. Beside the shallow blue-green lakes and lazy rivers, forest trees and climbing vines cloaked the shore. But farther from the water's edge, mahoganies and evergreens thinned out and grew in patches between clumps of woodland trees. And beyond the woodlands, across the rolling hills of East Africa, stretched an ocean of grass.[8]

Ancient kinds of elephants, ostriches, okapi, gazelles, zebras, wildebeests, bushbuck, elands, buffalo, even primitive horses, immigrants from Asia, strode across the plains. Their enemies, ancestral lions, cheetahs, and feral dogs, followed. At dawn, at dusk, through the day and night, these carnivores stole the weak from among the herds. Then vultures, hyenas, jackals, and other scavengers picked the fallen clean.[9]

It was into this landscape—the vast savanna plains—that our first ancestors were being pushed by the shrinking of the forests. The process had begun millennia before, when tree-dwelling, ape-like predecessors first ventured from the forests into the boulevards of grass that wove between more widely spaced woodland trees.[10] Perhaps small groups of males combed the woodlands for fresh meat. Three or four related females may have appeared in the woodlands together to look for termite mounds or ants. And sometimes whole communities, as many as thirty individuals—the old, the young, the adventuresome, and the fearful—congregated beneath these boughs when the forest branches were picked clean.

How many centuries our ancestors spent in this woodland habitat we will never know. But eventually they were pushed to the fringes of these spreading trees. Here they sat and studied the open countryside. The forest they left behind was full of safety zones. Even in the woodlands trees were spread out, but escape routes were still near. On the grassy plains there was nowhere to hide. But by roughly four million years ago our ancestors had no choice; they had to eat. So they probably moved cautiously into the open grass, sticking close to one another as they marched along.

If they came upon a cashew grove or field of seeds, they hooted, calling the less courageous onto the sun-soaked plains. And the timid came, driven by a curiosity born of need. At first our ancestors probably ventured into the grasslands only in the dry season, when forest and woodland fruits and buds were hard to find. But hunger and competition must have pushed them on. Then, like mice, like rhinos, like many other ancient forest species, they forayed into the uncharted grass. On the baked savannahs our first ancestors probably grabbed and tasted ostrich eggs, nestling birds, shrews, baby antelopes, or even unsuspecting baboons—anything that looked edible, even dead animals.

Man the scavenger. Several anthropologists have recently proposed that "opportunistic collecting" and scavenging preceded the hunting of large game—that our ancestors arrived on the grasslands of the ancient world to collect small animals and scavenge for a living.[11]

Meat Pirates

Anthropologist Gary Tunnell recently tested this hypothesis; he used bushcraft to see whether our ancestors could have survived by opportunistic hunting and scavenging millennia ago.[12] Tunnell set up his tent on the Serengeti Plains of East Africa in 1984. He chose an area of six square kilometers in southwestern Kenya, part of the Serengeti ecosystem. He shared his turf with nine lions. The trick would be to scavenge from their dinner rather than becoming part of it.

At night Tunnell slept below two high cliffs amid the sleeping-trees of the local baboon troop. These neighbors alerted him when the largest lion made his nightly visit to smell Tunnell and mark the pride's range beside his tent. Through the night, again at dawn, Tunnell listened. This way he established where the lions made their nightly kill. Then, at 9 A.M., after the lions were asleep, he set out on a specific route in search of meat.

Tunnell always found edible protein—an unwary warthog, a crippled topi, three sleeping bats, several glutted vultures, ten catfish in a dying pool, a three-foot lizard in a tiny canyon, or the carcass of a buffalo, wildebeest, or Grant's gazelle killed by lions or cheetahs hours earlier. Tunnell did not eat any of his discoveries. But he concluded that with no more than a sharpened rock and pointed stick just one human scavenger and a comrade to help butcher flesh could easily feed a group of ten—as long as they stayed out of the territories of hyenas, humankind's major competitor for flesh.

Like Tunnell, the modern Hadza of Tanzania sometimes scavenge in the dry season. They listen to the night calls of the lions and watch the vultures fly. On the next morning they find the kill, move in, drive away the carnivores, and collect the meat with simple tools.

It is unlikely that our first ground-dwelling ancestors used tools the way the Hadza do; at least we have no evidence of tools. So these first human forebears could not have broken through the skin, chopped off joints, or scavenged huge chunks of meat four million years ago. But other primates occasionally scavenge—and they don't use tools.[13]

Moreover, lions and cheetahs often leave their meals unfinished. Leopards even leave their kills unattended, hanging in the tree where they have eaten.[14] Perhaps our ancestors waited until the last of the cats had staggered off to sleep, then crept back to the carcass to smash the skull, collect the brains, pull off skin and tendons, and harvest scraps of flesh. Sometimes they may have thrown stones instead, terrifying the feeding carnivores just long enough to dart in, grab bits of meat, and flee.

Our first ancestors undoubtedly also lived on fruits and vegetables, as well as seeds and roots and rhizomes.[15] As you recall, among the !Kung gatherer-hunters of southern Africa women collected over ninety varieties of fruits and vegetables, contributing more than 65 percent of the band's daily caloric intake.[16] And !Kung women generally went gathering only two or three days a week, taking the rest off to relax, play games, plan rituals, and gossip. Domestic chores took about four hours every day.[17] In fact, because of the largess the grasslands provided, anthropologist Marshall Sahlins has called our gathering-hunting ancestors "the original affluent society."[18]

With just a stick and stone our first forebears could have eaten a rich variety of fruits, nuts, and berries too.

Their dinners must have been interrupted frequently, however. In the open countryside it is impossible to eat unnoticed. Eating takes time. The big cats, primordial enemies of the primates, were at eye level. And gone was the safety of the branches. So, like Tunnell, our first hominid ancestors probably stayed in the short grass, kept trees and cliffs in sight, and avoided tall grass, thickets, and the forest fringe where lions snooze. They probably also kept an eye on the local baboon troop. When these creatures got nervous, they became even more vigilant. Then, when a lion stalked, our ancestors bunched up back-to-back, rose onto their hind legs, waved their arms and branches, hurled rocks, and screamed.

They made one last adjustment—an adaptation that would irrevocably change the course of human history and eventually life on earth. At some point our ancestors began to pick up and *carry* in their arms what food they could collect and cart it to a clump of trees, a cliff, a sandy spit beside a lake—a place where they could eat unmolested by predators. Tunnell is convinced they never lingered at a kill or carted food to where they slept; instead, they collected, carried, and "dined out."

And to carry with your hands and dine out, you have to walk erect.

"Man alone has become a biped," Darwin wrote in 1871.[19] He conjectured that our ancestors rose from four feet onto two in order to use their hands to hurl stones and branches at enemies and attack their prey. Man the hunter; man the protector of women too.

Since Darwin's day generations of scientists have elaborated on this view. In the 1960s it was popular to believe that our male forebears stood to carry weapons to hunt big game like giraffes and zebras and strode to wield weapons in order to shield their mates. In response to this male-oriented hypothesis, female anthropologists of the 1970s and 1980s argued that our ancestors probably walked bipedally to collect and carry vegetables instead.[20] Woman the gatherer. Now scholarly sentiments have changed again. Today many anthropologists propose that the first hominids walked on two legs to collect and scavenge meat.[21]

Probably all of these theories are correct. Carrying a simple sharpened stick, early men and women could pry roots and tubers from the soil. Carrying stones, they could stun a warthog, a baby antelope, or a baboon. Carrying branches, they could scare a jackal or a vulture from its meal. Carrying a rudimentary pouch of leaves and cord, they could tote meat *and* vegetables to a safe spot atop a cliff or in the trees. Bipedalism also permits a metabolically efficient gait for moving long distances slowly. The head is elevated, good for seeing food and predators. Last, when early humans used their hands to carry, they could use their mouths to holler at a predator, to warn a friend, to signal plans.

What a transformation our ancestors must have undergone! At first they probably rose onto their hind limbs, stood, swayed, and staggered a few yards—the way chimpanzees do—before resuming a quadrupedal stance. With time, however, their big toes rotated to lie parallel to the others. They developed an arch from heel to toe and a second arch across the ball of the foot that together acted as a trampoline, stretching, then springing with each step to propel the body forward. With strong new muscles in the buttocks, a pelvis that had became broad and flat, knees aligned below their hips, and sturdy ankle bones, they no longer waddled when they walked. Instead, they almost effortlessly caught themselves as they fell forward—the human stride.

With walking, collecting, and carrying, Lucy's grandmother's grandmother's grandmother's ancestors had found their savannah niche.

But bipedalism, I propose, would start a sexual revolution.

When our forebears lived in the trees and females walked on all four limbs, the newborn had clung to mother's abdomen; as the infant aged, it rode on mother's back as the female walked along unimpeded by her child. But in the grass women walked erect. Now they had to carry the infant in their arms instead.

How could a female carry sticks and stones, jump to catch a hare, dart after a lizard, or hurl stones at lions to drive them from a kill— and carry an infant too? How could a female sit in the dangerous grass to dig for roots, collect vegetables, or dip for ants—and protect her child? In the forest children played among the trees. Safety was everywhere. On the plains children had to be carried and watched constantly, or they would end up in a lion's belly.

Could you survive in the Australian desert carrying a heavy, noisy basketball for several years? With the beginning of bipedalism mothers needed protection and extra food, or they and their infants would not survive. The time was ripe for the evolution of the husband and the father.[22]

Fatherhood

Pair-bonding is rare in nature. The Nile crocodile, American toad, damsel fish, starfish-eating shrimp, wood roach, dung beetle, horned

beetle, and some desert wood lice are all monogamous. Ninety percent of all birds make pair-bonds. But only about 3 percent of all
mammals form a long-term relationship with a single mate. Among
them are some muskrats, some bats, Asiatic clawless otters, beavers,
deer mice, dwarf mongooses, the klipspringer, the reedbuck, the
dik-dik and a few other antelopes, gibbons and siamangs, some seals,
a few South American monkeys, and all of the wild dogs. Foxes,
wolves, coyotes, jackals, the maned wolf of South America, and the
raccoon dog of Japan all form pair-bonds and raise their young as
"husband" and "wife."[23]

Monogamy is rare in mammals because it is not normally to a
male's genetic advantage to remain with one female when he can
copulate with several and pass more of his genes on to posterity. So
males of most species, like gorillas, try to accumulate a harem.

They do this in several ways. If a male can defend an asset, such as
the best place to eat or breed, several females will simply gather on
his territory; male impalas, for example, compete to win rich grazing
pastures where roaming herds of females linger. If resources are so
evenly distributed across the landscape that they are not defensible,
a male may try to attach himself to a group of females traveling
together and guard his entourage against intruding males—as lions
do. And when a male cannot sequester a harem one way or another,
he may establish a large territory and scramble to mate with several
females living within his range—rather like the milkman who visits
house to house. Male orangutans do this.

So it takes very special circumstances before a male will travel with
a *single* mate and help her defend her young.

From a feminine perspective, pair-bonding is not normally adaptive either; a male can be much more trouble than he is worth.
Females of many species prefer to live with female relatives and
copulate with visitors; female elephants do this. And if a female
needs a male for protection, why not travel in a mixed group and
copulate with several males—the common tactic of female chimps?
A host of ecological and biological conditions must be present in the
right proportions before perquisites exceed expenses, making monogamy the best—or only—alternative for both males and females
of a species.

A proper mixture of these conditions occurs in the lives of monogamous red foxes and eastern robins, though. And studying the sex lives of these creatures gave me my first important clue to the evolution of monogamy and divorce in humankind.[24]

Female red foxes bear exceedingly helpless, immature babies, a trait known as altriciality.[25] Kits are born blind and deaf. Not only does the vixen bear infantile young, but she often delivers at least five of them. Moreover, unlike mice that have rich milk and can leave their altricial newborns in a nest while they forage elsewhere and return, the female fox has milk that is low in fat and protein, so she must feed her kits constantly for several weeks. She cannot maroon her pups.

What an ecological conundrum. The female fox will starve to death if she does not have a mate to bring her food while she attends to her helpless kits.[26]

Monogamy is suitable to the male fox, however. These animals live in territories where the resources are spread out. Under normal conditions a male is not able to acquire a piece of property so rich in food and breeding sites that two females are willing to reside on his land and share one mate. Polygyny is rarely an alternative. But a male can travel with a female and guard her from other males during her peak of estrus (assuring paternity for the litter), then help her raise their altricial young in a small home range.[27]

Monogamy is thus the best alternative for both sexes, and red foxes form pair-bonds to raise their young. But here's the clue: foxes do not bond for life.

In February the vixen begins her mating dance. Typically several suitors dog her heels. At the peak of estrus one becomes her mate. They kiss and lick each other's faces, walk side by side, mark their territory, and build several dens as winter wanes. Then, after giving birth in spring, the vixen nurses her pups for almost three weeks while her "husband" returns nightly to feed her a mouse, a fish, or some other delicacy. Through the vibrant summer days and nights, both parents guard the den, train the kits, and hunt for the voracious family. But as summer dies, father returns to the den less and less. In

August mother's maternal temper changes too; she drives her kits from the lair and departs herself.

Among foxes a pair-bond lasts only through the breeding season.[28]

Monogamy for the length of the breeding season is also common among birds. Most birds form a pair-bond for the same reasons foxes do. Because territories generally vary little in their quality of food and breeding sites, a male eastern robin, for example, can rarely acquire a particularly elegant homestead and attract several females to his real estate. But he can defend a small territory and help a single mate. Equally important, female eastern robins deliver several altricial young—eggs that need incubating, chicks that need feeding and protecting. Someone must remain with these infants constantly. And since baby eastern robins do not suckle from a teat, males are just as qualified at parenting.

As a result of these and other circumstances, eastern robins and some 90 percent of over nine thousand other avian species form pair-bonds to raise their broods.[29]

But here's the clue again: like red foxes, eastern robins do not mate for life. They pair up in the spring and raise one or more broods through the torpid summer months. But when the last of the fledglings fly in August, mates split up to join a flock. Ornithologist Eugene Morton estimates that in at least 50 percent of all monogamous avian species, males and females pair *only through a breeding season* —just long enough to raise their young through infancy.[30] The next year a couple may return to the same spot and pair again; more often one dies or disappears, and individuals change mates.

A Theory on the Nature of Monogamy and Desertion

Our first hominid ancestors had several things in common with red foxes and eastern robins. In the cradle of humanity our forebears survived by walking, collecting, scavenging, and moving on; nuts, berries, fruit, and meat were spread across the grass. A male nomad could not collect or defend enough resources to attract a harem. Nor could he monopolize the best place to breed because our ancestors had coitus when they rested, then moved along; there was no best place to breed. And even if a male could attract a group of females, how could he protect them? When lions were not stalking his herd of "wives," bachelors would have lurked behind to steal his "brides." Under normal circumstances polygyny could not work.[31]

But a male could walk beside a single female, try to guard her during estrus from other males, and help her raise her young— monogamy.

The female's plight was even more compelling. It is unlikely that our first female ancestors bore highly infantile, altricial babies the way women do today (see chapter 12) or that they delivered litters. None of the apes bear litters, babies that would tumble from the branches. But, as mentioned earlier, when our ancestors rose onto two legs from four, females became burdened by their young.

So as pair-bonding became the *only* alternative for females—and a viable option for males—monogamy evolved.

But why did these early pair-bonds need to be permanent? Perhaps like foxes and robins, our ancestors only needed to form pair-bonds long enough to rear their young through infancy.

What made me think of this was a remarkable correlation between the length of human infancy in traditional societies, about four years, and the length of many marriages, about four years. Among the traditional !Kung, mothers hold their infants near their skin, breast-feed regularly through the day and night, nurse on demand, and offer their breasts as pacifiers. As a result of this constant body contact and nipple stimulation, as well as high levels of exercise and a low-fat diet, ovulation is suppressed and the ability to become pregnant is postponed for about three years.[32] Hence !Kung births are about four years apart. Four years is the usual period between successive births among continually breast-feeding Australian aborigines[33] and the Gainj of New Guinea.[34] Infants are generally also weaned around the fourth year among the Yanomamo of Amazonia,[35] the Netsilik Eskimos,[36] the Lepcha of Sikkim,[37] and the Dani of New Guinea.[38]

Although birth spacing varies among populations of hunter-gatherers, and maternal age and number of children previously born to a woman affect birth intervals, these data have led anthropologist Jane Lancaster[39] and others to conclude that a four-year pattern of birth spacing—caused by frequent exercise and the habit of continual nursing through the day and night—was the regular pattern of birth spacing during our long evolutionary past.[40]

Thus the modern worldwide divorce peak—about four years— conforms to the traditional period between human successive births—four years.

So here is my theory. *Like pair-bonding in foxes, robins, and many other species that mate only through a breeding season, human pair-bonds originally evolved to last only long enough to raise a single dependent child through infancy, the first four years, unless a second infant was conceived.*

There certainly must have been variations on this theme. Some couples did not conceive for months or years after mating. Often a baby must have died in infancy, triggering a return to cycling, extending the relationship. Some couples probably remained together regardless of infertility because they liked one another or because no other mates were available. A host of factors must have affected the length of primitive pair-bonds. But across the seasons, as decades turned into centuries, those first hominid forebears who remained together *until their child was weaned* survived disproportionately, selecting for serial monogamy.

The seven-year itch, recast as a four-year human reproductive cycle, may be a biological phenomenon.

Special Friendships

How serial monogamy evolved can only be surmised. Our earliest ancestors probably lived in communities much like modern chimps.[41] Everyone copulated with just about everybody else, except with mother and close siblings. Then gradually serial monogamy emerged. The life-styles of olive baboons provide a fascinating model, however, for how pair-bonding, the nuclear family, and divorce could have evolved in these primal hordes.[42]

Olive baboons travel in troops of about sixty animals through the grasslands of East Africa. Each troop is composed of several female-centered families, each headed by a matriarch surrounded by her children and often her sisters and their young. Sons leave home at puberty to join nearby groups. Like human families in many small towns, one baboon "matriline" dominates local social life; another family holds second rank, and so forth. And everyone knows who is who.

A male baboon takes part in this web of social life by way of his "special friendships" with specific females. First of all, these friendships gain him entrance to the troop. Ray, for example, was a healthy, handsome male who appeared at the periphery of one baboon troop, the "Pumphouse Gang," soon after anthropologist Shirley Strum began to hunker at the edge herself. Ray remained on the fringe of group activities for several months, a loner. But gradually he made friends with Naomi, a low-ranking female. Every day Ray came closer to Naomi, until finally they sat side by side to eat and slept near each other every night. Through Naomi, Ray made friends with other females and eventually he became welcome in the troop.

These special friendships have other payoffs. At the height of her monthly estrus, a female baboon forms a consort with a single partner—often with a "special friend." Other males follow the pair, harass them, and try to distract the male and steal the "bride." But if consort partners are also special friends, the female tends to stick close to her "lover," making it difficult for other males to interrupt the pair. If her special friend catches a baby gazelle hidden in the grass, she is the first to get a bite. His vigilance also provides a "buffer zone"—space where she can relax, play with her offspring, and eat undisturbed.

A male in a special friendship gets payoffs too. Often this companion becomes the social father of a female's young. He carries, grooms, cuddles, and protects them. But he uses these infants too. If another male threatens him, a male grabs the infant and holds it to his chest. This instantly stops attack. Among baboons, special friends are teammates that exchange favors, tit for tat.

Our ancestors probably made special friendships long before they descended from the trees; As you recall, chimpanzees sometimes go on safari with a consort. But when bipedalism obliged females to carry young through the dangerous grass, thus requiring them to gain male protection, these friendships could well have turned into deeper, longer-term relationships—the primitive beginnings of human marriage.

How our ancestral hominid forebears met a "spouse" is relatively easy to explain. Parties of four or five females, their special friends, and their children, a group large enough to protect itself yet small enough to move quickly, undoubtedly traveled together.[43] Most likely the territories of these bands overlapped. This way a meal missed by one group of these first "people" was collected by the next that wandered by.

In many primate species either males or females leave their natal group at puberty, so it seems probable that when groups met, adolescents occasionally switched residence. On the scorching plains of Africa four million years ago, individuals probably grew up within a large, loosely connected network of several different bands. From among these individuals the young made special friends and then developed pair-bonds—primitive hominid marriages.

Females were probably attracted to males who were friendly, attentive, and willing to share their food, while males may have been drawn to sexy females from high-status families. During a female's estrus, her mate undoubtedly tried to guard her from the advances of other males, perhaps not always effectively—males and females probably sneaked into the bushes with other lovers when they could. But together a mated pair roamed the grass. Together they collected and shared their food. Together they protected and raised their child. Then one morning either he or she left the band to travel with a new special friend in a different group.

Caveats

I am not suggesting that our first forebears abandoned each other casually. "Divorce" must have caused chaos, just as it does today. Around the world people argue before they separate. Some commit homicide or suicide. Children get confused, frightened, and dis-

placed. Relatives battle. Sometimes whole communities get involved. Even among other primates, rearrangements in the social
order often lead to vicious fights.

Nor am I suggesting that primitive children were independent by
age four, either nutritionally or emotionally. But children in modern
hunting-gathering communities begin to join multi-age play groups
at about this age. Older siblings, relatives, friends, and just about
everyone else in the community take a greater role in caring for the
child as well. In other species these older siblings are called helpers at
the nest, whereas the mother's adult relatives and friends who help
with child care duties are known as "alloparents." Undoubtedly
these extra mothers, seen in a host of other species and all human
cultures, existed in prehistoric bands.

So once the mother no longer needed to carry her infant continually at her side or nurse her baby day and night, her urgent depen-
dency on a protector-provider was reduced. Her incipient "husband"
was less dependent on her too. To safeguard his genetic future, he
had been obliged to protect his offspring until others could begin to
help him with the task. As the child grew out of infancy, however, he
could again respond to his biological imperative to sire further
young. Ancient lovers probably did not *need* to remain pair-bonded
past the infancy of a newborn, unless a second dependent baby was
born.

Finally, I am not suggesting that *all* males and females in our early
prehistory abandoned each other as soon as their offspring began to
toddle out of infancy. In fact, modern divorce data show several
striking circumstances under which lifelong monogamy regularly occurs—circumstances that undoubtedly led some of our forebears to
practice lifelong pair-bonding as well.

One circumstance associated with stable pair-bonds in people is increasing chronological age. As you recall, around the world divorce
continues to decline dramatically after age thirty. Perhaps four million years ago aging couples remained together in order to support
each other and to grandparent the growing young—selecting for
this modern human tendency.

Second, lifelong monogamy *appears* to be common today among couples in the United Nations sample who have three or more dependents—a pattern that *is* common in traditional societies.[44] Hence the more children you bear with a mate, the more likely you probably are to stay together. This tendency may also stem from the early days of humanity when parents with several offspring could not desert a large family. Why should they? If parents were compatible—and the mateship was conducive to raising several young—it was genetically advantageous to both partners to mate for life.

Third, lifelong monogamy occurs for an ecological reason. You may remember that divorce is less common in societies where men and women are economically dependent on one another—most notably in societies that use the plow for agriculture. Divorce is also low in herding cultures and other societies where men do the majority of the heavy labor and control important resources that women depend on to survive. So if either gender was totally dependent on the resources of the other in these early days of humanity, lifelong monogamy was probably the norm.

I doubt this was the general case, however. Before farm life, before the bow and arrow, before "people" made stone tools, our first ancestors traveled in small nomadic groups of four or five mated pairs, their offspring, and sundry single relatives and friends. Meat was a shared luxury. Women were efficient gatherers. And as you will see in coming chapters, the sexes were probably relatively economically autonomous. Thus when partners became caught in a quarrelsome "marriage," either she or he picked up a few belongings and walked out; serial monogamy was probably the norm.

So the monogamous life-styles of some birds and mammals, the conduct of nonhuman primates, the daily lives of people in hunter-gatherer societies like the traditional !Kung, and modern patterns of marriage and divorce around the world all lead me to propose that Lucy and her friends who walked through the muck below Mount Sadiman some 3.5 million years ago had already adopted our basic human mixed reproductive strategy.

This reproductive strategy had several parts. Young and childless couples tended to form pair-bonds, desert each other, and bond again. Couples with one or two children tended to remain together at least long enough to raise their young through infancy; then they "divorced"; then they picked new mates. Couples with three or more children tended to bond for life. Aging couples tended to stay together. And some males and females were adulterous along the way. Not everyone followed this reproductive script; many still do not. But because these patterns appear across the continents, they probably evolved with genesis.

They were probably adaptive too.

Nature Red in Tooth and Claw

When asked why all of her marriages failed, Margaret Mead replied, "I have been married three times, and not one of them was a failure." Mead was a rugged individual. But most Americans idealize lifelong marriage; they equate divorce with failure, as many peoples do. From a Darwinian perspective, however, there were advantages to serial monogamy millennia ago.

Foremost, variety. If offspring varied in their talents and abilities, a few would survive nature's unremitting drive to kill off poor strains. Equally important, an ancestral male could pick a younger female more capable of bearing healthy babies,[45] and a female could choose a mate who provided better protection and support.[46] Today these patterns still prevail. Men and women often have a child with one mate and then more young by a second spouse. Men still remarry younger women, and women still remarry men they think are more caring, more supportive. Although all this recycling can lead to painful social tangles, from a Darwinian perspective having children with more than one partner often makes genetic sense.

But was it to a male's genetic advantage to abandon his biological offspring to mate again and possibly acquire responsibilities for stepchildren? Likewise, was it reproductively logical for an ancestral female to subject her children to the whims of a "stepfather"? Darwinian wisdom says it's not adaptive to desert one's own DNA to nurture the protoplasm of another.

The answers to these questions, I think, are simple. The vicissitudes of stepparenting have increased in modern times. Today

Western parents raise their children largely by themselves, and the costs of education and entertainment are high. Children want bicycles, stereos, computers, and college educations. Hence stepparenting can have considerable economic disadvantages. But in our prehistoric past, a child joined a multi-age play group soon after being weaned, and older siblings, grandparents, and other community members helped nurture all these youths. The *isolated* nuclear family did not exist. Day care was free. And the costs of education and entertainment were low. So stepparenting (after the infancy of the offspring) was considerably less taxing in the past. In fact, stepparenting is exceedingly common in traditional societies today, probably for these reasons.

Ancestral children probably did not suffer severely from primitive divorce either, as long as a stepfather appeared after the child had entered a play group and joined the community at large. If a stepfather appeared while the infant was still suckling, however, the consequences for the infant may have been disastrous—due to another harsh reality of nature best illustrated by lions.

When a new group of male lions overtake a pride and drive out its former male leaders, they kill all new infants; from the Darwinian perspective it is not to their advantage to raise offspring they have not sired. The females of the pride quickly return into estrus after their infants die, the new leaders mate, and thus these male lions raise cubs with their own DNA.[47]

This pattern of infanticide has its ghastly counterpart in modern people. Today in the United States and Canada male stepparents kill more infant stepchildren; after the stepchild is past age four, however, the rate of infanticide reduces.[48] Here, then, was another reason an ancestral female probably felt freer to switch partners after her child had learned to walk and talk and join community affairs.

There may also have been cultural advantages to primitive "divorce" and "remarriage." Edward Tylor, a founding father of anthropology, observed in 1889, "Among tribes of low culture there is but one means known of keeping up alliances, and that means is inter-marriage."[49] Today many gardening peoples of New Guinea, Africa, Amazonia, and elsewhere marry off their children in order to make or keep friends. But these first marriages tend not to last very long.[50] Apparently nobody gets very upset about these divorces either. The marriage agreement has been honored. The alliance between adults has been reinforced. The offspring have returned undamaged. No grandchildren have been produced. And parents are delighted to see their young again.

If these attitudes prevailed millennia ago, why not "marry" more than once? With each new pair-bond social ties would be extended to a band nearby. Customs, ideas, and information would be circulated too.

Undoubtedly our first forebears were not thinking of their DNA when they deserted one another; people are still largely oblivious of the genetic consequences of their sexual and reproductive lives. But those ancestral males and females who abandoned one another some four million years ago survived disproportionately—establishing primitive patterns of marriage, divorce, and remarriage that were passed across the eons to you and me.

In the movie *The African Queen,* Katharine Hepburn remarks to Humphrey Bogart, "Nature, Mr. Alnutt, is something we were put on this earth to rise above." Can we rise above our natural heritage?

Of course we can. Our contemporary marriage patterns are a testament to the triumph of culture and personality over natural human tendencies. Almost half of all American marriages last for life; about half of all marital partners are faithful to their spouses. The world is full of people who marry once and forgo adultery. Some men have harems; some women have harems. Just about every reproductive strategy known—except random promiscuity—is practiced by someone somewhere. Some of us even choose celibacy or childlessness—genetic death. So malleable an animal is man.

But we have whisperings within: during reproductive years we were built to mate and mate again. What a world this sexual imperative would forge.

⌐ 8 ⌐

Eros

Emergence of the Sexual Emotions

We are never so defenseless against suffering as when we love.

—Sigmund Freud

To see her smile, to hear his voice, to watch her walk, to recall a charming moment or witty remark—the slightest perception of one's sweetheart sends a tidal wave of exhilaration through the brain. "This whirlwind, this delirium of Eros," wrote poet Robert Lowell, one of millions, if not billions, of people who have experienced the engulfing storm of infatuation. What a great equalizer this passion is—reducing poets and presidents, academics and technicians, to the same stuttering state of anticipation, hope, agony, and bliss.

Then, as infatuation wanes, a new sensation saturates the mind—attachment. Perhaps this is the most elegant of human feelings, that sense of contentment, of sharing, of oneness with another human being. As you walk together holding hands, when you sit next to each other reading in the evening, as you laugh simultaneously at a movie or stroll through a park or on the beach, your souls are merged. All the world's your paradise.

Alas, even attachment sometimes dulls, replaced by leaden indifference or a cloying restlessness that slowly eats one's love and leads to adultery, separation, or divorce. Then, after a relationship has finally ended, and both partners are free of the emotions that tied them up like puppets, some people feel that old sense of hope and intense excitement as they fall in love again.

The human craving for romance, our drive to make a sexual attachment, our restlessness during long relationships, our perennial optimism about our new sweetheart—these passions drag us like a kite upon the wind as we soar and plunge unpredictably from one feeling to another. These emotions must come from our ancestry. So I shall propose that they evolved with genesis, to drive our ancestors in and out of relationships some four million years ago.

Love Is Primitive

Indeed, there is some evidence that infatuation and attachment are very old emotions. As you recall, psychiatrist Michael Liebowitz theorizes that the euphoria and energy of attraction are caused by a brain bath of naturally occurring amphetamines that pool in the emotional centers of the brain. This is why infatuated lovers can stay awake all night talking, why they become so optimistic, so gregarious, so full of life.

With time, however, the brain can no longer tolerate this continually revved-up state. The nerve endings become either immune or exhausted, and exhilaration wanes.[1] Some people sustain that smitten feeling for only weeks or months. Those who have a barrier to the relationship, like a marriage to a third party, can sometimes maintain elation over their beloved for several years. But most partners who see each other regularly feel the euphoria of attraction for some two to three years.[2]

Then, as the excitement and novelty subside, the brain kicks in new chemicals, the endorphins, natural morphine-like substances that calm the mind. And as the endorphins surge along the brain's primeval pathways, Liebowitz maintains, they usher in the second stage of love—attachment—with its sensations of security and peace.

Not only are these sexual emotions housed in the human brain, suggesting the antiquity of attraction and attachment, but they occur in people around the world. Nisa, the !Kung woman of the Kalahari Desert that I have spoken of, succinctly described this two-phase progression of romance, saying, "When two people are first together, their hearts are on fire and their passion is very great. After a while, the fire cools and that's how it stays. They continue to love each other, but it's in a different way—warm and dependable."[3]

Few others have so accurately observed these stages of romantic love. But the vast majority of people acknowledge that romantic passion exists. In fact, a new study of 168 societies found that 87 percent of these vastly different cultures displayed direct evidence that people knew this madness.[4]

So infatuation and attachment have physiological components, and these emotions are common to humankind. Moreover, Liebowitz has proposed that these two distinctly different chemical systems in the brain evolved in the human animal for a simple reason: "For primitive man two aspects of relating to the opposite sex were important for survival as a species. The first was to have males and females become attracted to each other for long enough to have sex and reproduce. The second was for the males to become strongly attached to the females so that they stayed around while the females were raising their young and helped to gather food, find shelter, fight off marauders and teach the kids certain skills."[5]

I'll go one step further: perhaps our drive to leave a mate also has a physiological component that evolved some four million years ago when our first hominid ancestors were beginning to pair up and then part from each other as they raised successive young.

My thinking on this was stimulated by the work of an ethologist, Norbert Bischof. In trying to explain why birds abandon their nests at the end of the breeding season to join a flock and why creatures leave the safety of their natal home after infancy, Bischof suggests that an animal gets an "excess of security," to which it responds by withdrawing from the object of attachment.[6] This retreat he calls the surfeit response.[7] I suspect the same phenomenon might occur in humankind. At some point in long relationships the brain's receptor sites for the endorphins probably become desensitized or overloaded and attachment wanes—setting up the body and the brain for separation or divorce.

Planned obsolescence at nerve endings to stimulate serial monogamy in bygone days? Perhaps.

Westerners adore love. We symbolize it, study it, worship it, idealize it, applaud it, fear it, envy it, live for it, and die for it. Love is many things to many people. But if love is common to all people everywhere and associated with tiny molecules that reside at nerve endings in the emotional centers of the brain, then love is also primitive.

I suspect these chemical systems for infatuation and attachment (and perhaps detachment) had evolved by the time that Lucy and her comrades were walking through the grasslands of East Africa some 3.5 million years ago. Those who felt the passion of infatuation formed more secure partnerships with special friends. Those who sustained the pull of attachment long enough to raise a child through infancy nurtured their own DNA. Those males who crept away occasionally with other lovers spread more of their genes, whereas those females who philandered reaped additional resources for their growing young. And those who left one partner for another had more varied babies. The children of these passionate individuals survived disproportionately, passing the brain chemistry for infatuation, attachment, and restlessness during long relationships along to you and me.

What consequences this brain chemistry would produce. The "husband," the "father," the "wife," and the "nuclear family," our myriad conventions of courtship, our human celebrations of marriage, our divorce procedures, humankind's many punishments for adultery, cultural mores for sexual comportment, patterns of family violence stemming from desertion—countless customs and institutions would burgeon from our ancestors' simple drive to make and break pair-bonds millennia ago.

Most crippling of these legacies, however, are all of the emotional upheavals this romantic wiring still causes. Love sickness. We seem emotionally unfinished. Attached lovers, for example, tend to suffer during a period of separation such as a business trip or school vacation. Liebowitz thinks that, while apart, neither partner is getting his or her daily dose of natural narcotic drugs. Levels of the endorphins plunge. Then, as withdrawal sets in, lovers deeply miss, even crave, each other.

This romantic wiring is probably also partly responsible for the psychological and physical abuse that some men and women are willing to endure. Some rebuffed lovers make ridiculous compromises or accept hideous battering for fear of losing "him" or "her." Liebowitz proposes that these "attachment junkies" are suffering from low levels of these natural narcotic drugs, so they cling to a partner rather than risking a drop in these opiates. Like heroin addicts, they are chemically wedded to their partners.[8] What is equally compelling, some battered partners have learned to associate the pain inflicted on them with pleasure.[9] So as they receive abuse, levels of endorphins may actually rise—driving them to return for more pain and its corresponding high.

Psychiatrists also think that pining has a physiological component connected to the brain's attachment system. People become listless when they grieve for a deceased mate. Some hardly work or eat or sleep. As the psychiatrist John Bowlby put it, "Loss of a loved person is one of the most intensely painful experiences any human being can suffer."[10] The loneliness some people feel when unattached must also be caused, in part, by molecules in the mind.

Homosexual Love

So strong are these feelings of attachment, so basic to human nature, that they occur in all of us—whether our "love object" is a member of the opposite sex or of the same gender.

Scientists know very little about the causes of homosexuality, either male–male or female–female love. Some researchers report that male homosexuals more regularly come from homes where the father was absent, or cold and detached, while the mother had an intimate, smothering, primary relationship with her son.[11] Others maintain that the family life of homosexuals and heterosexuals show no basic differences.[12]

Currently some scientists think that homosexuality is associated, in part, with changes in the fetal brain instead. A few weeks after conception fetal hormones begin to sculpt the male and female genitals. And it is now thought that these hormones may also map the male and female fetal brain. Any tangle in this hormonal bath, however, changes one's sexual orientation in later life.[13]

An enormous amount has been written on homosexuality, but as yet no consensus has been reached. I can only add that homosexuality is exceedingly common in nature.[14] Female cats housed separately from males display all of the behavior patterns of homosexual arousal. Wild female gulls sometimes mate as lesbian couples. Male gorillas band together and exhibit homosexuality. Female pygmy chimpanzees have regular homosexual interactions. Even male stickleback fish occasionally act like females, as do mallard ducks and other birds. In fact, homosexuality is so common in other species— and it occurs in such a variety of circumstances—that human homosexuality is striking not in its prevalence but in its rarity.

I suspect that both hormones and environment have important effects on sexual preferences in humankind and other animals. But there is only one point that is important to this book: homosexual men and women fall in love, many form pair-bonds with mates, many break up, and many bond again. Homosexual men and women experience all of the same sensations of romantic love that heterosexual people report, and they struggle with all of the same problems of this romantic wiring.[15] These emotions clearly evolved long ago.

Jealousy

"The green-eyed monster which doth mock the meat it feeds on." So colorfully did Shakespeare describe jealousy—this intense human affliction, this combination of possessiveness and suspicion. Jealousy can arise at any time in a relationship. When persons are head over heels in love during the attraction phase, when they are snugly attached, while they are themselves philandering, even after they have departed or been abandoned, the green-eyed monster can come calling.

Psychological tests of American men and women show that neither gender is routinely more jealous than the other—although the sexes handle their attacks differently. Women generally are more willing to pretend indifference in order to patch up a sullied partnership. Men, on the other hand, more often leave a mate when they feel jealous; they are apparently more intent on repairing their self-esteem and saving face.[16] People who feel inadequate, insecure, or overly dependent on their partners tend to be more jealous.

Male jealousy is a leading cause of spousal homicide in the United States today.[17] And it is not unique to Westerners; in other cultures it is as prevalent as the common cold. Even where adultery is condoned, people suffer from jealousy when they hear about the dalliances of a beloved.[18] An aboriginal man of Arnhem Land, Australia, summed it up this way: "We Yolngu are a jealous people and always have been since the days we lived in the bush in clans. We are jealous of our wife or husband, for fear she or he is looking at another. If a husband has several wives he is all the more jealous, and the wives are jealous of each other. . . . Make no mistake, the big J is part of our nature."[19]

Whether other creatures feel jealous we will never know. But male and female animals of many species behave very proprietarily toward their mates. Male gibbons, for example, drive other males from the family territory, and females drive off other females. On one occasion Passion, a female chimp at the Gombe Stream Reserve, Tanzania, solicited a young male. He ignored her sexy gestures and began to copulate with her daughter, Pom. Looking incensed, Passion rushed up and slapped him hard.[20]

Better examples come from birds. In a test of "cuckoldry-tolerance," anthropologist David Barash interrupted the annual mating ritual of a pair of mountain bluebirds which had just begun to build their nest. While the cock was out foraging, Barash placed a stuffed male bluebird about a meter from their home. The resident male returned and began to squawk, hover, and snap his bill at the dummy. But he also attacked his "wife," pulling some primary feathers from her wing. She vanished. Two days later a new "wife" moved in.[21] Wife beating by a jealous male bluebird?

This possessiveness has genetic logic. Jealous males of any species will guard their partners more assiduously; thus jealous males are more likely to sire young and pass on their genes. Females who drive off other females, on the other hand, acquire more protection and gratuities; because of their jealousy, they have acquired additional resources—so their young are more likely to survive. In this way possessive creatures bred disproportionately across the ages, selecting for what we call jealousy—as well as modern male/female variations in jealousy: American men tend to be more jealous if a mate is sexually unfaithful, women are more jealous if a mate makes an emotional commitment to another.[22]

Jealousy had probably taken its human form by the time Lucy and her girlfriends began to chase boys and form pair-bonds some 3.5 million years ago. If a "husband" returned from scavenging and suspected adultery, he might have become enraged and attacked his rival with sticks and stones and shrieks and growls. And if Lucy caught her husband with another female, she perhaps assaulted both of them with words, then tried to ostracize the female from the group. Jealousy helped curb philandering in females and desertion by males—selecting for whatever it is in the male and female brain that contributes to the power of a jealous rage.

Breaking Up Is Hard to Do

What turbulence hath evolution wrought. The craving for a partner, the emotional dependence on a mate, the tolerance of physical and psychological abuse, pining, grieving, jealousy—such powerful emotional reactions can be elicited when the body's attachment system is threatened. Most compelling, however, is the emotional cyclone some people feel when a lover leaves for good.

Sociologist Robert Weiss, a divorcé, began to study marital separation among members of the organization Parents without Partners. Then, from discussions with 150 people who attended his "Seminars for the Separated," he began to see a pattern to detachment.[23] First, he confirmed that a feeling of attachment persists for the deserted partner. Despite all of the bitter disappointments, failed promises, vicious battles, and rank humiliations, home continues to be where one's mate is; anywhere else is exile. More interesting, this tie dissolves in a pattern—a specific configuration that could have evolved across the millennia.

If the relationship ends abruptly, shock is the first sensation the rejected person feels. Dumbfounded, he or she responds only with denial for several days, sometimes for as long as two weeks. But eventually reality sets in. "She" or "he" is gone.

Then the "transition" phase begins. Time hangs heavy. Many of life's daily rituals have evaporated, and one hardly knows what to do with all the blanks. Anger, panic, regret, self-doubt, and a desperate, consuming sadness overcome the rejected individual. Weiss says some rejected people feel euphoria or a sense of freedom too. But this joy cannot last. Moods swing relentlessly, so a decision made today vanishes tomorrow. Some turn to alcohol or drugs or sports or friends; others rely on psychiatrists, counselors, or self-help books; many just lie in bed and cry.

And as they mourn, they begin to review the relationship—obsessively. Hour upon hour they rewind old memories, playing out the cozy evenings and touching moments, the arguments and silences, the jokes and snide remarks, listening endlessly for clues to why "he" or "she" departed. "What went wrong?" "How could I have acted differently?" As the tormented person recalls the events leading to the separation, he or she develops an "account" of who did what to whom.

Themes and key incidents dominate this mental narration as the individual fixates on the worst humiliations. But with time he or she builds a plot with a beginning, a middle, and an end. This account is a little like a description of an auto accident; perceptions are garbled. But the process is important. Once in place, the story can be addressed, worked on, and, eventually, discarded.

Sometimes the transitional phase lasts a year. Any setback, such as an unsuccessful reconciliation or a rejection by a new lover, can hurl the sufferer back into shattered anguish. But as he or she develops a coherent life-style, the "recovery" phase begins. Gradually the abandoned individual acquires a new identity, some self-esteem, new friends, fresh interests, and some resiliency. The past begins to loosen its stranglehold. Now he or she can proceed with living.

But there are two provocative results of Weiss's study, data suggesting that our emotions have physiological components and that the chemistry of attachment and abandonment evolved long ago in a specific evolutionary design. Weiss noticed that none of the 150 "separated" men and women who joined his seminars had been married less than a year; few had separated within two years after wedding. To account for this, he surmised "that it takes about two years after marriage before individuals fully integrate the marriage into their emotional and social life."

I suspect that brain chemistry also plays a role. As you recall, it generally takes a couple of years before the infatuation high wears off and the attachment drugs set in, tightly binding partners to each other. Perhaps this is also why so few couples that divorced within two years of marrying joined Weiss's seminars. Since they never reached the attachment stage, they didn't need help with the process of parting.

Even more interesting, Weiss noted that the entire process of separation normally takes two to four years, "with the average being closer to four than to two." The number four has come up again. Not only do we tend to form pair-bonds for about four years, but it often takes about four years to dissolve the relationship.

The human animal seems driven by a tide of feelings that ebb and flow to an internal beat, a rhythm that emerged when our ancestors descended from the fast-disappearing trees of Africa and developed a tempo in their relationships that was in synchrony with their natural breeding cycle, about four years.

"Fresh Features"

"The chains of marriage are heavy and it takes two to carry them—sometimes three," Oscar Wilde once said. He put his finger on another emotion that probably has a physiological component and evolved in human evolution: our human craving for sexual variety. Psychologists, psychiatrists, sex therapists, and family counselors regularly see patients who are struggling with stale partnerships and many more who turn to new individuals for sexual release. What motivates people to philander?

There are countless reasons. Some adulterers apparently need a companion when they are on business in a foreign city. Some like to sleep around with members of a different ethnic group, class, or generation. Some want to solve a sex problem. Some are looking for intimacy, excitement, or revenge. Chapter 4, on adultery, lists many psychological reasons why men and women climb into bed with auxiliary lovers. But it seems likely that there is also a biological component to infidelity, one that evolved through time and countless trysts.

Evidence for the physiology of adultery comes from the work of psychologist Marvin Zuckerman and his colleagues, who point out that people respond very differently to novelty. Many avoid it. But sensation seekers come in four varieties.[24] Some crave outdoor sports and activities that feature speed and danger. Others seek inner experiences through drugs, travel, the arts, and avant-garde life-styles. Swingers like reckless parties, sexual variety, gambling, and quantities of alcohol. Last, some individuals cannot tolerate predictable people or routine of any kind.

These men and women score higher on tests for susceptibility to boredom and psychological tests show that they suffer less from anxiety and lack of nurturance. So Zuckerman thinks that the brains of these thrill seekers are more wired to seek sensation, experience, theater and adventure—variety of any sort.

Monoamine oxidase, or MAO, may be the biological accomplice. Adults with low levels of MAO, an enzyme in the brain, tend to be gregarious, drink heavily, indulge in drugs, like fast cars, and seek out the excitement of rock concerts, bars, and other places of public entertainment. People with low MAO also pursue an active, varied sex life.[25] They seem to be physiologically wired to create drama and excitement. This may begin in infancy; newborn babies with low levels of MAO are more excitable and crankier.

Human beings are not the only creatures that seem to vary in their love of risk. Some cats, dogs, monkeys, wolves, pigs, cows, and even fish seek more novelty than others do; some consistently approach new things, while others flee. Shyness is an inborn trait.[25]

Why would anyone in a relatively happy relationship risk family and friends, career, health, and peace of mind to pursue a casual affair? Americans disapprove of infidelity—yet they engage extramarital lovers regularly. So there must be something in the brain that fuels this madness. Whatever its underlying brain physiology is, the genetic component of philandering probably began to evolve soon after our first forebears turned down the road toward humankind.

Are we alone in our drive to court and love and leave each other? Or is the stallion that paws the ground, fills his nostrils with the scent of a receptive female and mounts this mare feeling infatuation too? Does the dog fox feel attachment as he nudges an appetizing dead mouse toward his hungry vixen in their den? Do Nile crocodiles that raise infants as a team feel fondness for one another? Are the bluebirds that desert the nest in autumn glad to part? Have billions of animals over millions of years felt the ecstasy of infatuation, the peace of attachment, the tension of philandering, the agony of abandonment?

Several things suggest that a wide range of creatures are capable of feeling the sensations of love. All birds and mammals have a hypothalamus deep in the center of the brain. Sometimes called the hub of the emotions, this little gland plays a major role in steering sexual behavior. Because this nodule has evolved very little in the last seventy million years and is so similar across species, it suggests continuity between man and beast.[27]

The limbic system in the brain, which governs feelings of lust, rage, fear, and ecstasy, is rudimentary in reptiles but is well developed in birds and mammals, also suggesting that other creatures are capable of intense emotions.[28] Last, it is generally accepted that the basic emotions of fear, joy, sadness, and surprise are linked with specific facial expression. And since humans and other animals share several of these facial expressions, such as the snarl, it is possible that they share some of these emotions too.[29]

Perhaps all of the world's birds and mammals are servants of a few chemicals that surge through their various nervous systems, directing the ebb and flow of attraction, attachment, and detachment to fit their breeding cycles.

And if animals love, Lucy loved.

She probably flirted with the boys she met when bands convened at the beginning of the dry season and became infatuated with one who gave her meat. She might have lain beside him in the bushes and kissed and hugged, then stayed awake all night, euphoric. As she and her special friend wandered together across the plains in search of melons, berries, and fresh antelope, she must have felt exhilaration. When they curled up to dream, she probably felt the cosmic warmth of attachment. Maybe she became bored as they passed their days, and felt a thrill when she sneaked into the woodlands to copulate with another. Probably she mourned when she and her partner split up one morning to join separate groups. Then she fell in love again.

I am not surprised we feel with such intensity. *After all, reproduction is the primary purpose of any organism. Nature would have done shoddy work had she not produced powerful mechanisms to make us breed and breed again.*

What an incredible plot. The crippling passion of infatuation, the deep closeness of attachment, the seductive craving to philander, the torment of abandonment, the hope to mate anew—Lucy's children's children's children's children would pass these kernels of the human psyche through time and chance and circumstance along to you and me. And from this evolutionary history would arise an eternal struggle of the human spirit—the drive to marry, to philander, to divorce, and to pair again.

No wonder love is cherished. No wonder so many people have suffered from a broken heart. If love is a cyclic process of the human brain that evolved to produce variety in our species, then romantic passion is powerful—and fleeting.

Our restive, churning temperament would create more than the sexual emotions. It also led to the evolution of our human sexual anatomy—physical attributes designed to lure prospective mates into the siren's web.

~9~

The Siren's Web
Evolution of Human Sexual Anatomy

Why were we crucified into sex?
Why were we not left rounded off,
and finished in ourselves,
As we began,
As he certainly began,
so perfectly alone?

—D. H. Lawrence, "Tortoise Shout"

Vermilion noses, crimson chests, puffy buttocks, strips and spots and dapples, tufts, crowns, manes, horns, and hairless patches, such are nature's decorations; sexual beings are like ornamented Christmas trees, bearing an arsenal of accoutrements to win their fortunes and their futures through copulation and reproduction. We human beings have a fantastic array ourselves. Among them are large penises, beards and fleshy breasts, everted reddened lips, continual female sexual receptivity, and other beguiling male and female traits that are like a siren's web, sex lures that evolved over millennia of seductions.

How did we come to be decorated so?

Sexual Selection

Over a hundred years ago Darwin proposed a solution to many of the riddles of human sexuality. He wanted to explain why stags have antlers and lions manes, why male peacocks sport brilliant tails and male elephant seals are twice a big as females. Because these traits were cumbersome, of little value to daily living, even apparently maladaptive, Darwin could not believe they had evolved by means of natural selection, survival of the fittest in the struggle for existence. So in *The Descent of Man and Selection in Relation to Sex* (1871), he detailed a corollary to natural selection—sexual selection.

The theory: these peculiarities evolved by a slightly different, closely related form of selection—reproductive selection, the mating game.[1]

Darwin's argument was elegant. If a mane made a lion more threatening to other males, or more attractive to females, those males with longer manes bred more often and bore more young, and the young passed along this otherwise unnecessary trait. Likewise, if large, strong male elephant seals fought off smaller, weaker ones and then lured a harem during the short, synchronized breeding season, large males bred more often. So through these endless battles and courtship rituals, the stag evolved its antlers, the peacock its brilliant tail, the elephant seal its lumbering size and excessive weight.

Darwin was fully aware that sexual selection could not account for all of the differences between the sexes. But the eternal struggle of who will mate and breed with whom—the mating game—is the only explanation for the evolution of some of nature's more bizarre sexual accoutrements, including the human phallus.

Men have big penises, larger than those of gorillas, a primate with three times a man's body bulk. Gorillas apparently have small phalluses because they do not compete with their genitals. These creatures live with stable harems. Males are twice the size of females, and they impress competitors with their large body size; large genitals are not part of their display. As a result, a gorilla's erect penis is only two inches long.

We do not know why men have conspicuous genitals, but a male chimp solicits a female by opening his legs, displaying an erect penis and flicking his phallus with a finger as he gazes at a potential partner. A prominent, distinctive penis helps broadcast one's individuality and sexual vigor, which may lure female friends. In many species of insects and primates, males have exceptionally elaborate penises, and scientists think these evolved specifically because females *chose* those males with elaborate, sexually stimulating genitals.[2] So perhaps as Lucy's ancestors became bipedal some four million years ago, males began to parade their genitals in order to make special friends with favored females—selecting for those with large organs.

Two factors work together to make a penis conspicuous, however—thickness and length, and these separate assets may have evolved by slightly different means of sexual selection.

Human penises are relatively thick, and this may have emerged in human evolution simply because Lucy and her girlfriends liked thick penises. A fat phallus distends the muscles of the outer third of the vaginal canal and pulls on the hood of the clitoris, creating exciting friction, making orgasm easier to achieve. Indeed, if early females *chose* males with thick phalluses, as they must have done, then those who had thick penises had more special friends throughout their lives and more extra lovers too. These males produced more children. And thick penises evolved. As Darwin wrote ". . . The power to charm the female has sometimes been more important than the power to conquer other males in battle." Indeed penis thickness may be a result of this.

Sperm Wars

Long penises may have evolved for a different reason, though, another form of sexual selection known as sperm competition. The theory of sperm competition was first developed to explain the mating tactics of insects.[3] Most female insects are highly promiscuous; they copulate with several partners, then either eject the sperm or store it for days, months, or even years. So males compete inside the female's reproductive tract.

A male damselfly, for example, uses his penis to scoop out the sperm of previous suitors before he himself ejaculates. Male insects also try to dilute the sperm of competitors or push it out of place. Some insert a "mating plug" in the female's genital opening after copulation; whereas others guard the female until she has deposited her eggs.[4] Perhaps the long human phallus is the result of sperm competition too, designed to give the swimmers a head start.[5]

Men's averaged-sized testicles are probably also the result of jousting in the vaginal canal. This reasoning is based on data from chimpanzees. Male chimps have large testicles for their body size, as well as long penises, and it is thought that they sport these factories because male chimps are promiscuous. In a chimpanzee horde, males are quite tolerant of one another, even lining up to copulate. So as the reasoning goes, in the past those chimp males with large testicles and numerous speedy sperm deposited more copious quantities of highly motile sperm in a female's reproductive tract. These chimps conceived more young—selecting for large testicles in chimps. Gorillas, on the other hand, have very small testicles, and, as is to be expected, they copulate infrequently and with little competition from other males.[6]

These facts led scientist Robert Smith to propose that men's medium-sized testicles and copious ejaculate evolved for the same reason that they arose in chimps: ancestral men with vigorous seed bags and more sperm produced more conceptions, selecting for men's average-sized testicles and their abundant energetic seed. Even nocturnal emissions and male masturbation, Smith thinks, are the result of sperm competition between males, a pleasurable way to replace old sperm with new.[7]

Male–male competition. Female choice. Scientists generally emphasize these two aspects of sexual selection because in nature females should be choosy about their lovers, whereas males should fight among themselves for the privilege of breeding.[8]

In fact, this reasoning shows impeccable genetic logic: for females of many species, the costs of reproduction are high. Females conceive the embryo, tote the fetus for days or months, and often raise the children largely by themselves. And females are limited in the number of offspring they can produce; it takes time to bear and raise each infant, brood, or litter. So it is to a female's advantage to pick her partners carefully; she hasn't many opportunities to reproduce.

For males of most species the costs of reproduction are much lower. Males just donate sperm. Even more important, males can conceive offspring much more regularly than females—as long as they can fight off other suitors, attract females, and withstand sexual exhaustion. So it is to a male's reproductive advantage to copulate relatively indiscriminately.

Because of these differences in "parental investment," it is generally males of the species who *compete* among themselves for females and regularly females who *choose* between males. But the alternative forms of sexual selection, males who choose between females and females who compete among themselves to breed, are also seen in nature. People are no exception. Just go to any bar or club or party, and watch women compete with one another while men choose between them. As H. L. Mencken summed it up, "When women kiss it always reminds one of prize fighters shaking hands."

In fact, several important female traits are probably the consequence of female–female competition and males who chose between them in yesteryear. Among the most conspicuous are permanently enlarged female breasts.

Why Did Big Breasts Evolve?

In 1967 ethologist Desmond Morris proposed that when our ancestors became bipedal, the sexual signals that initially ornamented the rump evolved to decorate the chest and head instead.[9] Hence women evolved everted reddened lips to mimic the lips of the vagina and dangling fleshy breasts to mimic puffy buttocks. Ancestral males were attracted to women with these signs of sexual readiness, so women with bulging breasts bore more young—spreading this trait across the centuries.

Several scientists have added alternative hypotheses. Perhaps breasts evolved to signal "ovulatory potential." Because women of prime reproductive age have more voluptuous breasts than do subadults or postmenopausal women, ancestral men may have seen these swellings as signs of likely fertility.[10] As another hypothesis goes, among primates breasts swell only while a female nurses, so maybe these flags evolved to advertise a woman's ability to reproduce and feed her young[11] — the "good-mother" signal — or as a deceptive sign to trick males into thinking a female was a good reproductive bet.[12] A last interesting theory holds that breasts were primarily storehouses of fat, crucial reserves that could be drawn on during pregnancy and lactation if food was scarce.[13]

All these theories make genetic sense.

But what a bad design. These protuberances around the mammary glands seem poorly placed. They bobble painfully when a woman runs. They flop forward to block vision when she leans over to collect food. And they can suffocate a suckling child. Moreover, breasts (of any size) are sensitive to touch. Why? A woman's nipples harden at the slightest touch. And for many, fondling the breasts stimulates sexual desire.

So I do not wish to overlook Morris's original theory for the sexual purpose of the female breast: for whatever genetically adaptive reasons (and there were probably several), ancestral males *liked* females with these sensitive, pillowy appendages and bred more often with sexually responsive, big-busted women — selecting for this decor.

As females picked their lovers and men chose between women, as all our early ancestors jockeyed for prized spouses and lovers, other fundamental aspects of human sexuality probably emerged.

Men have beards; women have smooth complexions; men develop deep voices at puberty, while women retain mellifluous tones. How come? Of facial hair Darwin wrote, "Our male ape-like progenitors acquired their beards as an ornament to charm or excite the opposite sex. . . ."[14] Perhaps beards signaled strength and maturity to women. Darwin also referred to the high female voice as a musical instrument, concluding, "We may infer that they first acquired musical powers in order to attract the opposite sex."[15] Maybe to men the sweet voice was childlike, unthreatening.

For whatever reasons, in Lucy's day some males and females bore more young than others did, selecting for the peculiar body ornaments of these individuals — thick long penises, permanently enlarged breasts, men's beards, and women's dulcet tones.

We are indeed naked apes, and the loss of body hair could have been, at least in part, another result of sexual selection. Actually we did not lose our body hair; we have the same number of hair follicles as do the apes, but the hair itself is less developed.

Explanations of this trait, our puny pelage, have cost a lot of ink and paper. The classic explanation is that it evolved as part of a revision in the body's heating and cooling system. The sweaty jogger. In order for our hunting-scavenging ancestors to lope long distances in search of game, insulating hair was replaced by body fat and sweat glands that poured a cooling liquid film across an exposed chest and limbs when they got too hot. Some argue instead that our ancestors lost their body hair to reduce the frequency of parasitic infestations. Still others think that our hairlessness may have evolved in conjunction with our human trait of being born exceedingly immature (see chapter 12).[16]

But Morris has proposed that these human hair patterns served as sex attractants too. With a diminutive pelage, the tender areas of the chest and around the groin became more visible, more exposed, more sensitive to touch. Not coincidentally, women evolved less hair around their lips and breasts—places where stimulation can easily lead to intercourse. And where our ancestors retained hair seems just as much a stimulant to sex as where they lost it. Hair in the underarms and crotch holds the aromas of sweat and sex—odors that are sexually exciting to many people.

Like beards, deep voices, smooth chins, and high voices, some of these modern hair patterns also appear at puberty—the beginning of the sex season. So the simplest explanation is that all these traits evolved for several reasons—among them, to dazzle mates and paramours when our hominid ancestors first emerged from the shrinking forests of Africa to mate and raise their young as "husband" and "wife."

Of all our sexual habits, the most striking and pleasurable to both men and women are three bizarre traits of human females: their ability to copulate face-to-face, their intense but fickle pattern of orgasm, and their remarkable ability to copulate around the clock.

About these feminine lures men have rhapsodized for centuries, if not millennia.

Did Lucy copulate face-to-face? I think she did. All modern women have a downward-tilted vagina rather than the backward-oriented vulva of all other primates. Because of this tipped vulva, face-to-face copulation is comfortable. In fact, in this position the man's pelvic bone rubs against the clitoris, making intercourse extremely stimulating.

Not surprisingly, face-to-face coitus in the missionary position is the preferred copulatory posture in most cultures, although variations abound.[17] The Kuikuru of Amazonia sleep in single-person hammocks strung around a family hearth, so lovers have little privacy. Moreover, one false move and both partners are pitched into the night fire. Because of these inconveniences, spouses and paramours make love in the forest, where the ground is uneven and often wet. Here a woman cannot lie on her back to copulate. Instead, she squats, leans back, and holds her buttocks and back above the ground with flexed arms and legs. Still, she makes love while looking at her partner. People have invented dozens of other positions for intercourse. But face-to-face copulation is depicted around the world; it is probably a badge of the human animal.

The downward-tilting human vaginal canal could have evolved via sexual selection.[18] If Lucy had a tipped vagina and encouraged face-to-face coitus, her partners could see her face, whisper, gaze, and pick up nuances of her expressions. Face-to-face copulation fostered intimacy, communication, and understanding. So, like those ancestral females with pendulous sensitive breasts, those with tipped vaginas perhaps forged stronger bonds with their special friends and bore disproportionately more young—passing this trait to us.

Multiple Orgasm

Another dazzling female trait is "multiple orgasm." Unlike her mate's, a female's genitals do not expel all the fluid during orgasm, and—if she knows how—she can climax again and again. Why do women have the capacity for multiple orgasm while men do not?

That's a good question. In males, orgasm is critical to insemination; the pulsations push sperm into the vagina. But a woman's egg pops naturally from her ovary once a month regardless of her sexual response. In fact, anthropologist Donald Symons thinks that, because female orgasm is of no direct use to conception, female orgasm is an unnecessary anatomical and physiological phenomenon which was retained through evolution in women only because it was of such importance to men. He compares female orgasm and the clitoris to the nipples on the breasts of men—useless appendages decorating the body of one sex only because they are of such vital use to the other. Hence Symons concludes that female orgasm is not an adaptation at all.[19]

Wait a minute. The clitoris is not a relatively inert patch of tissue like the male nipple but a remarkably sensitive clump of nerves that produce orgasm—a violent, pounding physical sensation and tumultuous emotional experience. Moreover orgasm signals something: satisfaction. Men like women to climax because it reassures them that their partner is gratified and perhaps less inclined to seek sex elsewhere. Female orgasm boosts the male ego.[20] Why else would women fake orgasms?

And for a woman orgasm is a journey, an altered state of consciousness, another reality that escalates to chaos, then elicits feelings of calm, tenderness, and attachment—which tend to cement a relationship with a partner.[21] Orgasm also satiates a woman, and that motivates her to remain lying down; hence sperm is less likely to flow out of the vaginal canal. Last, female orgasm most likely stimulates a woman to seek more coitus, which inevitably facilitates conception too.

I cannot agree with Symons; I think female orgasm evolved for genuine purposes: to encourage females to seek sex, to make an intimate connection with a reproductive mate or extra lover, to signal enjoyment to this partner, and to aid fertilization.[22]

And it probably evolved long before our ancestors descended from the trees. All female primates and higher mammals have a clitoris. A chimp's clitoris is larger than that of women, both relatively and absolutely, and once a female becomes sexually excited, she begins to copulate at a fevered pitch—suggesting that female chimps climax several times. Females of many species experience changes in blood pressure, respiration, heart rate, muscular tension, hormonal levels, and vocal tones that resemble the human female response during orgasm. So orgasm probably occurs in many other creatures.[23]

Multiple orgasm also would have been adaptive for ancestral arboreal females, whose livelihood depended on forming good relations with several males. So Lucy probably inherited the ability for multiple orgasm from her ancestors living in the trees and passed it along to us.

Women do not climax all the time, however. And even this characteristic may have been selected millennia ago. Women tend to climax when they are relaxed, with men who are sexually attentive, and with longtime, committed partners. Women achieve orgasm much more regularly with husbands, for example, than with secret lovers. And streetwalkers who copulate with strangers climax less frequently than do call girls with better-paying, more-considerate customers. Perhaps this orgasmic fickleness is a mechanism women unconsciously evolved to distinguish a caring, patient Mr. Right from a cavalier, restive Mr. Wrong.[24]

Take your choice. Female orgasm may be no more than a functionless accoutrement, the consequence of embryonic growth so crucial to male sexuality that it was retained through evolution in women, or a highly adaptive feature in a complex female strategy to win the mating game.

Will She or Won't She?

Of all the sexual ploys women have acquired from the past, none is so captivating to scientists—and so enjoyable to men and women—as the female's remarkable ability to copulate when she wants to. As you recall, to males or females of almost any other living species, sex is not constantly available. Why? Because females of sexually reproducing genera have a period of heat, or estrus, and when they are not in heat they generally refuse to accept a male.

There are exceptions, of course.[25] But women fall at the far end of a long continuum of behavior: they regularly can and do copulate throughout their entire monthly menstrual cycle; they can engage in intercourse throughout most of pregnancy; and they can and often do resume coitus as soon as they have recovered from childbirth—months or years before a child is weaned.

Critics say that continual female sexual readiness exists only in the fears of old men and the hopes of young boys. This is not the point. If a woman *wants* to, she *can* copulate anytime she pleases. American married women copulate, on average, one to three times a week, depending on their age.[26] In many cultures women reportedly make love either every day or every night, except when rituals of war, religion, or other local customs intercede.[27] Sex does not end with menopause or aging either.[28] This is not to say that a woman always has a high libido. But the human female has lost her period of heat.

Several theories have been offered for the loss of estrus periodicity.[29] The classic explanation holds that ancestral females lost estrus in order to cement a pair-bond with a male. With the ability to copulate at any time, a female could keep her special friend in perpetual attendance. This is an interesting idea. But many birds and some mammals are monogamous, and none except women display continual sexual availability. There must be a richer explanation for this remarkable human female trait.

Perhaps adultery selected for the loss of estrus. If clandestine copulations provided Lucy and her female compatriots with extra protection and support, then it would have been to their advantage to copulate on the side whenever the opportunity arose. But in order to philander, you have to seize the moment. If your special friend is away scouting and scavenging and his brother appears to collect nuts with you, you cannot wait until your period of heat returns; you must make love then.

Continual sexual receptivity enabled females to pursue *both* of their fundamental reproductive strategies: securing a pair-bond with a mate and allowing for ancillary copulations with additional lovers too.

Ecological factors undoubtedly also contributed to the loss of estrus. It would have been adaptive for our ancestors to bear young throughout the year so that infants were not born all at once, burdening the band, inviting the lions to a lovely lunch. Loss of estrus would have facilitated year-round births. Maybe estrus was also ex-cess baggage, part of a hormonal system females had to shed in order to incorporate other physiological adaptations. Most important, loss of estrus may have been a meal ticket. When male chimps kill an animal and everyone congregates to beg for pieces, estrous females get extra portions.[30] Early women may have needed these gratuities as well.

So if Lucy had a slightly longer monthly period of sexual receptiv-ity, lasting, let's say, twenty days as opposed to ten, she would have maintained a longer sexual relationship with her special friend and clandestine lovers, garnering more protection, more of their sca-venged meat. She would have lived. Her young would have lived. And the propensity for longer and longer periods of sexual receptiv-ity evolved.[31] Likewise, those females who copulated throughout more of pregnancy and sooner after delivering a child also received extra gratuities and survived disproportionately, passing on to mod-ern women the trait of continual sexual availability.

Silent Ovulation

So magnificent is this bizarre trait, continual sexual availability, that it must have been the culmination of several environmental and reproductive forces. But did women lose estrus or acquire perpetual estrus?

They lost estrus. Women exhibit almost no signs of midcycle ovulation. Shortly before the egg pops from the ovary, the tacky mucus on the cervix becomes slippery, smooth, and stretchable. Some women feel cramping. A few bleed slightly at this time. Others have unusually oily hair, their breasts become sensitive, or they have more energy than usual. A woman's body temperature rises almost a full degree at ovulation and remains normal or above until the next menstruation. And as her body voltage goes up, she becomes more electrically charged as well.[32] With these exceptions, ovulation is silent.

Women do not become sex crazed at midcycle either.[33] Not all primates flash puffy, conspicuous genitals at estrus. But one and all flaunt ovulation with alluring aromatic scents and persistent court-ing gestures. Hence the word *estrus,* derived from the Greek for "gadfly." On the contrary, most women do not even know when they are fertile. In fact, a woman must copulate regularly in order to get pregnant and take precautions if she does not want to bear a child. For women ovulation is concealed.

What a dangerous inconvenience "silent ovulation" is. It had led to millions, perhaps billions, of unwanted pregnancies. But it is easy to speculate on the advantages of silent ovulation in Lucy's day.

If Lucy's partner did not know when she was fertile, he was obliged to copulate with her regularly in order to bear a child. Silent ovulation kept a special friend in constant close proximity, providing protection and food the female prized. Paramours did not know whether Lucy was fertile either. She could count on their attentions too. And because primate males that consort with a female are often solicitous toward her young, these ancillary lovers may have doted on her children. Silent ovulation got the female more of what she needed—males.

Males got more sex. With the loss of estrus, a female mate was continually available sexually. Lovers were consistently ready too. With silent ovulation a "husband" did not have to fight off other suitors either, because his "wife" and lovers never signaled fertility. Silent ovulation probably also kept the peace.[34]

Of all the payoffs of this magnificent female trait, however, the most staggering was choice. Unchained from the ovulatory cycle of all other animals—and a sex drive that peaked and waned—Lucy could finally begin to *choose* her lovers more carefully.

Though female chimps definitely have favored sex partners and sometimes deflect intercourse with those they dislike by moving inappropriately at key moments or refusing to get into a mating pose, female chimps cannot conceal their receptivity, feign tiredness, or drive off suitors with nonchalance or insults. They are propelled by chemistry to copulate. Freed from this monthly hormonal flood, ancestral females gained more *cortical* control of their sexual desire. They could copulate for myriad new reasons too—including power, spite, lust, companionship, and love. "Will she or won't she?" came into vogue.

From large penises and dangling breasts to face-to-face copulation and continual sexual receptivity—all of the restless rivalry, the love affairs, and the recycling of partners started to change our bodies. As ancestral men and women paired and worked together, selection would also build the male and female brain.

Now the human psyche would take flight.

~ 10 ~

Why Can't a Man Be More Like a Woman?

Development of the Human Sexual Brain

Man is compos'd here of a two-fold part;
The first of Nature, and the next of Art.

—Robert Herrick, "Upon Man"

"**M**an is more courageous, pugnacious and energetic than woman, and has a more inventive genius. . . . Woman seems to differ from man . . . chiefly in her greater tenderness and less selfishness." Darwin wrote these words in 1871. Man the aggressor, woman the nurturer: he believed these gender qualities were the "birthright" of humankind, acquired from our distant past.

Darwin also thought men were naturally smarter. This superior male intelligence, he proposed, arose because young men had to fight to win mates. Because ancestral males had to defend their families, hunt for their joint subsistence, attack enemies, and make weapons, males needed higher mental faculties, "namely, observation, reason, invention or imagination." So, through ancestral competition among males and the survival of the fittest, intelligence evolved—in men.

An aggressive, intelligent Adam, a gentle, simple Eve; proof of this gender inequality Darwin saw everywhere around him. The poets, merchants, politicians, scientists, artists, and philosophers of Victorian England were overwhelmingly men. Moreover, Paul Broca, the eminent nineteenth-century French neurologist and authority on race, had confirmed the belief in feminine intellectual inferiority. After calculating the brain weights of over a hundred men and women whose bodies were autopsied in Paris hospitals, Broca wrote in 1861, "Women are, on the average, a little less intelligent than men, a difference which we should not exaggerate but which is, nonetheless, real."[1]

Broca had not corrected his calculations for the smaller body size of women. He had used an impeccable "correction formula" to prove that the French were just as capable as the Germans. But he did not make the necessary mathematical adjustments on his female skulls. Everyone knew that women were intellectually inferior anyway; such was the climate of the times.

This sexist credo saw a bitter reaction after World War I. Margaret Mead was among the intellectual leaders of the 1920s who emphasized the predominance of nurture over nature. The environment, she said, molded personality. As she wrote in 1935, "We may say that many if not all the personality traits which we have called masculine and feminine are as lightly linked to sex as are the clothing, the manners and the form of headdress that a society at a given period assigns to either sex."[2]

Mead's message spelled hope for women—as well as for ethnic minorities, immigrants, and the poor—and helped usher into scientific dogma the concept of "cultural determinism," the doctrine that people are essentially all similar.[3] Strip men and women of a few cultural ornaments, and you have basically the same animal; society and upbringing make women behave like women and men act like men. Biology begone.

The 1930s and following decades saw a rash of scientific treatises proclaiming that men and women were inherently alike. But now the tide has turned again. A host of new data have emerged, and today many scientists think that the sexes are quite different and that these differences begin to be established in the human brain during development in the womb.

When egg meets sperm and conception occurs, the embryo has neither male nor female genitals. But around the sixth week of fetal life a genetic switch flips and chromosomes direct the precursors of the gonads to develop into testes or ovaries. Now the die is cast. The differentiating gonads, if testes, begin to produce fetal testosterone. And as this powerful male hormone surges through embryonic tissues during the third month of life, it builds the male genitals. These fetal hormones also pattern the male brain. If the embryo is to be a girl, it develops without the stimulus of male hormones, and female genitals emerge—along with the female brain.[4]

So hormones "sex" the fetal brain. And several scientists think that this brain architecture plays a role in creating the gender differences that appear in later life. I will add that these gender differences came across the centuries, out of our distant past when ancestral men and women began to pair and raise their young as "husband" and "wife."

The Gift of Gab

In tests of verbal abilities among Americans, it is becoming clear that, on average, little girls speak sooner than boys. They speak more fluently, with greater grammatical accuracy, and with more words per utterance. By age ten, girls excel at verbal reasoning, written prose, verbal memory, pronunciation, and spelling. They are better at foreign languages. They stutter less. They exhibit dyslexia four times less often than boys. And far fewer girls are remedial readers.[5]

This is not to say that boys are inarticulate or that *all* boys have weaker verbal skills than *all* girls. Men vary; women vary. In fact, there is more variation within each gender than there is between them.[6] Proof lies in our Western heritage. For the past four thousand years, Western culture has suppressed women's opportunities to be orators, writers, poets, or playwrights and cultivated male geniuses. Not surprisingly, the vast majority of our public speakers and literary giants have been men. But scientists are beginning to agree that, on average, women exhibit more verbal skills than men.

These gender differences could be purely learned. Some argue, for example, that because infant girls are born more mature than boys, girls enter life with a slight edge in language ability that parents and the school system then cultivate as they age.[7] In fact, a host of arguments have been marshaled for the possibility that verbal skills are instilled more regularly in girls than in boys.[8] But data now suggest that these sex differences have an underlying biological component as well.

Women are more verbally fluent not only in the United States but in places as diverse as England, Czechoslovakia, and Nepal.[9] The International Association for the Evaluation of Educational Achievement recently reported that in some 43,000 writing samples of students in fourteen countries on five continents, girls expressed their thoughts more clearly on paper. The most compelling argument for women's verbal superiority, however, is the link between estrogen, the female hormone, and female verbal skills.

In a recent study of two hundred women of reproductive age, psychologists showed that during the middle of the monthly menstrual cycle, when estrogen levels peaked, women were at their best verbally.[10] When asked, for example, to repeat the tongue twister "A box of mixed biscuits in a biscuit mixer" five times as fast as possible, they performed particularly well at midcycle. Directly after menses, when estrogen levels were much lower, these women's speed declined. Even at their worst, most of these women outstripped men on all verbal tasks.

The Math Gap

Men excel, on average, at higher mathematical problems (not at arithmetic). And they are generally better at reading maps, solving mazes, and completing several other visual-spatial-quantitative tasks.[11]

Some of these skills appear in childhood. Little boys take toys apart and explore more of the space around them. They are better at tracking objects in space, and they see abstract patterns and relationships more accurately. By age ten, more boys can rotate three-dimensional objects in their mind's eye, accurately perceive three-dimensional spaces on flat paper, and begin to score higher on some other mechanical and spatial problems. Then at puberty boys begin to outstrip girls in algebra, in geometry, and in other subjects involving visual-spatial-quantitative skills.[12]

In one test of nearly 50,000 seventh-graders who took the standard Scholastic Aptitude Test, 260 boys and 20 girls scored over 700 (out of 800) on mathematical problems—a ratio of 13 to 1.[13] In the United States three out of four Ph.D.'s in math are awarded to men. And these gender differences in spatial acuity and interest in mathematics are seen in several other cultures.[14]

Like verbal skills in females, these abilities observed in many boys and men clearly have a large cultural component. But there is also a link between the predominant male hormone, testosterone, the male Y chromosome, and excellence in math and certain visual-spatial-quantitative tasks. Girls who receive abnormally high doses of male hormones in the womb (because of fetal malfunctions or drugs that the mother took while pregnant) exhibit tomboyish behavior in childhood—and do better on math exams in teenage. Conversely, pubescent boys with low levels of testosterone do poorly on spatial tasks. Moreover, men with an extra Y chromosome (XYY) score higher on visual-spatial tests, and those with an extra female X chromosome (XXY, or Klinefelter's syndrome) have a poorer spatial aptitude.[15]

I am not suggesting that women have developed no superior spatial skills. On the contrary, scientists Irwin Silverman and Marion Beals recently uncovered an intriguing feminine spatial aptitude. They displayed several dissimilar objects in a room and drawn on a piece of paper and instructed men and women to memorize the objects that they saw. Then they asked the participants to recall what they had memorized. The results: women were able to remember a great many more of these stationary objects and their locations.[16]

So each gender has specific spatial talents.

Does society train women to fail at math and men to fail at English?

Several cultural explanations have been proposed to explain these gender differences: teachers' assumptions and their treatment of students, parents' attitudes toward their children and how they train boys and girls to be adults, society's perception that math is masculine, the different games and sports that boys and girls play, each gender's self-perception and ambitions, the many social pressures on adolescents, even the way that tests are designed and how scientists interpret the results all undoubtedly affect test scores.[17] Scholastic Aptitude Test scores, for example, vary as much with social class and ethnic background as with gender. And the gap between male and female performance on standardized math tests has declined since the 1970s.

Is biology destiny?

Not at all. No one denies that culture plays an enormous role in molding human action. But it is unscientific to overlook some equally significant facts: the body of data on gender differences in infants, the persistence of male/female differences on tests other than the SATs, the fact that adolescent girls do not fall behind on *other* tasks because of social pressure, the corroborative data from other countries, and the literature linking testosterone with spatial skills and estrogen with verbal aptitude all support the view that the sexes do indeed exhibit gender differences in some spatial and verbal abilities—and that these gender differences stem, at least in part, from male/female variations in biology.

I can add only that, from an anthropological perspective, these gender differences make evolutionary sense. As ancestral males began to scout and track and surround animals millennia ago, those males who were good at maps and mazes could well have survived disproportionately. Ancestral women needed to locate vegetable foods within an elaborate matrix of vegetation instead, so they developed a superior ability to remember the locations of stationary objects, a different spatial talent. And for women whose job it was to rear the young, verbal skills may have been critical as well.

Hence I will argue that as pair-bonding emerged and the human hunting-gathering-scavenging tradition took shape, so did these subtle gender differences in aptitude.

Other variations between the sexes could have a biological foundation and may also have evolved during our long nomadic past.

Woman's Intuition

"It is generally admitted," wrote Darwin, "that with woman the powers of intuition . . . are more strongly marked than in man."[18]

Science is beginning to prove Darwin right. Tests show that, on average, women read emotions, context, and all sorts of peripheral nonverbal information more effectively than men.[19] A slight twist of the head, lips pulled taut, shoulders hunched, a shift of body weight, a change in tone of voice—any of these subtle movements can lead a woman to feel that her guest is uncomfortable, fearful, angry, or disappointed. Could this aptitude stem from brain anatomy? Perhaps.

The bundle of nerve fibers that connect the two sides of the brain, the corpus callosum, thickens and bulges toward the rear in women but is uniformly cylindrical in men.[20] Hence the two sides of a woman's brain are better connected. The sections within each hemisphere may be better connected too.[21] And from several hundred experiments on stroke victims, on patients with brain tumors or injuries, and on normal subjects, it now appears that women's skills are more widely distributed throughout the cortex, that men's skills are more localized and more compartmentalized and that their hemispheres operate slightly more independently.[22]

This brain circuitry suggests an explanation for women's intuition. Perhaps women absorb cues from a wider range of visual, aural, tactile, and olfactory senses simultaneously. Then they connect these ancillary bits of information—giving women that ready insight that Darwin extolled.

And it is not illogical to suggest that *if* there is a biological component to women's intuition, it evolved in large part to help women detect the needs of their growing infants millennia ago.[23]

Female verbal skills, male excellence at math and some spatial problems, and feminine intuition are not the only differences between the sexes that appear to have a biological component and could well have developed during our long prehistory.

Women of all ages have better "fine" motor coordination, manipulating tiny objects with ease. (No wonder they are better at sewing! They would also be better with a surgeon's scalpel.) This feminine dexterity even increases during the middle of the menstrual cycle, when estrogen levels are at their highest—suggesting that there is a physiological element to this fine manual prowess.[24] Boys and men are, on the average, more dexterous at gross motor skills requiring speed and force, from running and jumping to throwing sticks and stones and balls.[25]

Once again, these gender differences make evolutionary sense. As ancestral women picked more seeds and berries and more regularly picked the grass and dirt and twigs off their young, those with superior fine motor dexterity may have survived disproportionately—selecting for this trait in modern women. On the other hand, it seems likely that as men hurled more weapons at predators and moving beasts, a male aptitude for gross motor coordination emerged.

Boys Will Be Boys

A last trait distinguishes men and women: just as Darwin said, men are, on average, more aggressive and women do more nurturing.

In a telling study of aggressiveness in villages in Japan, the Philippines, Mexico, Kenya, and India, as well as in "Orchard Town," an anonymous New England city, anthropologists Beatrice and John Whiting found that boys were more aggressive in each culture.[26] Psychologists confirm this for Americans. Boy toddlers grab and scratch. Nursery school boys chase and wrestle. Teenage boys like contact sports. Rough-and-tumble play is almost exclusively a male preoccupation throughout childhood, as it is in other primates. More men are drawn to the violent acts of war. And the vast majority of homicides around the world are committed by men, often by young men with high levels of testosterone.[27]

I am not suggesting that women are unaggressive. We all know that women can be exceedingly tough-minded, sometimes physically violent—and they are very protective of their young. Just threaten a baby to see a mother's vicious rage. But some scientists think that in females the environment may play a larger role in aggressive interactions whereas male aggression is more governed by hormones instead.[28]

This aggressive spirit certainly would have served men well as they strode forth to confront their predators and enemies on the grasslands of Africa a few million years ago.

Nurturing is often considered to be the female counterpart to male aggressiveness. Women of every ethnic group and culture around the world (and every other primate species) show more interest in infants and more tolerance of their needs. Moreover, in every society on record, women do the majority of daily infant-rearing tasks.[29]

Some would like to attribute feminine nurturance to learned behavior. But data indicate that this, too, may have a biological foundation.[30] Infant girls chatter, smile, and coo to people's faces, while boys are just as likely to babble at objects and blinking lights. Infant girls are more sensitive to touch, high sounds, loud noises, voice inflection, tastes, and smells. Little girls have longer attention spans and devote more time to fewer projects; boys are more distractible, more active, more exploratory. Girls are more attracted to new people, while boys are drawn to novel toys. And girls are better at discerning your emotional state from your tone of voice. All of these traits are useful to rearing young.

In her 1982 book, *In a Different Voice,* psychologist Carol Gilligan proposes that women also have an outstanding sensitivity for interpersonal relationships. In interviews with over a hundred men and women, boys and girls, she and her colleagues found that women cast themselves as actors in a web of attachments, affiliations, obligations, and responsibilities to others. Then they nurture these ties— another attribute helpful to raising babies in a group.

As male aggressiveness is linked to testosterone, so female nurturing also seems to have a physiological component. Individuals born with only one X chromosome, or Turner's syndrome, are "extremely feminine"; they show less interest in sports and childhood fighting and are more interested in personal adornment than are normal girls. They also score extremely low on tests of mathematical and spatial tasks. But these girls are very interested in marriage and are strongly drawn to children.[31]

Perhaps women's sensitivity to interpersonal relationships, their need for affiliation, their natural interest in people's faces, their heightened sense of noise and smell and touch and taste, and their longer attention span are yet more aspects of the feminine psyche that evolved as ancestral females nurtured their young millennia ago.

"If it's true we are descended from the ape, it must have been from two different species. There's no likeness between us, is there?" said a man to a woman in August Strindberg's 1887 play, *The Father*. The misogynistic Swede was, of course, exaggerating. But men and women, on average, seem to be endowed with varying spatial, verbal, and intuitive skills, different kinds of hand-eye coordination, and dissimilarities in aggressiveness and nurturing behavior that appear to have a biological component. And logic holds that they emerged with the evolution of the human hunting-gathering tradition.

Nevertheless, neither sex is more intelligent than the other.

Here Darwin was wrong. Intelligence is a collage of thousands of separate abilities, not a single trait. Some people excel at reading maps or recognizing faces. Others can mentally rotate objects, fix a car, or write a poem. Some people reason well at thorny scientific problems, while others reason well in difficult social situations. Some people learn music rapidly; others can learn a foreign language in weeks. Some remember economic theories; others recall philosophical ideas. Some people just remember more of everything but can't express what they know or apply it meaningfully; others know far less but express themselves creatively and have a greater capacity to generalize or use their knowledge or ideas. Hence the magnificent variety in human sagacity, wit, and personality.

The sexes are not identical, however. Some women are brilliant mathematicians, composers, or chess players; some men are the world's finest orators, playwrights, and interpreters. But a good deal of data suggests that, on average, each gender has an undercurrent, a melody, a theme.

Why can't a man be more like a woman?

Why can't a woman be more like a man?

Selection for spatial and verbal skills, for female intuition, for gross versus fine motor coordination, for aggressiveness and nurturing behavior, may have begun even before our female and male forebears emerged on the grassland of the ancient world to start scavenging, hunting, and collecting for a living.

"Darwinian Man, though well-behaved, / At best is only a monkey shaved." So goes the ditty written by the English librettist W. S. Gilbert. Indeed, modern scientists are not the first to think there is continuity between man and beast. Confirming it, however, is anthropologist William McGrew who has found rudiments of the human hunting-gathering tradition among modern chimpanzees.[32]

As you recall, male chimps that live along Lake Tanganyika, in East Africa, hunt. They stalk, chase, and kill animals. These are spatial, quiet, aggressive tasks. Males also scout along the border of their range and guard the community territory—occupations that are more spatial, silent, and aggressive. And male chimps throw more foliage and rocks—gross motor habits.

Female chimps gather. They engage in termite fishing and ant dipping three times more often than males do. These tasks require minute manual dexterity. Female common chimps also engage in more social grooming, using fine motor dexterity to pick tiny specks from one another for hours at a time. And while they forage and groom one another, female chimps interact with their young, touching and vocalizing. This has spurred their verbal skills. Like their counterparts among many higher primates, male chimps tend to bark, growl, and roar, to make strident aggressive sounds, while females make more "clear calls," appeals for affiliation.[33]

These data suggest that some of the modern differences between the genders *preceded* our descent onto the grasslands of Africa. Then, as our forebears began to collect small game, to hunt, to scavenge, and to forage for seeds and berries on the open plains, these gender roles must have become critical to survival—selecting for today's male/female differences in spatial and verbal skills, as well as intuition, hand-eye coordination, and aggressiveness.

"The Gorge"

We have, of course, no physical evidence of male scavenging and hunting or female gathering among Lucy and her relatives who strolled across the savannas of Africa almost four million years ago. We have only footprints and a few old bones. But the fossil record becomes more abundant by two million years ago. And some peculiar archaeological remains suggest that human gender roles—and gender differences in the brain—had started to emerge.

The data come from Olduvai Gorge, Tanzania, a barren, desiccated canyon land where over the last 200,000 years a river has cut a deep seam between the rocks, exposing a layer cake of ancient geological strata. Since the 1930s Mary and Louis Leakey had been digging in this crevasse, looking for evidence of early man. And in 1959 Mary discovered a site at the bottom of the gorge, Bed I, that exposed life as it had been between 1.7 and 1.9 million years ago.

The area had been a shallow, brackish, emerald-colored lake surrounded by marsh, bush, and trees. Pelicans, storks, herons, and hippos had waded through the tranquil pools. Crocodiles had floated in the brine. And ducks and geese had nested in the papyrus reeds at the water's edge. Sloping off the lake, the brush merged into high open countryside, dotted here and there with acacia trees. At the horizon were forests of mahoganies and evergreens that stretched up mountain slopes toward volcanic peaks.

On the eastern edge of the extinct lake, where salty marshes were once fed by freshwater streams, Mary Leakey unearthed over twenty-five hundred ancient tools and fragments of worked stone.[34] Someone with "a good eye" had made these tools. Some were big chunks of lava, quartzite, or other stones that had a few edges whacked off to make a sharpened edge. Others were fragmentary flakes that had been chipped from larger rocks. "Débitage," small slivers of sharp stone, and manuports, hunks of unfashioned stone, were strewn along the shore. Some of these tools were of local stone; others came from outcroppings, stream channels, and lava flows kilometers away. Some had been made elsewhere and then been left whole beside the lake. Others had been chipped or worked at the marsh and carried off, leaving only their detritus behind. Here, then, was a tool factory and depository.

Known as Oldowan tools, these primitive choppers and scrapers are not the oldest ever found. Two and a half million years ago someone left tools in Ethiopia. But these utensils at Olduvai, Bed I, were special.

Around them lay some sixty thousand bits of animal bones. Elephants, hippos, rhinos, pigs, buffalo, horses, giraffes, oryx, elands, wildebeests, kongoni, topis, waterbucks, bushbucks, reedbucks, Grant's gazelles, Thompson's gazelles, and impalas made up the larger species. The remains of turtles, elephant shrews, hares, and ducks, and the bones of hundreds of other smaller animals and birds lay here as well. In the 1960s and 1970s the Leakeys uncovered five more sites along this ancient lake. At one, an elephant had been butchered.

Like palimpsests, these assemblages at Olduvai are blackboards half erased. But the brand-new field of taphonomy has begun to establish what happened beside this lake so long ago.

Bone Puzzles

Taphonomy is the ingenious science that studies fossilized bones by working backward.[35] By looking at how modern people butcher meat, how other carnivores such as lions or hyenas chew on bones, and how water and wind spread bones across the landscape, taphonomists establish how ancient bones arrive in the positions and conditions that they are in. For example, taphonomists have watched hunters cut up carcasses and they report that when hunters remove the flesh, they leave cut marks in the center of the long bones; to harvest skin and tendons they etch distinctive cut marks at the ends of bones instead. Hyenas, on the other hand, chew the feet and ends of bones, leaving quite different marks on bone refuse.

Using these and many other taphonomic clues, anthropologists have tried to piece together what happened at Olduvai some two million years ago. Most convincing is the work of Henry Bunn and Ellen Kroll.[36]

After studying all of these ancient bones, these anthropologists proposed that our ancestors caught the turtles, shrews, herons, and other little creatures with cord traps or with their hands. They surmise that, because lions would have dragged off the entire carcass, our forebears hunted and killed the middle-sized animals like gazelles. The larger animal bones without carnivore teeth marks on them probably were those of animals our ancestors collected at the end of the dry season, when animals collapse. And the bones with carnivore tooth marks on them our forebears undoubtedly scavenged.

Maybe they drove their carnivore competitors from a meal, just long enough to steal joints, the "bully sneak" strategy. Perhaps they picked over the remains after their rivals had wandered off to snooze instead. They could also have stolen the carcasses that leopards dragged into trees.[37]

Our ancient forebears not only collected, scavenged, and hunted animals, but they must have butchered these beasts. Some of the tools have microscopic scratches that come from cutting meat. Many of the bones have parallel cut marks in the middle of the shaft where someone must have sliced off chunks of flesh. And other fossil bones have tool cut marks at the joints where someone disarticulated limbs and carried these long bones to the shore.

Last, the disproportionately large number of meaty limb bones from middle-sized animals like wildebeests suggests that our ancestors had enough meat for "cooperative group sharing." "People" had begun to butcher, carry, and share meat almost two million years ago.[38]

But why are the bones and stones in discrete heaps? After lengthy analysis of the bones, the tools, and the sites and of computer simulations combining all these data with factors like energy expenditure, time of travel, and other variables, anthropologist Richard Potts has theorized that these piles of bones and stones at Olduvai were "stone caches," places where our ancestors stashed their tools and stone raw materials.[39] Here they made tools, left tools, and brought animal parts to be processed quickly. Then, after chopping off meat, extracting marrow, and harvesting skin or tendons, they abandoned the butchery station before the hyenas arrived. When they were in the area again with meat in hand, they revisited one of these stone caches.

Year upon decade upon century the bones and tools and raw materials accumulated. Then Mary Leakey found these garbage heaps.

These refuse dumps say something important about women, men, and the evolution of gender skills. If our ancestors two million years ago had stone caches spotted along the landscape, complete with tools and raw materials to butcher meat, then clearly these early peoples coordinated their activities, engaged in the dangerous pursuit of getting meat from middle- to large-sized animals, delayed eating it, carried joints to specific shared locations beside the lake, butchered meat, and had enough food to share it with relatives and friends. And it is highly unlikely that many ancestral females, often burdened with small children, engaged in the dangerous activities of hunting or scavenging even medium-sized beasts.

For decades after Darwin initiated the "man the hunter" concept, academics ignored the roles of early females. But in the early 1980s revisionist anthropologists began to set the record straight.[40] And today most think ancestral women engaged chiefly in the far more productive, dependable activity of collecting nuts, berries, vegetables, and delicacies like eggs and fruit.

Unfortunately the principal tools of gathering—the digging stick and the pouch—do not normally fossilize. But scientists have recently found broken long bones of antelopes in the cave at Swartkrans, in southern Africa, that had polished ends. Microscopic wear patterns near the tips indicate that someone had used these implements for digging vegetables too. Ancient teeth from this era suggest that our ancestors also ate a lot of fruit.[41] In fact, Potts suggests that meat composed less than 20 percent of the diet.

So if men did more of the hunting and scavenging whereas women did the bulk of the collecting of vegetables, women had essential jobs two million years ago.

With time, these gender roles would select for men's knack for maps and mazes and other spatial skills, their aggressiveness, and their gross motor coordination. And as days turned into centuries, women's spatial memory for stationary objects, their verbal acuity, their facility for nurturing, their fine motor abilities, and their uncanny intuition would become firmly established as well.

The Nature of Intimacy

These gender traits may explain some misunderstandings between the sexes. We struggle, you and I, with intimacy. In poll after book after article women express their disappointment that their mates do not talk out their problems, do not express their emotions, do not listen, do not share—verbally. Women derive intimacy from talking. No doubt this form of intimacy comes from their long prehistory as nurturers.

Sociologist Harry Brod reports that men often seek intimacy differently. "Numerous studies," he writes, "have established that men are more likely to define emotional closeness as working or playing side by side, while women often view it as talking face to face."[42] Men, for example, derive intimacy from playing and watching sports. I am not surprised. What is a football game but a map, a maze, a puzzle, spatial action, and aggressive competition—all of which engage skills that appeal to the male brain. In fact, watching a football game on television is not very different from sitting behind a bush on the African veldt, trying to judge which route the giraffes will take. No wonder most women do not understand why men get such pleasure from watching sports; these pastimes don't ring a chord in their evolutionary psyches.

Psychologists have even begun to capitalize on this gender variation in intimacy. One Iowa psychologist advertises his kind of therapy, "For men only," in the yellow pages of the telephone book. He offers help to men by means of sports activities, dance, and drama. Talking, he maintains, is a female approach—inappropriate for men. The rest of us would do well to remember this male/female distinction. A woman should probably adopt at least one nonverbal, side-by-side leisure activity that her spouse enjoys, whereas men could improve their home lives if they took time out to sit face-to-face with their mates and engage in talk and "active listening."

Another possible gender variation in standards of intimacy may stem from our ancestry. Psychologists maintain that women more regularly seek to feel included, connected, and attached, while men more often enjoy space, privacy, and autonomy.[43] As a result, women say they feel *evaded* by a husband, and men report they feel *invaded* by a wife. Could a woman's drive to be included come from a time when women's roles as nurturers selected for those who felt comfortable in a group? Perhaps men's need to seek autonomy harks back to those days, too, when men made their living as solitary, stealthy scouts and trackers—selecting for those individuals who enjoy space and unconnectedness today.

We may have some sexual tastes that come from our distant past as well. Some men are voyeurs. Some like to look at visual porn. Others have an indefatigable love for erotic underwear, nighties, and sex gadgets. In fact, men's sexual fantasies are regularly aroused by visual stimuli of all sorts.[44] Perhaps these partialities are, in part, directed by their more spatial brains. Women like romance novels and soap operas on television—tepid verbal porn. Maybe these inclinations arise from their sensitivity to language.

This is not to say that *all* men are voyeurs, that *all* men feel invaded by their wives, or that *all* men derive intimacy from sports or are verbally unexpressive. Nor do *all* women read romance novels, shun television football, or derive a feeling of intimacy from talking face-to-face. The mixture of appetites in any one human personality is vast; I marvel at how strikingly different people are. But these gender differences in conduct have been recorded.

And one must admit that men puzzle over the age-old question "What do women want?" Women, on the other hand, regularly say, "They just don't understand." I suspect our ancestors had begun to mystify one another by two million years ago, when males and females began to split up to forage around the emerald lake at Olduvai and our fundamental human gender skills had started to emerge.

Who were these "people" at Olduvai?

The bones of two separate species of early hominids have been recovered from Bed I, the bottom sedimentary layer of the gorge. Individuals with enormous cheek teeth and buttressed skulls known as *Australopithecus boisei* lived along the lake, then died out about a million years ago. Although these creatures had expanded cranial capacities of 430 to 550 cubic centimeters and related specimens had hands capable of making tools to fell and butcher prey,[45] their monstrous jaws and the structure and wear patterns on their teeth suggest that they sat in the reeds instead and chewed enormous quantities of tough, fibrous vegetables, nuts, and seeds. These probably were not hunters.

"Handy Man," or *Homo habilis*, lived here too. These people had gracile skulls and smaller cheek teeth. The original four fossil specimens found were nicknamed Twiggy (a crushed cranium with seven teeth), George (teeth and skull fragments), Cindy, and Johnny's Child (more bits of ancient jaws and teeth). All had died near streams where fresh drinking water tumbled into salty marsh on the eastern margin of the lake some 1.9 million years ago. Recently the partial skeleton of a woman was also recovered; she stood only three feet tall.[46]

To the north at Koobi Fora, a parched, desolate spit of land that extends into today's Lake Turkana in northern Kenya, were Twiggy's relatives. Here Richard Leakey, the son of Mary and Louis Leakey, has uncovered over three hundred specimens since 1968. A mother lode. The most famous fossil was a skull that has acquired the name 1470, after its catalog number. Why is 1470 so important?

Because this individual had an expanded brain volume of 600 to 800 cubic centimeters. Moreover, like Twiggy and the other specimens of Handy Man, 1470 had a cranial volume well above that of his or her contemporaries, the australopithecines, and about half the cranial capacity of modern people.

Our gang was getting smarter. Anthropologist Ralph Holloway has exposed the contours of their brains by making latex casts of the insides of these fossil skulls. He reports that the frontal and parietal areas of the cortex—the portions of the brain used to discriminate, categorize, reflect, and reason—had begun to assume a modern shape. Twiggy and her relatives could well have developed the ability to plan ahead.

They may have discussed their plans too. Holloway's endocasts show a slight bulge in Broca's area, named after the nineteenth-century neurologist I mentioned in the beginning of this chapter. Broca's area is a portion of the cortex above the left ear that directs the mouth, tongue, throat, and vocal cords to produce speech sounds. In the brain of 1470, as well as in other speciments of Handy Man, this language section had begun to swell.[47]

Language is the hallmark of humanity. Although there are over ten thousand works on the origin of language, no one has been able to explain how or when our ancestors first began to arbitrarily assign words to objects (like *dog* for the tail-wagging, four-legged creature we play with in the yard), to break down these words into separate sounds (like d-o-g), or to recombine these tiny noises to make novel words with novel meanings (like g-o-d). But with all our meaningless little squeaks and hisses, clicks and hoos, strung together to make words, with all our words linked to one another according to grammatical rules to make sentences, humankind would eventually dominate the earth.

Twiggy may have crossed this threshold of humanity.

Did Twiggy call hello to her lover as she returned from collecting nuts? Did she verbally describe the animal tracks she had seen on the plains or whisper that she loved her mate as she curled up to sleep? Did George and 1470 reprimand their infants, tell jokes, weave tales, lie, give compliments, discuss tomorrow and yesterday—with words? Certainly not the way you and I do. Postures, gestures, facial expressions, and intonations were probably critical to the message too. But since Broca's area was indeed expanding in the brain, Twiggy probably conversed with primitive, prehuman language.

Man the scout, tracker, explorer, scavenger, hunter, and protector. Woman the gatherer, nurturer, mediator, and educator. We may never know which early peoples first began to do separate tasks. But someone carted chunks of meat into the reeds and stripped these bones two million years ago.[48] And I do not think that females with small children were the hunters or the butchers.

At the same time, there is no reason to think that either sex had rigid, formal roles. Probably females without children joined and even led scavenging and hunting parties. Certainly men often gathered plants and nuts and berries. Probably some couples beat the grass together to catch small animals. But our ancestors had begun to collect, butcher, and share meat. The sexes had started to make their living as a team.

Freud called the female psyche the "dark continent" for good reason. For decades, if not centuries, scientists in search of an understanding of human nature have used male behavior as a bench mark and compared all data on females with this standard. Hence we have known almost nothing about the biological tendencies of women. Times have changed. And from what we now know of the feminine psyche, it is becoming evident that the sexes were designed across the millennia to put their heads together.

This hunting-gathering life-style would produce an intricate balance between women, men, and power.

~11~

Women, Men, and Power
The Nature of Sexual Politics

Everything is the sum of the past, and nothing is comprehensible except through its history.

—*Pierre Teilhard de Chardin*

Tens of thousands of women, their faces smeared with ashes, wearing loincloths and wreaths of ferns, poured from villages across southeastern Nigeria one morning in 1929 and marched to their local "native administration" centers. There the district's British colonial officers resided. They congregated outside these administrators' doors and shook traditional war sticks, danced, ridiculed them with scurrilous songs, and demanded the insignia of the local Igbo men who had collaborated with this enemy. At a few administration centers women broke into jails to free prisoners; at others they burned or tore apart native-court buildings. But they hurt no one.

The British retaliated, opening fire on protesters in two centers, slaughtering sixty women. So ended the insurrection. The British "won."

History often records the words of victors, and this "Women's

War," as the Igbo called it, soon acquired its British name, the Aba Riots.[1] But the British never comprehended what this war was all about—that it was orchestrated entirely by women and for women; the notion of a violation of women's rights was beyond their grasp. Instead, most of the British officers were convinced that Igbo men had organized this demonstration, then directed their spouses to revolt. Igbo wives had rioted, colonial officials reasoned, because they thought the British would not fire on the weaker sex.[2]

A colossal cultural chasm stretched between the British and the Igbo—a gulf that gave rise to the Igbo Women's War and symbolized a profound European misunderstanding about women, men, and power in cultures around the world.

For centuries these Igbo women, like women in many other West African societies, had been autonomous and powerful, economically and politically. They lived in patrilineal villages where power was informal; anyone could participate in Igbo village assemblies. Men engaged in more of the discussions and normally offered the final settlement on disputes. Men had more resources, so they could pay the fees and hold the feasts that brought them more titles and prestige. And men controlled the land. But at marriage a husband was obliged to give his wife some property to farm.

This soil was a woman's bank account. Women grew a variety of crops and took their produce to local markets run entirely by women.[3] And women came home with luxury goods and money that they kept. So Igbo women had independent wealth—financial freedom, economic power. Thus, if a man let his cows graze in a woman's fields, mistreated his wife, violated the market code, or committed some other serious crime, women did what they would do to the British administrators: they assembled at the offender's home, chanted insults, sometimes even destroyed his house. Igbo men respected women, women's work, women's rights, and women's laws.

Enter the British. In 1900 England declared southern Nigeria a protectorate and set up a system of native-court areas; each district was governed by a British colonial officer from a district seat, the native court. This was unpopular enough. Then the British appointed one representative from each village, a warrant chief, to membership in each district's native court. Often this was a young Igbo who had curried favor with the conquerors rather than a respected village elder; always it was a man. Steeped in the Victorian belief that wives were appendages of their husbands, the British could not conceive of women in positions of power. So they excluded women, one and all. Igbo women lost their voice.

Then, in 1929, the British decided to take inventories of women's goods. Fearing impending taxation, Igbo women met in their market squares to discuss this crippling economic action. They were ready to rebel. And after a series of flare-ups between women and census takers in November, they dressed in traditional battle garments and went to war, an uprising that erupted over six thousand square miles and involved tens of thousands of women.

After the British quashed the revolution, Igbo women requested that they, too, serve as village representatives in the native courts. To no avail. As far as the British were concerned, a woman's place was in the home.

"It's a Man's World"

The Western conviction that men universally dominate women passes like a deleterious gene from one generation to the next.[4] Is this true? Has it always been so? To explore the long evolutionary history of women, men, and power, let me first unravel what we know of gender relations in societies around the world today.

Before the women's movement of the 1970s, American and European anthropologists simply assumed that men were always more powerful than women, and their research reflected their convictions. Accounts of the Australian aborigines provide a striking example.

Several academics—mostly men—wrote that these people's marriage system, in which infant girls were married to men thirty years their senior and men had several wives, was the crowning example of male rule. From their perspective, aboriginal women were pawns, commodities, currency in the marriage manipulations of men.[5] They explained the aborigines' separate men's and women's religious ceremonies as evidence of women's subordination too. And as for women's work, Ashley Montagu summed it up in 1937, calling the women no more than "domesticated cows."[6]

Today we know that this picture of aboriginal life is distorted. Women ethnographers have gone into the Australian outback and talked to women. From conversations during gathering expeditions, at swimming parties, across the firelight, these scholars have established that Australian aboriginal women politick avidly in the betrothal poker game and begin to choose their own new husbands by middle age. Women regularly engage lovers. Some tribes have a *jilimi*, or single women's camp, where widows, estranged wives, and visiting women live or visit, free of men. Far from being a battered wife, a woman sometimes hits a lazy husband with her "fighting stick." Women hold some rituals that are closed to men. And women's economic contributions are vital to daily life. In short, although women's and men's activities are often segregated, Australian aboriginal women appear to be every bit as powerful as men.[7]

Neither sex dominated—a concept that was apparently foreign to Western scholars. An obsession with hierarchy, in concert with deeply ingrained beliefs about gender, colored scientific analyses of other peoples.

This changed during the women's movement when feminist anthropologists began to challenge the dogma of universal female subordination. They argued that because men had done most of the fieldwork, spoken mostly to male informants, and primarily observed men's activities, many anthropological reports were biased; the voices of women had not been heard.

Some charged, moreover, that male anthropologists had misconstrued what they saw, denigrating women's work as "housework," women's conversations as superficial "gossip," women's artistry as "crafts," and women's participation in ceremonies as "nonsacred," while aggrandizing hunting, men's arts, men's religious rituals, men's oratory, and many other male pursuits.[8] Because of selective blindness, androcentrism, or sexist bias—call it what you wish—women's work and women's lives had been ignored, tainting anthropological reports.

These accusations are not entirely true. Sociologist Martin Whyte recently compared gender roles in ninety-three traditional societies and noted that in some of these studies, data on women's roles were neglected or minimized; in others, aspects of men's power were disregarded. These omissions were random, however, rather than systematically biased against women. Moreover, these oversights were not linked specifically to male or female authors. Androcentrism may not be as pervasive as some feminists report.[9]

Nevertheless, even a casual reader of the literature can point to some classic ethnographies in which women look like faceless drones. And the ubiquitous articles about "man the hunter" have only recently become balanced by literature on "woman the gatherer." So the feminist era turned the tide, adding a necessary lens to scholarly investigations of other peoples, women as well as men.

This new focus on women's lives has uncovered a reality of extreme importance: like the Igbo women of Nigeria, *women in a great many other traditional cultures were relatively powerful—before the coming of the Europeans.*[10] Some survived Western influence with their power intact. But many others, like the Igbo, fell victim to European mores.

Anthropologist Eleanor Leacock arrived at this conclusion while studying the Montagnais-Naskapi Indians of eastern Canada. Most instructive to her were the journals of the Jesuit Paul Le Jeune. Le Jeune took up his post as superior of the French mission at Quebec in 1632. Here he wintered with the Montagnais-Naskapi. To his horror, he saw indulgent parents, independent women, divorced men and women, men with two wives, no formal leaders, a peripatetic, relaxed, egalitarian culture in which women enjoyed a high economic and social status.

This state of affairs Le Jeune resolved to change. He was convinced that discipline for children, marital fidelity, lifelong monogamy, and, above all, male authority and female fealty were essential to salvation. As he told the Indians, "In France women do not rule their husbands."[11] Within months Le Jeune had converted a handful of these "heathens." Ten years later some had started to beat women.

How many women have colonialism and Christianity tethered? It's impossible to say. But the Igbo Women's War was no fluke of history. As one scientist summed up the situation, "The penetration of Western colonialism, and with it Western practices and attitudes regarding women, has so widely influenced women's roles in aboriginal societies as to depress women's status almost everywhere in the world."[12]

Power Plays

Knowing, then, that women have indeed been powerful in many traditional societies around the world, what can we infer about life in Africa during our long nomadic prehistoric past—millennia before European guns and gospels skewed power relations between men and women? We have two ways of gaining insight: by examining daily life in modern traditional societies and by dissecting power relations among our close relatives, the apes. Let's begin with the power plays of people.[13]

Anthropologists generally agree that power (the ability to influence or persuade, as opposed to authority, formal institutionalized command) regularly resides with those who control valued goods or services and have the right to distribute this wealth outside the home.

The gift. If you own the land, rent the land, give away the land, or distribute resources on the land, like water holes or fishing rights, you have power. If you have a special service, like doctoring, or a connection with the spirit world that others need, you have power. If you kill a giraffe and give away the meat or make baskets, beads, blankets, or other products for trade, you can make friends—alliances that bring economic ties, prestige, and power. So who collects what, who owns what, and who gives, rents, sells, or trades what to whom matters in the power dance between the sexes.[14]

The traditional north Alaskan Inuit (or Eskimos) offer a good example of this direct relationship between economic resources and social control. In the barren north, where only moss and grasses appear above the permafrost for much of the year, there were no plants to gather. As a result, women traditionally did not leave home for work as gatherers or bring back valuable goods to trade. Men did

all the hunting. Men left the house to chase seals or whales throughout the winter months and fished or hunted caribou during the long
Arctic summer days. Men brought home the blubber for the candle
oil, the skins for parkas, trousers, shirts, and shoes, sinew for cord,
bone for ornaments and tools, and every scrap of food. Women
depended on these supplies. Eskimo men depended on their wives to
tan the hides, smoke the meat, and make all the heavy clothing. So
the sexes needed each other to survive.

But men had access to the fundamental resources. And Eskimo
girls realized early in life that the way to succeed was to "marry
well."[15] Young women had no other access to power.

Traditional !Kung Bushmen women of the Kalahari Desert, on the
other hand, were far more economically powerful. And they did not
marry as a career. As you know, when anthropologists first recorded
their lifeways in the 1960s, women commuted to work and came
home with much of the evening meal. !Kung women had economic
power; they also had a voice. But !Kung wives, unlike their husbands,
did not distribute their food within the larger social group.

This distinction is important. When men returned from a successful hunting trip, they divided the precious meat according to rules as
well as with fanfare. The owner of the arrow that killed the animal
got the prestigious task of distributing the catch. The man who first
saw the beast got certain choice sections, those who tracked it got
others, and so forth. Then each hunter in turn gave steaks and ribs
and organ meats to his family and other kin. These were "invest-
ments," however, not offerings. !Kung hunters expect to be reim-
bursed. For when the hunter gave his neighbors these hunks of meat,
he garnered honor and obligations—power. And although women
"had a formidable degree of autonomy," both !Kung men and
women thought that men were slightly more influential than their
wives.[16]

"It's better to give than to receive," the adage goes. The !Kung
and many other peoples would agree. Those who hold the "purse
strings" have substantial social power—an economic formula that
suggests that ancestral women had a good deal of social pull.

But power, of course, is not always a matter of economics. Can anyone be sure, for example, that economically powerful women or men are persuasive in the bedroom too? It ain't necessarily so.

Inuit women may marry well to get ahead, but there's no saying these Eskimo wives feel subordinate to their husbands. And who's to know whether the farmer who presides at the dinner table dominates private conversations with his wife as well. In fact, in peasant societies today where men monopolize all the positions of rank and authority and women tend to act deferentially toward men in public, women have a great deal of *informal* influence. Despite men's strutting and public posturing in these cultures, anthropologist Susan Rogers reports, neither sex actually thinks men rule women. She concludes that the sexes sustain a rough balance of power, that male dominance is a myth.[17]

So economics undoubtedly played an important role in the power relations of men and women millennia ago. But the sexes were actually engaged in a much more complicated duel.

In an effort to unravel this subtle power dynamic between women and men, Martin Whyte mined the Human Relations Area File, a modern data bank that records information on over eight hundred societies.[18] From this file and from other ethnographic reports, he compiled a study group of ninety-three preindustrial peoples: one-third were nomadic hunter-gatherers; one-third were peasant farmers; one-third were peoples who herded and/or gardened for a living. Societies ranged from the Babylonians living around 1750 B.C. to present-day traditional cultures. Most had been studied by anthropologists since A.D. 1800.

Whyte then culled from these data the answers to a number of questions about each culture: What were the sexes of the gods? Which sex received more-elaborate burial ceremonies? Who were the local political leaders? Who contributed what to the dinner table? Who had the final authority to discipline the children? Who arranged the marriages? Who inherited valuable property? Which gender had the higher sex drive? Did people believe women were inferior to men? He cross-correlated these and many other variables in order to establish the status of women in societies around the world.

Whyte's findings confirm some widely held beliefs.[19]

There was *no* society in which women dominated men in most spheres of social life. Myths of Amazon women, tales of matriarchs who ruled with a velvet fist, were just that—fiction. In 67 percent of all cultures (mainly agricultural peoples), men appeared to control women in *most* circles of activity. In a fair number of societies (30 percent) men and women appeared to be roughly equal—particularly among gardeners and hunting-gathering peoples. And in 50 percent of all these cultures, women had much more informal influence than societal rules accorded them.

Whyte uncovered an even more important fact: there was no single constellation of cross-cultural factors that together added up to *the* status of women. Instead, each society revealed a series of pluses and minuses. In some cultures women made an enormous economic contribution but had less power over their marital and sex lives. In others they could divorce easily but had little say in religious matters or held no formal political offices. Even where women owned valuable property and had considerable economic power, they did not necessarily have extensive political rights or religious sway. *In short, power in one sector of society did not translate into power in the next.*

This fact is nowhere more obvious than in the United States. In 1920 women won the right to vote; their political influence increased. But they remained second-class citizens on the job. Today women's power in the work force is rising; many are highly educated as well. At home, though, married working women still do the vast majority of the cooking, washing, and cleaning up.[20] Because Americans assume that status is a single phenomenon, we cannot understand why working women still do most of the housework. But one's status in one sector of society does not necessarily affect one's position in another.

Whyte established that there is no such thing as *the* status of women—or of men. Instead, the power game between the sexes is like a crystal ball; turn the sphere a little, and it casts a whole new light. Hence ancestral women may have been economically powerful and have had a great deal of informal influence, yet not necessarily have been leaders of the group.

What else can a study of traditional peoples say about women, men, and power in the past? Well, class, race, age, sex appeal, accomplishments, and kinship ties also contribute to the mosaic we call power.

Under certain circumstances the most insipid member of a higher class or dominant ethnic group can reign over a smarter, more dynamic person of a lower station. And although we are inclined to make sweeping judgments about the miserable status of women in Asia, an elderly Chinese or Japanese woman can be just as dictatorial as any man. In many societies age counts. So do sex appeal, wit, and charm. A barmaid can rule a businessman with sex; a cartoonist can puncture a politician with pen and ink; a student may beguile her vastly better-educated teacher with a gaze.

Kinship also plays a part in who runs whom. In patrilineal societies, where men regularly own the land and children mark their descent from father, women tend to have little formal power in most sectors of society. On the other hand, women in matrilineal societies own more property and this gives them much more influence in the community as a whole.

Last, the genders derive power from their society's symbolic world. As a culture evolves, it develops a "sexual template" or social script for how the genders are to behave, as well as beliefs about the powers of each sex.[21] These scripts people carry in their minds. Mbuti pygmies of Zaire, for example, think women are powerful because only women give birth. The Mehinaku of Amazonia and many other people bestow power on menstrual blood; touch it, and you get sick. Westerners have immortalized women's power to seduce men in their fable of Adam, Eve, the serpent, and the apple. Ultimately what a society designates as symbolically powerful becomes just that.

Power, then, is a composite of many forces that work together to make one man or woman more influential than the next.

What, then, of Twiggy, George, 1470, and the other hominids discussed in the last chapter who left their bones beside a blue-green
lake at Olduvai two million years ago? Were those men and women
social equals?

Undoubtedly these early "people" did not have class or ethnic
distinctions. It is also unlikely that they had a cultural life rich with
symbolic associations of power. But we can say a few things with
some degree of certainty about Twiggy and her companions. They
did not live like the Inuit, whose men collected all of the food and
whose women stayed at home. There was no home. Twiggy was not
a farmer's daughter either. Instead, she was nomadic. No one stayed
in camp. And women worked.

Most important, Twiggy and her friends ate meat. And as I have
maintained, hunting and scavenging are not logical pastimes for
pregnant women or mothers with small children. So Twiggy probably let her lover collect the meat, the sinew and the marrow from
dangerous beasts, while she gathered fruit, vegetables, seeds, and
small game with her female friends. In this way Twiggy made an
enormous contribution to the evening meal. If so, she was economically powerful, as traditional !Kung women were and still are. The
more sexually active and charismatic females in Twiggy's world were
probably more powerful as well.

But how did Twiggy live? Who actually bossed whom?

Not only do traditional cultures give us a clue; so do other species.
In fact, we can glean a great deal of insight into Twiggy's daily power
plays by examining a fascinating colony of chimpanzees in the Arnhem Zoo, in Holland.[22] To these chimps, maneuvering for rank and
power is the spice of daily life.

Chimpanzee Politics

In 1971 more than a dozen chimps were introduced to their new
residence at the zoo. At night they slept in separate indoor cages;
then after breakfast the chimps were free to enter a two-acre outdoor
yard. It was surrounded by a moat and a high wall in the rear. About
fifty oak and beech trees, each cloaked in electric fencing, loomed
inaccessibly above them. Rocks, tree trunks, and a few dead oaks for

climbing spread across the pen. Here the chimps engaged in all of their political power plays—after the great escape.

On opening morning the chimps inspected their outdoor acreage inch by inch. That afternoon, after the last of the anthropologists, zookeepers, and trainers had departed, they staged their getaway. Some of them wedged a five-meter tree limb against the back wall. Then several chimps quietly scaled the fortress. Reportedly a few even helped the less surefooted with their climbing. Then they all descended nearby trees and availed themselves of the park's facilities. Big Mama, the oldest female of the group, made a beeline for the zoo cafeteria. Here she helped herself to a bottle of chocolate milk and settled among the patrons.

Since these chimps were enticed back into their cages, they have engaged in perpetual power struggles among themselves—maneuvers that shed light on Twiggy's life in ancient times and on the nature of modern human power plays.

Male chimps negotiate regularly for rank. A male begins his "intimidation display" by puffing up his hair, hooting, and swaying from side to side or stamping, often holding a rock or stick in his hand. Then he dashes past his rival, pounds the ground, and crows. This ritual is normally enough to persuade his adversary to defer. This deferential retreat is a distinctive gesture; the subordinate emits a short sequence of panting grunts as he bows deeply to his superior or crouches with his hair flat against his body to look small.

Aggressors enlist allies too. At the beginning of this threat display, the attacker often tries to get a companion to back him up, holding out a hand, palm up, toward a potential friend—inviting him to side with him. If he succeeds in recruiting a supporter, he may charge his opponent, pelting him with stones, screaming, pummeling him with fists, and biting him on the hands, feet, or head. But he also keeps an eye on his ally. If his deputy seems to waver in his allegiance, the aggressor renews his begging gestures to him.

"There is no such thing as a free lunch," they say, and it's just as true of chimpanzee politicians as of human ones. When one chimp backs up another, he expects his favor to be returned. In fact, chimps seem to feel obliged, rousing themselves from a perfectly peaceful doze to stand near an argument or join the fray. Alliances count. On one occasion at Arnhem, the male who was second in command groomed one female after the next, patting each and playing with her children. These rounds completed, he immediately threatened the number one male. Had he bribed these females to support his cause? Probably. Like politicians who kiss babies and speak out on women's issues, male chimps cultivate female friends.

Some male coalitions last for years; many more last only minutes; status-hungry male chimps make fickle friends. But when an individual gets into another scrape, he "pulls strings," hollering until allies come to root or join the brawl. Sometimes four or five males participate in the melee, a huge knot of yelling, tumbling, gouging apes.

Perhaps when Twiggy and her hominid comrades rested at midday, a male flaunted his high status, huffing, hooing, and swaying threateningly until a subordinate bowed to him. Occasionally fights must have broken out. And males probably cultivated Twiggy for her support and that of her female friends.

Networking

Curiously, male and female chimps at Arnhem arrange themselves in quite different power structures, a dissimilarity that could well be true of humans and may also hark back to Twiggy's times.

Male chimps are connected in a web of hierarchical intrigues with friends and enemies that add up to a flexible dominance ladder with one male at the top. These ranks are clearly demarcated at any one moment. But as a male wins more allies and more skirmishes, the dominance ladder slowly changes. Finally a series of confrontations or a single vicious fight swings the balance and a new individual emerges as king of the male hierarchy.

This ruler has an important job—sheriff. He steps into a brawl and pulls the adversaries from one another. And he is expected to be a nonpartisan referee. When this alpha male keeps fights to a minimum his chimp underlings respect him, support him, even pay him homage. They bow to him, plunging their heads and upper bodies rapidly and repeatedly. They kiss his hands, feet, neck, and chest. They lower themselves to make sure they are beneath him. And they follow him in an entourage. But if the leader fails to maintain harmony, his inferiors shift their allegiance, and the hierarchy slowly changes until peace is reached. Subordinates create the chief.

Female chimps do not establish this kind of status ladder. They form cliques instead—laterally connected subgroups of individuals who care for one another's infants and protect and nurture each other in times of social chaos. Females are less aggressive, less dominance oriented, and this network can remain stable—and relatively egalitarian—for years. Moreover, the most dominant female generally acquires this position by sheer personality, charisma, if you will, as well as by age, rather than by intimidation.

Female chimps quarrel, though, and, like males, they use their allies to settle scores. On one occasion a threatened female called on a male friend for help. Amid high-pitched "indignant" barks, she pointed with her whole hand (rather than a finger) toward the assailant, at the same time kissing and patting her male ally. When her pleas became more insistent, her male friend counterattacked the antagonist while the female stood by and watched approvingly.

Do human males naturally tend to form hierarchal ranks and then jockey for better positions, whereas females form more-egalitarian, stable cliques? This would be hard to prove. But if Twiggy was anything like the female chimps at Arnhem, she had a network of devoted friends. She also had embittered foes. And she could nurse a grudge for years.

Twiggy's most powerful role may have been as group arbiter, however. At Arnhem, Big Mama played this part. She broke up arguments between juveniles just by standing near them, barking, and waving her arms. It was always Big Mama who coaxed the vanquished from the dead tree in the center of the enclosure. And after any battle the loser always fled whimpering to her side. As time went by, Big Mama became the safety zone, the police, the judge, and jury.

Other females at Arnhem acted as mediators too. Once during a male's "bluff display," a female strolled up to him, peeled his fingers from around his rock, and walked away with it. When the male found a new rock, she took it away too; this confiscation process occurred six times in a row. Other mediators behaved differently. Some simply jabbed the victor's side with a hand, driving him until he sat down beside his enemy and began the grooming ceremony.

This grooming ritual has a pattern, and it suggests perhaps the single most important thing about power relations in our past: peacemaking was a staple of daily life. Within minutes after a brawl, or hours or even days later, chimp enemies walk up to one another, grunt softly, shake hands, hug, kiss one another on the lips, and gaze deeply into one another's eyes. Then they sit, lick one another's wounds, and groom each other. Chimp rivals also spend inordinate amounts of energy suppressing their animosity, grooming one another particularly furiously when they are very tense.

Chimps and all other primates work hard to mollify their companions. Violence is the exception; placating is the rule—as it must have been among our ancestors of Twiggy's day.

From the perpetual power struggles at the Arnhem Zoo, primatologist Franz De Waal established several things about power among these apes, principles that probably applied to our ancestors on the grasslands of Africa millennia ago and that have been carried across time to modern humankind.

First of all, power shifts. Ranks are formalized, but animals are part of a pliable network of relationships. Moreover, the ability to rule does not depend on strength, size, speed, agility, or aggressiveness; it depends on wits, on whom you know, and how you pay your social debts. Last, power can be either formal or informal. As supporters and arbiters, females are major players in the power game; under the right set of circumstances even a female can reign.

In fact, when visitors asked De Waal which were more powerful, male or female chimps, he shrugged and explained it thus. If you look at who greets whom, males dominate females 100 percent of the time. If you count who wins aggressive interactions, males win 80 percent of the time. But if you measure who takes food away from whom or who sits in the best spots, females win 80 percent of the time. And to emphasize the complexity of power, De Waal liked to add, "Nikkie (male) is the highest-ranking ape but he is completely dependent on Yeroen (male). Luit (male) is individually the most powerful. But when it comes to who can push others aside then Mama (female) is the boss."[23]

De Wall confirmed the two things that anthropologists have observed in human cultures: status is not a single, monolithic quality measured in a single way; and male dominance, if it implies power over females in every sphere of life, is a myth.

A final factor may have contributed to Twiggy's power—her family status. In several primate species, such as baboons, groups of related females usually stick together, while the males often switch from troop to troop. Within each troop, one "matriline" tends to dominate the next, and so forth down the line, a relatively stable hierarchy of dynasties, an "old girls" network.[24] Hence a juvenile of a high-ranking female clan can often dominate a mature female from a less prestigious family.

Moreover, children often assume their mother's rank. Among wild chimps at Gombe, where females are not organized into matrilines but form cliques instead, the children of the sovereign female, Flo, grew up to become influential in the community, whereas the offspring of a submissive peer became subservient adults.

Gender Relations at Ancient Olduvai

Power relations in traditional human cultures and politics among chimpanzees, our closest living relatives, certainly suggest how our ancestors could have lived and jockeyed among themselves for status at Olduvai Gorge some two million years ago.

Twiggy's first memory may have been that of looking across the waving grass as she rode on her mother's hip. By the time she was three or four, she knew where the cashews grew and how to dig for roots. She probably played at water holes as her mother collected crabs and lolled below the fig trees when grown-ups gathered blossoms or sweet fruit. If her mother was powerful, like Big Mama, Twiggy probably rested in the shady spots. If mother's lover was a

good scavenger, she dined on tongue and other delicacies of wildebeest. And maybe when all lined up to slurp water trickling from a
rock, Twiggy went first.

Whether these ancestors traveled in groups of related males or
related females, we will never know. But every morning some ten to
fifty members of Twiggy's band must have awakened, chattered,
drunk, relieved themselves, and abandoned their night nests to wander along the lake or out into the grass. Sometimes a few males split
off to scout or scavenge and return later in the day. Then they all
settled in early evening to share their food and sleep in a clump of fig
trees, on a grassy cliff, or in a dried-up streambed on the ground. The
next morning they began again.

As the days passed, Twiggy probably became used to seeing other
males and females bow and scrape to her mother as they marched
along. When she grew older, she probably tagged along beside her
older sister, formed a clique with other girls, and spent her time
grooming them, playing tag and tickle, and chasing boys. Undoubtedly Twiggy knew her place in the social network and grinned,
bowed, and kissed the hands and feet of her superiors. When Twiggy
got into battles with other children, her mother (or father) defended
her and she won. And by wits and charm, Twiggy made friends with
boys, then coaxed them into sharing bits of meat.

After Twiggy reached puberty, she must have formed a pair-bond
with a special friend. Maybe he was someone from a different group
she met when her band made its annual pilgrimage in the dry season
to camp beside the blue-green lake. Together Twiggy and her lover
walked through the open plains; together they shared their food and
bore a child. If the partnership became acrimonious, she probably
waited until her infant had stopped suckling, then picked up her
digging stick and pouch and joined a neighboring band. Economic
autonomy enabled Twiggy to leave her mate as soon as her infant
was on his feet.

She may have been powerful in other aspects of daily life as well. If
Twiggy consistently remembered where to find honey and prized
vegetables, she was admired. Perhaps she was an arbiter, too, taking
rocks and sticks from her husband's hand as he swayed and shouted
at a rival. Undoubtedly she had one or two girlfriends who always

defended her in a quarrel. And if Twiggy was charismatic, bright, respected, and clever at keeping friends, she could well have become a leader of the group. Among primates the law of the jungle is not strength but brains.

These brains soon harnessed fire and invented new tools and weapons. Then like a rocket our ancestors shot into "almost human" social life.

~12~

Almost Human
Genesis of Kinship and the Teenager

It is indeed a desirable thing to be well descended, but the glory belongs to our ancestors.

—*Plutarch*, Morals

F.ire.

Ever since our ancestors descended from the trees, they must have fled to lakes and streams when volcanoes disgorged balls of molten rock or lightning licked the prairie and flame spread across the grass. While the plains still smoldered, they probably picked their way back through the embers to collect hares, lizards, fallen bee's nests, and seeds, then gorged on the roasted food.

At the mouths of caves, where the dung of owls, bats, saber-toothed tigers, and other cave dwellers collected in rich deposits, the embers may have flickered on for days or even weeks, and gradually ancients learned to sleep beside these coals, even to feed the thirsty flame with dried branches until passing game, the promise of distant flowering fruit trees, or lack of water moved a tiny band to abandon the warm, protective glow.

Fire was humankind's companion—an enemy when it raged, a

friend when it subsided. But when our ancestors first learned to control flame, to carry embers in a baboon skull or wrapped in fleshy leaves, fire became their greatest strength. With fire they could harden wood to make more-deadly spears. With burning moss they could smoke out rodents from their burrows or drive rabbits toward their snares. With hearths they could ward off stealthy nighttime predators from carcasses they had half consumed. And with burning branches they could drive hyenas from their lairs, then usurp these cave homes and sleep within the halo of the flame. Now injured band members, older men and women, pregnant females, and small children could stay in camp. There was a camp. No longer servants of the sun, our ancestors could stoke the embers and lounge about in morning, mend their tools at dusk, and reenact the day's events late into the night.

This innovation was but part of the advances our ancestors had made by a million years ago—ushering in vast changes in human sexuality as well.

We may never know exactly when humankind first began to control flame. Anthropologists certainly do not agree.[1] But what could be the oldest evidence of campfires comes from the Swartkrans cave, in South Africa, where anthropologists C. K. Brain and Andrew Sillen recently collected 270 charred bits of ancient animal bones.[2]

These fossils, they report, had been burned at between 200 and 800 degrees centigrade. This is within the temperature range created today by a campfire of stinkwood branches. Someone may have collected dead limbs from the many white stinkwood trees that have covered this area for eons and enjoyed fire about one to one and a half million years ago. And once our ancestors began to make campfires, they built them over and over again. More than twenty separate levels of fire-burned debris at Swartkrans suggest our ancient love of flame.

What "people" warmed their hands and burned these bones at the Swartkrans cave?

Primitive *Australopithecus robustus* creatures, who died out about a million years ago, left parts of their skeletons here among the debris. But *Homo erectus* individuals lived here, too. And Brain thinks these more advanced hominids fed these ancient flames. Why? Because *Homo erectus* hominids were far more intelligent and well on their way toward humanity.

These "people" appear in the fossil record at Olduvai Gorge, Tanzania, at Koobi Fora, Kenya, and in the Omo River valley in southern Ethiopia by 1.8 million years ago. But the most telling early *Homo erectus* site is Nariokotome III.[3]

Here, in arid sediments near the western shore of Lake Turkana, Kenya, a youth died in a marsh almost 1.6 million years ago. The robustness of the face and shape of the hips indicate that the creature was most likely a boy.[4] He was about twelve years old and somewhat less than five feet six inches tall the day he passed away; had he lived, he would have grown to be about six feet. His hands, arms, hips, and legs were very much like ours. His chest was more rounded than the chest of modern people, and he had one more lumbar vertabra. But if this young man had walked, fully clothed, down your street on Halloween wearing a mask, you would not have noticed him at all.

Had he removed the disguise, you would have fled. His rugged, protruding jaw and huge teeth, the heavy brow ridges above his eyes, his sloping flattened forehead, his thick skull, and his bulging neck muscles would have stunned even the corner cop. Nevertheless, the child was reasonably smart. He had a brain volume of 900 cubic centimeters, much larger than that of Twiggy or her australopithecine contemporaries and just below the range of 1,000 to 2,000 of modern men and women. Later *Homo erectus* skulls show even larger cranial capacities—reaching as high as 1,300 cubic centimeters.

Interestingly, chimpanzees like to smoke cigarettes, and they are adroit at lighting a match and blowing out the flame.[5] So it is likely that *Homo erectus,* with a brain a great deal bigger than that of chimps, understood how to manage fire and fanned flames at Swartkrans cave over a million years ago. With their advanced "thinking caps," these creative individuals would also start to build our modern human social and sexual world.

Foremost, *Homo erectus* developed sophisticated tools.

While former residents of the Swartkrans cave had made simple

Oldowan pebble tools—no more than waterworn rocks with a few edges whacked off to make a sharpened edge—ingenious *Homo erectus* people had begun to separate delicate flakes from larger stones. They probably used these small flakes to cut, slice, scrape, or dig. More impressive, however, were their large, six- to seven-inch stone hand axes, called Acheulean hand axes because they were first discovered in St. Acheul, France. With a rounded butt end and careful flaking along both edges to make a tapered point, these tools looked like large almonds, pears, or teardrops of stone.

Like golf balls in a water trap, these hand axes have been found strewn along ancient streams and rivers, on channel bars, at lake margins, in swamps and bogs and marshes across South and East Africa, as well as along watercourses in Europe, India, and Indonesia. So although some must have been used to dig for vegetables that grew along the banks, it has long been thought that early *Homo erectus* peoples used these massive streamlined tools mainly to skin and disarticulate carcasses at the shore, then chop meat from bone, cut sinew, and crack bones for marrow.

This may well have been the fate of a baby hippo whose remains were found at Lake Turkana, in what had been a shallow, muddy lake some 1.5 million years ago. Acheulean hand axes lay nearby. And seven footprints of a *Homo erectus* individual were imprinted nearby in the mud.[6] Perhaps the individual, who stood about five and a half feet tall and weighed some 120 pounds, had waded silently into the water and slain the wallowing beast.

Fire. Fancy tools. Hunting large animals. Anthropologists now think these ancestors also had home bases, campsites they returned to for days or weeks.[7] In short, *Homo erectus* men and women had started to perfect the basic elements of the hunting-gathering way of life. With these developments, our fundamental human style of life and sex and love would soon emerge. Our expanding brain created a complication, however, that sped our journey along that path.

Born Too Young

Since the early 1960s, anthropologists have reasoned that at some point in hominid evolution the brain became so large in proportion to the mother's pelvic birth canal that a woman began to have difficulty bearing her large-brained young. In short, with its growing head, it couldn't get out. This tight squeeze is known as the obstetrical dilemma.[8] Nature's solution: to bear young at an earlier (smaller) stage of development and extend fetal brain development into postnatal life. As Ashley Montagu summed it up, "If he weren't born when he is, he wouldn't be born at all."[10]

Indeed, we are born too soon; the human newborn is really just an embryo. All of the primates bear immature (altricial) young, and the degree of altriciality (immaturity) increases from monkeys to apes to humans. But human babies are born even more immature than those of our closest relatives, a characteristic known as secondary altriciality.[9] Not for six to nine months does the human infant acquire the chemical responses of the liver, kidneys, immune system, and digestive tract, the motor reactions, or the brain development displayed by other primates shortly after birth.

Scientists estimate that our ancestors began to bear exceedingly immature helpless babies when the brain reached an adult cranial capacity of 700 cubic centimeters—about a million years ago, among *Homo erectus* people.[12]

What an impact this single adaptation had on human patterns of marriage, sex, and love. Foremost, these helpless young must have dramatically increased the "reproductive burden" of *Homo erectus* females, further stimulating selection for infatuation, attachment, and monogamy. Now a steady consort was even more critical to the survival of the helpless child.[13]

Anthropologist Wenda Trevathan thinks that the complications of this tight squeeze at birth also stimulated women's first specialized occupation—midwifery. In her book *Human Birth: An Evolutionary Perspective*, Trevathan looks at human parturition from the viewpoint of an animal behaviorist. She proposes, for example, that when a human mother strokes her newborn, this gesture stems not just from a psychological need to bond but also from the mammalian practice of licking one's young to stimulate breathing and other bodily functions. Because human newborns are covered with a creamy fluid known as the vernix caseosa, perhaps new mothers also evolved their patting habit to rub in this fatty gel, lubricating the skin, protecting the infant from viruses and bacteria. Trevathan also notes that, regardless of their "handedness," new mothers hold their infants in the left arm—directly over the heart, probably because the heartbeat soothes the child.

More important to our story, Trevathan thinks that by *Homo erectus* times birthing had become so difficult that women needed a helper to "catch" the baby. Thus the human tradition of midwifery emerged. Perhaps these helpers became bonded to the newborn, too, widening the circle of adults who felt responsible for the child.[14]

Our *Homo erectus* ancestors spawned another monstrous burden— the teenager. From characteristics of ancient teeth, anthropologists have surmised how fast our ancestors grew up. It appears that at some point between a million and 200,000 years ago the human maturation process slowed down; not only did women now bear exceedingly helpless babies, but childhood also became extended.[15]

Hail the origin of teenage, another hallmark of the human animal, another distinct divergence from our relatives, the apes. A chimpanzee has an infancy quite similar to that of people in hunting-gathering societies—about four years. But among chimps the first molar tooth emerges at about age three, and chimps reach puberty at about ten. Our human first molar doesn't appear until age six. And girls in hunting-gathering societies often do not reach menarche until age sixteen or seventeen; boys go through a prolonged adolescence too. In fact, humans do not stop growing physically until about age twenty.

Even more remarkable, human parents continue to provide food and shelter for their teenagers. After a chimp mother has weaned her infant, the youngster feeds itself and builds its own nest every night. The juvenile chimp still stays near its mother much of the time. But once an ape infant has stopped suckling, the mother no longer feeds or shelters her offspring. Not so humankind. At five the human child can barely dig a root; even the most sophisticated youngster in a hunting-gathering society could not forage and survive until late teenage. So human parents continue to rear their offspring some ten to twelve years after these children have been weaned.[16]

Human childhood thus became almost twice as long as that of chimps and other primate.

Why did the human maturation process became so extended? To gain time, I think—time in childhood to learn about an increasingly complex world. Boys needed to learn where to quarry flint and other stones, how to hit these rocks at the precise angle to remove a flake and fashion their weapons to be just right for throwing. Boys had to watch the animals, learn when and where the females bore their young, which creatures led the herd, how the winds and seasons changed, which prey to track, how to track, where to surround and fell their quarry, and how to cut the game and divide the spoils.

Girls had even more to learn: how to carry flame, where the low-lying berry bushes grew, what bogs to avoid, where to find birds' eggs, what the life cycles of hundreds of different plants were, where small animals burrowed or reptiles sunned, and which herbs were best for colds, sore throats, or fevers. All this took time, trial, error, and intelligence. Perhaps the young also had to commit to memory long tales, stories like morality plays that taught them about the weather and the habits of the plants and animals around them.

Equally important, they had to learn the nuances of the mating game. With the evolution of teenage came all of those extra years to experiment at courting, sex, and love—crucial parts of life in a social world where men and women needed to pair up to share their food and raise their children as a team.

Brotherly Love

As the brain expanded and women began to bear helpless young with a long teenage, pressures on parents must have mounted even more—stimulating the evolution of another human hallmark: kinship.

A great many animals, including all of the higher primates, recognize biological kin and tend to favor aunts, nephews, and even more distant blood relatives. So the roots of human kinship lie deep in our mammalian past. But when our ancestors began to produce helpless young that took almost twenty years to mature, these new pressures must have hastened the evolution of one of humankind's greatest social inventions: formal relatives with specific roles—the glue of traditional human social life.

One might argue that with the origin of dependent teenagers, parents became obliged to remain together longer in order to provide for their adolescent young. But as I pointed out in chapter 5, divorces tend to cluster around the fourth year of marriage—about the duration of human infancy. Nowhere in the world do people characteristically remain together to raise their young through their teenage years, then systematically depart.

Since our ancestors did not adopt the reproductive strategy of extending their partnerships to rear their adolescents, nature took a creative tack: human kinship evolved. What an ingenious twist, a web of related *and unrelated* individuals locked in a formal network of ties and obligations, an eternal unbreakable alliance dedicated to nurturing their mutual offspring, their shared DNA. How did this come about; what does it have to do with the evolution of marriage, adultery, and divorce?

The nature of the first human kin groups and the evolution of our unique kinship systems are subjects of some of the oldest arguments in anthropology. Basic to the debate is the question: which came first, matriliny or patriliny; did our ancestors trace their heritage through mother or through father? I review this controversy in chapter 15. For now I want to make only one simple point.

Among common chimpanzees, related males tend to remain together to defend their community, whereas females typically leave the group at puberty to seek mates elsewhere; hence brothers live together in adulthood, and sisters tend to disperse. Here are the seeds of patriliny, the kinship system based on male ties. Among savanna baboons the reverse is true. Groups of related females travel as a unit, whereas males depart for other troops as they mature—the kernal of matriliny. My point: because kinship structure varies among primates, it is impossible to make an informed guess about the kin networks of these early hominid bands.

With one exception. As I have proposed, I think ancestral males and females began to bond and move through the plains together almost as soon as they descended from the trees, some four million years ago. Now I can add that couples were beginning to travel within a wider group whose members were welded together through formal kinship ties.

How vague visceral notions of kinship actually evolved into concrete rules is open to speculation. As a child, an ancient girl probably expected her mother's special friend to share his meat, protect her, and hold her when she cried. With him she had a specific tie that would become "daughter–father." She was obliged to help care for her younger male sibling, a defined obligation that would evolve into "sister–brother." And some females who were more often in the vicinity of mother, she would eventually know as "aunts."

With the escalation of big-game hunting, the intensified division of labor between the sexes and the vicissitudes of raising helpless babies through a long teenage, early people began to see *categories* of individuals, each with distinct obligations, duties, and unspoken social roles. And with the evolution of kinship systems, our ancestors must have begun to define who was permitted to mate with whom. As you will see in the next chapter, rules of sexuality emerged.

Out of Africa

Our *Homo erectus* ancestors also began to spread across the globe. Some anthropologists think early hominids moved into Europe as early as two million years ago.[17] At a few sites north of the Mediterranean Sea are found tools dating to possibly a million years ago. By this time our forebears had also unquestionably moved eastward into Java. By some 500,000 years ago they had reached northern China too. In fact, their skulls, their bones, and tools are found at sites across Eurasia dating to about half a million years ago.

Why our ancestors left Africa, we do not know. Perhaps because they could. By a million years ago the earth's temperature had taken another dramatic plunge. To the north, in Europe and Asia, snow piled in the high country during the longer colder winters, and less snow melted during the chilly summer days and nights. Century upon century, ice sheets grew into mile-high glacial crusts. Then gravity pulled these ice fortresses from the mountain peaks, carving valleys, moving rocks, felling trees, extending the bitter weather to the south. Each cold spasm lasted several thousand years.

With each bout of freezing weather, more and more of the ocean's water became locked in ice. So almost imperceptibly the sea level dropped some four hundred feet, exposing wide land bridges, highways to the north.

Not only could our ancestors now walk north; maybe they had to. As they grew more efficient at hunting game, they probably needed to look farther afield for prey.[18] Moreover, with fiery torches with which to hunt and protect themselves, as well as efficient tools with which to butcher game, they could probably collect more meat— enabling more children to survive. So when a tiny band appeared at the Swartkrans cave, another had already moved in, or the fig groves and crabbing pools were picked clean when a band arrived. Last, skirmishes with neighbors or quarrels among themselves might have driven splinter groups or whole communities out of their native lands.

Whatever the reasons for the migration, our ancestors gradually explored new river valleys and new trails that led them out of Africa. Moving no more than ten miles every generation, they would have reached Beijing in less than twenty thousand years.

They did just that.

The biggest cache of evidence is at Dragon Bone Hill, a site about thirty miles from Beijing, well known to anthropologists as Zhoukoudian. Here Chinese fossil hunters had been collecting ancient bones for centuries, treasures they sold to local chemists who ground the fragments into a sour-tasting powder that they peddled as medicinal elixirs. After hearing of these expeditions, Canadian anatomist Davidson Black launched his own pilgrimage in 1927.

Since then, over a dozen skulls, some 150 teeth, and parts of over forty *Homo erectus* individuals have been unearthed at Dragon Bone

Hill—along with the bones of wild pigs, elephants, rhinos, horses, and hundreds of stone tools. Curiously, some of the hominid skulls had been smashed at the base, as if the brains had been extracted.

Cannibals?

This has been the standard explanation. *Homo erectus* men and women camped here, perhaps in the autumn when the mammoths and mastodons, rhinos, deer, and ancient horses lumbered past their campsites heading south to warmer, wetter weather. Here some *Homo erectus* people fed on others some 500,000 years ago—either as a ritual of reverence for dead friends or to desecrate their enemies.[19]

While some of our forebears followed reindeer, musk ox, bison, giant elk, and other massive beasts into northern China, others trickled south to Java where they left their remains along the steamy Solo River some 500,000 years ago. Still more ate near the Sea of Galilee around 700,000. And others camped and left their garbage in Hungary, France, England, Wales, and Spain at various times between 400,000 and 200,000 years ago.[20]

What, then, of sex, love, and life among the men and women who stalked hippos in Lake Turkana, those who ate and slept at Zhoukoudian, and all the other ancients who left their bones, tools, and refuse along the sand dunes of Algeria, the tundras of Spain, the plains of Hungary, the steppes of Russia, the forests of England, and the jungles of Java between 1.6 million and 200,000 years ago?

Men probably valued women for their work as gatherers and mothers. These women must have known every stand of yarrow, every honey tree, the tiniest berry shrub, every site where water dribbled from a rock, and every hillock, cave, and trail for over a hundred miles around them—even in plains as seemingly uniform as the Pacific Ocean. On most mornings women must have left camp carrying their infants in skin pouches on their backs. Every evening they returned with nuts, berries, firewood, and often information concerning the whereabouts of herds, water, enemies, and relatives. Men counted on their women to survive.

Women must have appreciated men for their bravery in the hunt, for their gifts of steaks and roasts and chops, and for their protection against enemies. Women needed the skins of these slaughtered animals for shawls and blankets, the skulls for containers, the bones for tools, and the sinews for string and cord.

Surely men and women smiled and joked when they returned at night to feed the embers and recount the day's events. Undoubtedly they flirted as they sucked on bones and berries across the smoky haze. And most likely they slipped in next to one another as the campfire faded and sometimes kissed and held each other long into the night. But what these people dreamed, who they loved, or what they thought as they drifted off to sleep is gone with the firelight.

These were not ancient replicas of modern people. They painted no pictures of bears or bison on cave walls. No small bone needles suggest they made tailored coats. No amulets indicate they worshiped the sun, the stars, or a god. They left no graves. But they were *almost* human beings. They had big brains. They nurtured flame. They bore very helpless babies, as we do today. Immature teenagers trailed along with one or both parents and other members of the band. Old and young were all intertwined in an elaborate network of related kin. And the fireside had become synonymous with "home."

By 300,000, some from among these ancestors of ours had begun to emerge into archaic forms of modern men and women. Now our world of sex would take its completely human form.

~13~

The First Affluent Society

A Flowering of Conscience

Two things fill the mind with ever-increasing wonder and awe, the more often and the more intensely the mind of thought is drawn to them: the starry heavens above me and the moral law within me.

—*Immanuel Kant,* Critique of Pure Reason

Beneath the quiet towns of southwestern France, the Pyrenees, and northern Spain, restless ancient torrents carved out a labyrinth of caves. Here, in the windless chasms deep below the ground, stalagmites and stalactites attend like ghostly ivory soldiers. Bullets of dripping water make a metallic ping in the utter quiet. The sounds of bats dance off craggy pits and hollows. And the roar of still-living rivers rushes up through chutes, funnels, and "cat holes," then vanishes into stillness at some hairpin turn.

What nature built, our ancestors came to decorate between twenty and ten thousand years ago, leaving behind thousands of cave paintings and engravings, evidence that modern humanity had burst onto earth.

In the giant underground rotundas in the cave at Lascaux, near Les Eyzies, France, someone painted dozens of stampeding herd animals. In a recess of the cave of Les Trois Frères, in the Pyrenees, another artist incised a magical beast—with the head of a man, the antlers of a stag, and the body and tail of a horse. In the La Juyo cave, in Spain, our forebears carved a monstrous stone head, half man, half cat. In over thirty caves giant bison, reindeer, mammoths, ibex, bears, and other beasts are outlined in red or black, their fur and muscles filled in with carefully placed strokes that use the natural fissures and protrusions of the rock.

And where real figures give way to magical ones, headless horses, duckbilled people, wolf-headed bears, disembodied hands with missing fingers, floating arms and legs, snake patterns, and dots and dashes dance along the walls and ceilings. Some of these paintings appear in large galleries; others are painted in culs-de-sac so remote that professional spelunkers have fainted from claustrophobia trying to gain access to these crypts.

In these sunless tunnels, amid heightened sounds and cool, stagnant air, something of significance was going on. No one lived here. Our ancestors came to paint and gather for communal purposes instead. Perhaps they held ceremonies to ensure a good hunting season, to celebrate the birth of a son or daughter, to cure the sick, to fulfill a ritual in a myth, or for a host of other purposes.[1] John Pfeiffer, in his book *The Creative Explosion,* proposes that they may have held complex initiation rituals as well.

Pfeiffer thinks it possible that young initiates were left in isolated tombs in the bowels of the earth until fear, isolation, and monotony stripped them of their normal senses and put them in a trance-like state of receptivity. Then their elders, using trickery and illusion, led these spellbound youngsters through convoluted alleys while they told them important clan traditions, clan history, and clan legends, the accumulated wisdom of the tribe.

To emphasize an incident in an encyclopedic tale, these sorcerers may have held a lamp beneath a painting. The flickering torch lit a hand or bird or fish, then suddenly a dancing snorting elk or swimming stag to animate a specific point in the story line. Then after each meandering trek, these priests assembled their disoriented students in large subterranean theaters where the brainwashed youths underwent more ordeals and repetitions that permanently etched these "textbooks" in their minds.

What were the elders saying? Why this first flowering of human art? What does this outpouring of artistic expression say about human sexuality twenty thousand years ago?

Pfeiffer thinks these people were experiencing an "information explosion," produced by vast changes in technology and expanding social networks. And because the footprints of children are prevalent in many of these caves, he theorizes that these young were taken into these surreal mazes to participate in initiation rituals designed to teach them all these new facts.

Even today this strategy is common. Human beings around the world store concepts and data in art form. One look at a swastika can elicit a panoply of remembered information about Hitler and the Nazis, while a cross has tremendous symbolic power to a Christian. The Australian aborigines use their myths and arts as mnemonics (as well as for many other purposes), and it was the inventiveness of these people that led Pfeiffer to his theory about the cave art.

The Australian aborigines live in the world's most barren desert. If they are to find water regularly, they are obliged to remember every rise, every dip, every tree, rock, and hole in an area of several hundred miles. So every physical feature of the landscape is woven into elaborate tales of mythical ancestral beings. The dots, squiggles, and figures they paint on their tools, on walls, and on themselves often symbolically depict the water holes and rock formations where these apparitions visit. Thus the myths, songs, and art are actually maps of the Australian outback. As one memorizes the escapades of the gods, the smallest details of the desert become committed to memory too.

To teach their children all this lore, Australian aborigines put their young through excruciating ordeals. Traditionally, the Arunta of central Australia took their male initiates into the desert far from home and family, denied them food and clothing, and sang, danced, and acted out these survival tales.[2] On the final night of the ritual the youngsters were concealed under blankets beside a roaring fire.

And after the chanting, darkness, isolation, and fear engulfed the youths, their penises were slit from tip to base. A horrible experience. But these boys never forgot the script they had learned; and it would forever guide them from one water hole to the next.

The cave paintings of these early European peoples, Pfeiffer thinks, were just the same—cue cards for ancient epic tales, part of a "survival course" in an era of dangerous social change.

We will never know exactly what occurred in the bowels of the earth so long ago. But one thing is clear: humankind had metamorphosed from being simple hunting-scavenging-gathering creatures with fire and a few elementary tools into individuals who consciously sought out the depths of caves to paint on walls, primates richly endowed with abstract symbolic culture.

Anthropologists use the term *symbolic thinking* to mean the ability arbitrarily to bestow an abstract concept upon the concrete world. The classic example is holy water. To a chimpanzee, the water sitting in a marble basin in a cathedral is just that, water; to a Catholic it is an entirely different thing, holy water. Likewise, the color black is black to any chimp, while to you it might connote death. When our ancestors acquired the ability to create symbols for thoughts, ideas, and concepts and to use these symbols to express themselves, the truly modern human mind had emerged.

It is now debated whether the immediate precursors of these cave painters, the Neanderthals, engaged in symbolic thinking or whether symbolic thinking sprang into life among these modern human cave artisans instead.[3] This question is important to our understanding of the evolution of human sexuality. For it is only with this capacity for symbolic thought, and for formulating abstract ideas such as good/bad, right/wrong, and should/shouldn't, that humankind could fully evolve such essentially modern concepts as morality, conscience, and our vast store of culturally coded beliefs, rituals, taboos, and rules about sex and love.

To be expected, the fossil record offers a mixed bag of clues to the puzzle of when symbolic thinking actually appeared in human history.

Neanderthal Bashing

For over a million years before our ancestors began to paint the walls of caves in France and Spain, episodes of severe cold had gripped the northern climes in ice and struck the tropics with drought. Each Ice Age lasted several thousand years, followed by milder weather. During these intense glacial ages and warmer interglacial epochs, our ancestors crept north in small bands. By 100,000 years ago, *Homo sapiens neanderthalensis*—an archaic racial variant of modern people—lived in Europe as well as in the Near East and in Central Asia.[4]

The Neanderthals were a curious combination of physical traits. They had heavy brow ridges above their eyes, rugged teeth and jaws, and muscular, thick-boned bodies; if you saw one on a street in America today you definitely would think him brutish. Yet these people with beetle brows had skulls *larger* than ours—as well as brains organized just like yours and mine. We know this from studying the contours of their ancient crania, which is done quite easily by means of "endocasts."

These are ingenious inventions: you simply take some rubber, pour it into a Neanderthal cranium, let the latex set, and remove the lumpy blob. On the surface of this endocast are all the tiny impressions of the skull that the brain engraved when this protoplasm once squeezed against its bony helmet. So the design of seams, grooves, and fissures on the surface of the rubber shows how the brain's lobes were organized. These endocasts illustrate that the Neanderthal brain was constructed like ours today.[5]

These people thought.

They also spoke. The remarkable discovery of a Neanderthal hyoid bone, the tiny U-shaped bone that lies suspended in the throat and aids in speech, suggests that the Neanderthals had the physical ability to talk with modern human language.[6] But here disagreement festers. Some scientists report that the shape of the bottom of the Neanderthal skull, the basicranium, is not fully flexed (as is the modern human skull)—indicating that the larynx (or voice box) had not fully descended down the throat.[7] Hence Neanderthals may not have been able to produce the vowel sounds *i* or *u*. They may have sounded more nasal than modern people too.

Several anthropologists remain unconvinced by these data, however. The shape of the basicranium, they argue, may not be an accurate indicator of the shape of the oral cavities. Moreover, one does not need our full array of linguistic sounds to speak with human tones or make human grammatical constructions. Hawaiian tongues, for example, have far fewer linguistic sounds than English does, and Navajo has many more; yet all of these people use a modern human language.

I suspect that by the time the Neanderthals were roasting mammoth tongues and lying with one another in the snow-bound caves of ancient France some 100,000 years ago, they spoke much as we do today.

But did the Neanderthals "believe" in anything? Had they created the concept of the soul or plan for an afterlife? Did they have a symbolic world?

In several caves across Europe archaeologists have found what look like shallow graves where Neanderthals may have interred their dead, tucked in sleeping positions. Kin may have left grave offerings as well, for some of the skeletons were surrounded by stone tools, well-placed stones or bones or horns of animals. At the most controversial site, a cave high in the hills of northern Iraq, friends and lovers may have laid bouquets of flowers on the deceased some sixty thousand years ago. Around the bones were scattered the fossilized pollens of hollyhocks, grape hyacinths, bachelor's buttons, yellow-flowering groundsel, and other wildflowers of the area.[8]

If the Neanderthals believed in an afterlife, if they thought that human beings had souls, then they could symbolize. And if they could symbolize and think in abstract terms, they undoubtedly had developed beliefs and rules about such fundamental matters as sex and marriage too.

Skeptics do not accept that possibility. They maintain that sick people may have crawled into some of these caves to die, that others were buried simply to dispose of the bodies, and that still other corpses were carried into caves by feeding carnivores; then the artifacts appeared around the skeletons by accident at later dates.

Hence these burials were not intentional. As for the flowers, these pollens could have blown into the cave on winds or been carried into these shelters on rodents' paws or insects' wings. They conclude that there were no ceremonial burials, no grave offerings, no bouquets; the Neanderthals had not evolved the capacity for symbolic thought.[9]

Skeptics would probably argue that the red ocher found at several Neanderthal sites did not illustrate symbolic thinking either. People around the world use red ocher to color their faces, hands, figures, and regalia before a ceremony. But this red crumbly rock is also used to tan hides and repel vermin. Perhaps the Neanderthals used it for these purely functional reasons; perhaps they did not have the aesthetic symbolic sense to decorate themselves.

What Is Art For?

No one knows whether the Neanderthals had begun to adorn the burials of loved ones with grave offerings or decorate themselves and their belongings. But ethologist Ellen Dissanayake thinks they did. And she has an interesting proposal for the evolution of the human drive to create art and appreciate the arts.

In her book *What Is Art For?* Dissanayake traces all of the arts back to an apparent human need to shape, to embellish, to beautify, to make things and activities "special." Those who made an event or tool special with decorations or ritualistic fanfare remembered the occasion. And because the creating of tools and the performing of ceremonies were acts important to survival, those who produced art and appreciated the arts lived on. Hence our ancestors evolved the biological proclivity to make and enjoy paintings, sculpture, and all the other arts.

Dissanayake notes that some 250,000 years ago two individuals in today's England each chipped flint hand axes and both stone tools had a fossil shell prominently displayed at their center. These people had found the fossil and fashioned the tool around it—they had begun to recognize special things and make their tools special. At about the same time in prehistory someone left globs of red, yellow, brown, and purple ocher in a sea cliff cave in France; perhaps these people had begun to make themselves and their belongings special too.

The Neanderthals did not leave us much of their art, however, if they really had any. Someone marked some bear teeth with shallow grooves; another punctured a fox tooth; another perforated a reindeer bone. Only a few other questionable signs of artistic endeavor remain from this period of human prehistory—not an impressive inventory of aesthetic expression. But it was a beginning. So Dissanayake is convinced that the Neanderthals were indeed embellishing their grave sites and using ocher for decorative purposes, that by then an artistic predisposition was becoming part of human nature, encoded in our DNA.

The Neanderthals remain a mystery. We cannot be sure that they enjoyed abstract symbolic thought or had rules for sex and love. All we really know is that they lived in small nomadic hunting bands, made large stone tools, did some long-distance trading across Europe, hunted big game, and ate a great deal of meat. Several thousand bones of mammoths, woolly rhinos, reindeer, and bison have been excavated below sheer rock walls where these hunters drove the beasts from plateaus above. This "cliff fall" hunting marked an innovation—and it was organized, systematic, planned.[10]

How these people loved, whom they loved, where they loved—we can only wonder about these things. All the passion and pain, the jealousies and intrigues, the incidents and conversations, have vanished. Only ancient pollens on an ancient grave indicate that someone may have mourned another so long ago.

Then the Neanderthals mysteriously died out about 36,000 years ago, replaced in western Europe by modern *Homo sapiens sapiens*— men and women who looked just like you and me, totally modern people who began to paint the cave walls of France and Spain and perform ceremonies in a dank, still world beneath the ground.

These new individuals left all sorts of artifacts, however, clear signs that human beings had evolved the ability for abstract symbolic thought—as well as a conscience, a complex system of beliefs about right and wrong, and stringent rules about sex and love.

How and why modern humankind replaced the Neanderthals are questions that have captured the imagination of archaeologists, novelists, and laymen for more than a century. Traditionally scientists thought that *Homo sapiens* simply evolved from populations of Neanderthals then living in Europe; now many believe that these modern people originated in Africa at least 90,000 ago and swept into Europe from the Near East, killing off the Neanderthals instead.[11] Whatever their relationship, the hapless Neanderthals ceased to be and new modern Cro-Magnon individuals, named after the place in France where their bones were first discovered, appeared across Europe by 35,000 years ago.

Now human art and cultural life exploded.

Some think this remarkable creative outburst began with population pressure.[12] At this time the inclement weather of the most recent glacial age was raging in the north; the land where London is today lay under a mile-high rind of ice. But along what is now the Mediterranean stretched vast grasslands much like today's Serengeti. Here woolly mammoths, woolly rhinos, reindeer, ibex, bison, ancient horses, and hundreds of other hooved animals grazed in droves. Pushed by glaciers to the north and deserts to the south, our ancestors congregated on these savannas, too, in what is today France and Spain.

And as people became hemmed in by one another, they were forced to forge new social networks and create all sorts of new traditions to survive.

The cave art was only one of their innovations. About a dozen people must have worked a week stacking the jaw bones of ninety-five mammoths, one atop the next in a herringbone design, to build the sides of one oval hut found in the Ukraine dating to some 20,000 years ago.[13] Others in this ancient village painstakingly arranged the long bones of mammoths to make oval huts. Then these early architects threw skins over the bones or chinked each structure with mud and grass to keep out the winter winds. And near their houses they dug storage pits, indicating that our relatives had begun to settle down.

Cro-Magnon people also built houses of skin and wood at the fords of rivers where the great herds came to drink, atop hillsides with a vista, and on sunny floodplains that straddled migration trails.

Usually these homes faced south to take advantage of solar heat. By the time the cave art reached its height, 15,000 years ago, some were clearly living in large seasonal communities.

No longer could men and women pick up and leave when conflict surged. Instead, bands had to cooperate, thus setting the stage for social and political hierarchies with rules.

As populations rose and resources grew scarce, Cro-Magnon people were compelled to invent new tools and weapons too. Whereas Neanderthal folk had made only large stone tools, these modern human beings fashioned utensils of ivory, bone, and antler. Lightweight barbed harpoons, fishhooks, spear-throwers, and miniature projectile points—perhaps used in the first bows and arrows—became part of a vast new array of deadly weapons.[14] Big-game hunting of reindeer and wild cattle intensified.

Impressions of plaited strands found on a bit of clay in the Lascaux cave suggest they made cordage, probably rope, twine, netting, and fishing line. And because amber mined in the Baltic has turned up in their homes on the Russian plains and because seashells from the Atlantic are found over a hundred miles away in Les Eyzies, France, these people must have established networks of exchange and engaged regularly in long-distance trade for precious stones and lithic raw materials.[15]

Life took on gaiety. Cro-Magnon people invented the flute, the whistle, and the drum. They wore necklaces of bear and lion teeth, bone bracelets and pendants, and hundreds upon hundreds of ivory, shell, and stone beads.[16] Bone needles as small and sharp as any found in a modern sewing kit were used to sew hooded parkas and make shirts with collars and cuffs, tunics, leggings, boots, and other tailored clothing. Palm-sized portable figurines of big-busted, fat-buttocked women (known as Venus figurines) as well as sculptured animals of ivory, bone, and ceramics have been found in places ranging from the Pyrenees to the Urals. Perhaps these were fertility symbols, aids to divination, or good-luck charms.[17]

They may also have developed social strata. When two children were buried near Moscow, our Cro-Magnon ancestors bedecked the bodies with rings, anklets, spears, darts, daggers, and some 10,000 beads. These youngsters could not have earned fame as mighty hunters or leaders of any sort; were they of an upper class?

No wonder Pfeiffer thinks these people led their children through the belly of the earth and scared them half to death to train them for adulthood. Life had become vastly more complex. These people lived cheek by jowl in the world's first seasonal villages. They had myths, magic, rituals, and gods. They enjoyed music, dance, and song. They buried their dead with grave goods. They wore fox skin coats, braided their hair, donned jewelry, and styled their clothes. They used stone lamps with burning oil in order to paint in caves and light the night. They sat around well-built hearths, roasted large sides of beef, and talked with human language. They looked like us; they thought like us. And they had a whole corpus of traditions they embodied in their art. Theirs was the original affluent society.

These men and women must have had mores about sexuality, marriage, adultery, and divorce. What were these codes for love?

Forbidden Fruit

All human societies have some sort of incest taboo.[18] At times in history the Egyptians, Iranians, Romans, and others sanctioned brother–sister incest for special groups such as royalty. But with these few curious exceptions, mother–son, father–daughter, and brother–sister matings have been forbidden; the incest taboo is universal to humankind. Moreover, this stringent rule is the first sexual restriction children learn. Infringement sometimes brings severe punishment, even death, mutilation, or ostracism. And the taboo is never lifted—regardless of one's age or reproductive status.

It is fair to assume that the human incest taboo had emerged among Cro-Magnon peoples (or long before)—for several reasons. Foremost, incest would have been vastly impractical. If a Cro-Magnon girl mated with her brother or her father and produced a baby, the group then had a helpless new member and no new adult to help support the infant. What a dangerous economic burden. It was far more economically logical to breed with an outsider and enlist this foreigner as manpower to help rear the child.

Incestuous matings would have caused endless social conflict too. Humans are jealous, possessive creatures; we are not built to share a beloved sex partner. So incestuous sex would have caused serious domestic rivalry, undermining the fragile relationship between wife and husband, weakening friendships between kin, and disturbing social order.[19] Incest might have affected the child's social development as well. Children attach to parents. But if a parent has coitus with the youngster, this can weaken the authority of the adult, inhibit trust, and interfere with the psychological process of separation from family.

Cro-Magnon people could not afford all this discord.

Incest also carried political liabilities. As the old axiom goes, "It is better to marry out then to be killed out."[20] If your daughter leaves the group to mate with a man in the next valley, your relations with these people improve; they become kin. If she stays home and mates with you, you have forged no new trading, warring, or social ties.

Not surprisingly, the vast majority of human cultures prescribe that the young marry outside the family, the clan, sometimes even the community.[21] This does not necessarily preclude incest, but it does ensure the flow of adults, goods, and information between different social units, reducing the likelihood of incest as well as encouraging the "good neighbor" policy. "Breeding out" was also important in order to avoid dangerous physical effects.[22]

So for economic, social, political, and genetic reasons, it seems likely that Cro-Magnon people had rules that parents and siblings were not fair game. In fact, so important were helpers to raising the young, group harmony, band cohesiveness, political ties, and genetic health that our Cro-Magnon ancestors may even have inherited a *biological* distaste for incestuous relationships—a predisposition to mate and breed outside the nuclear family.

Incest

A genetic tendency to avoid sex with mother, father, or siblings? This is not a new idea. In 1891 Edward Westermarck first proposed this, saying that children develop a natural physical repulsion toward those they grew up with.[23] Since then this aversion has been confirmed by studies of sexuality in Israel.

Investigations began when Melford Spiro watched infants as they grew up together in a *kevutza*, a common living, sleeping, and bathing quarter where a group of age-mates lived throughout their juvenile years.[24] Here boys and girls played at sex, lying under bedcovers together, examining one another in a game they called clinic—which consisted of kissing, hugging, and touching one another's genitals. By age twelve, however, these children became shy and tense in one another's company; by fifteen they developed strong brother–sister bonds.

Although these unrelated youngsters were free to copulate and marry, to Spiro's knowledge not a single one either wed or even engaged in intercourse with another member of the same *kevutza* group.

Pursuing this investigation in the early 1970s, sociologist Joseph Shepher obtained records on all known kibbutzim marriages; of 2,769 weddings, only 13 occurred between individuals of the same peer group. And none of these marriage partners had entered their common childhood living arrangement until after the age of six. Shepher thinks there is a critical time in childhood between ages three and six when people develop a natural sexual aversion for those they see regularly.[25]

Chemistry seems to play a role in incest avoidance. And this physiological response must have evolved by the time our ancestors were wearing foxskin coats, playing flutes, and decorating the walls of caves in France and Spain—for incest avoidance has extensive correlations in the rest of the animal community.

Among birds, insects, and other mammals, opposite-sexed creatures reared together also prefer to mate with strangers. In fact, other species have developed so many ways to avoid inbreeding that biologists think the human incest taboo actually derives from our animal nature.[26]

Higher primates, for instance, recognize kin and rarely breed with close relatives, particularly mothers. One reason for this is nicely illustrated by young male rhesus monkeys on Cayo Santiago Island, just east of Puerto Rico, although it also applies to you and me. Here males grow up under the tutelage of their mother and her close female kin. As juveniles mature, they rarely approach their mother sexually, however. Instead, they see this female as an authority figure and a wailing wall. Rather than court her, they become infantile, climbing into her arms, cooing, and nuzzling instead; some even try to suckle.[27] Men and women occasionally regress, too, becoming quite childlike in the presence of their parents.

Brother–sister incest and father–daughter matings are rare in nature for a different reason. In many species, either the pubescent male or female leaves the social group. Chimpanzee siblings sometimes end up in the same community, however, and at the Gombe Stream Reserve, Tanzania, Goodall saw a few incestuous matings. During these copulations either the brother or the sister appeared extraordinarily bored or the two had a vicious fight. Fifi, for example, hung screaming from a branch as her brother, Figan, forced her into coitus.

These same natural antipathies to incest must have been present in our distant human past. Probably as early as four million years ago individuals saw those they grew up with as sexually unattractive; they sought their parents for succor, not for copulation, and boys or girls switched groups at puberty. Under "natural" conditions incest was rare. Then, when humankind evolved a brain capable of making, remembering, and following sexual rules, people readily sensed the economic, social, and political disadvantages of incest. *So what had been a natural tendency became a cultural dictum too.* [28]

When in human history this occurred we will never learn, but surely by the time Cro-Magnon women and men were learning the legends of their ancestors in eerie caverns beneath the Pyrenees, they knew whom they could court and marry and who was "forbidden fruit." Incest had become taboo.

Undoubtedly these people had other sexual prohibitions. Postpartum taboos are the most universal of these mores, existing in some 94 percent of all cultures on record.[29] Generally couples are supposed to abstain from sex for about six months after the birth of a child. These rules probably evolved so that mother—and father—could attend to their helpless infant.

In every known society sexual intercourse has spawned myriad beliefs, so there is every reason to think our Cro-Magnon ancestors had their own. But which ones? The Bellacoola of central British Columbia, for example, believe that chastity brings a man closer to the supernatural—as do many Christians. Many peoples think continence is critical before a hunt and some American football coaches are convinced their players do better if they avoid sex prior to a game.

Cro-Magnon couples probably avoided making love for a period of time after bearing a child and never had intercourse before they set out to stalk prey or attend a ritual in a cave. And they must have coupled in the dark or out of view. Nowhere in the world do people regularly have coitus in public.

In the vast majority of societies men and women bestow power on menstrual blood. Our European ancestors were steeped in superstitions about this. "In various parts of Europe," wrote Sir James Frazer, the great explorer of worldwide folklore, "it is still believed that if a woman in her courses enters a brewery the beer will turn sour; if she touches beer, wine, vinegar or milk, it will go bad; if she makes jam, it will not keep; if she mounts a mare, it will miscarry; if she touches buds, they will wither; if she climbs a cherry tree, it will die."[30] Until the 1950s American women still called menstruation "the curse" and avoided sexual contact when it occurred.

Our Cro-Magnon ancestors probably avoided making love during the woman's menstrual period as well.

Undoubtedly they also observed codes for sexual modesty. Even in the steamy jungles of Amazonia women and men wear clothing, although you might not recognize it as such. Yanomamo women wear no more than a thin cord around their waists. But if you ask a woman to remove her string belt, she shows just as much anguish as does an American woman if you ask her to take off her blouse. A Yanomamo man wears a string about his abdomen, and he carefully tucks the foreskin of his penis into it so that his genitals lie snugly against his stomach. When a Yanomamo man's penis slips from its mooring, he responds with the same embarrassment that a tennis player might if his penis flopped from the leg of his shorts.

Be it a string belt in Amazonia or a full-length dress in Victorian England, men and women give power to apparel. Without this sexual drapery they are nude, vulnerable, ashamed. Since our Cro-Magnon ancestors were wearing leather tunics and necklaces of lion's teeth, they undoubtedly had clothing codes for their genitals as well. And they were fastidious about their sexual decorum.

Last, our ancestors must have had precepts about adultery and divorce. As you recall, hunting-gathering and gardening peoples are generally less finicky about infidelity than are many Western industrial societies. Maybe the punishment for philandering in a Cro-Magnon community was no more than an afternoon of public ridicule, a mild beating, or a few fierce arguments. But surely by 35,000 years ago our ancestors had developed strictures about fidelity—and both men and women knew these rules.

Even the most hotheaded must also have honored basic customs for divorce. In small groups, where gossip is a perennial pastime and ostracism is tantamount to death, no one wishes to risk too much alienation. So long before a Cro-Magnon man or woman gathered a few belongings and stomped off to another valley, to another band, he or she must have spent many afternoons staring across the meadows, pondering, deliberating how to break the news, deciding when it was most appropriate to go and how to do it according to etiquette.

Origins of "Ought"

Rules, rules, rules. How did Cro-Magnon people curb their sexual desires and abide by all these strictures? Had they a conscience, feelings of morality, a sense of right and wrong?

Probably. "Of all the differences between man and the lower animals," Darwin wrote, "the moral sense or conscience is by far the most important." He defined conscience by saying, "It is summed up in that short but imperious word, 'ought.' "[31] I suspect *ought* was a well-used term by the time Cro-Magnon folk were terrifying and educating their children in magical caves deep below the ground.

How did this extraordinary thing, our human conscience, evolve?

In 1962 Michael Chance proposed a theory for the evolution of self-control that gives a clue to how conscience could have emerged in humankind.[32] Chance reasoned that in order to manipulate older, more powerful males and work their way up the dominance ladder, young male primates had to "equilibrate," to balance alternatives and control their sexual and aggressive drives. Those who could act from the head rather than the heart survived, selecting for the expansion of the brain in higher primates as well as for the ability to defer gratification and control one's sexual impulses.

Anthropologist Robin Fox then used this kernel to theorize about the evolution of conscience in people. He reasoned that as human social life emerged, young men had to follow stringent new rules concerning whom to court and whom to avoid, intensifying their need to restrain their natural sexual and aggressive drives. "The upshot of this selection process," Fox writes, "was to produce a creature who was capable of becoming extremely guilty about his sexuality."[33]

And Fox is convinced that our conscience is "soft-wired" in the brain. He describes this predisposition as "a syndrome of genetically determined behaviors which make the pubescent human, in particular, susceptible to guilt and other forms of conditioning surrounding the sexual-aggressive drives."[34] The seat of the conscience, Fox thinks, is the amygdala, a tiny gland connected to the primitive emotional center (the limbic system), as well as to the nearby hippocampus, which controls memory, and to the sophisticated neocortical thinking areas of the brain.

Welcome, the amygdala. Could this spare bit of protoplasm be among the culprits that keep you up at night when you try to resolve a moral problem? Some scientists think that the endorphins, the "feel good" chemicals in the brain, may also be involved; when one acts in accordance with the rules, one secretes these natural morphines and feels rewarded and secure.[35]

Fox may be onto something. Perhaps the proclivity for morality does reside in our DNA. Studies of infants certainly support this view. Scientists now believe that the potential for moral reactions is present when a neonate emerges from the womb.[36] An infant, for example, will begin to cry when it hears another sob. Known as global empathy, this generalized concern, this sympathy, this "foundation-stone," as Darwin called it, is the first twinkle of what will blossom into the child's moral code.

Then morality develops in stages.[37] Between the ages of one and two, children achieve a sense of "self" and "other" and begin to express specific care about those around them. A toddler will attempt to comfort a hurt friend, for example. Toddlers feel shame and, slightly later, guilt. They understand rules of right and wrong. And they try to adhere to convention, honoring secrecy, stealth, and social propriety.

From these beginnings, boys and girls continue to absorb their culture's moral rules and build their personal styles of adhering and cheating. Even these generalized styles have an adaptive component. Young children are exceedingly self-centered. Indeed, from a Darwinian perspective they *should* be self-centered; altruism is not logical for the very young, whose primary goal is to survive. On the other hand, it is to a teenager's adaptive advantage to make alliances with peers. And we all know that adolescents are highly sensitive to peer approval; their moral codes reflect this obsession with peer acceptance. Then as people age, they assume the moral systems of parents, obviously to prepare them to rear their own young.

"Far from knowing whether it is learned or inherited, I have no idea of what virtue is," Socrates once said. Certainly definitions of morality vary with age, with status, and from one individual and one culture to the next. What is virtuous behavior in New Guinea is not necessarily virtuous in the United States. But it appears that the human animal is born to construct beliefs of right and wrong; then we absorb our culture's mores; then we wrestle with our inner disposition to follow or bend the rules. Hence no one has to teach you to feel guilty; people just teach you *what* to feel guilty about.

The Unfolding Conscience

When this human predisposition for moral behavior evolved is another matter. Darwin noted that many animals exhibit "social instincts" such as defending their young, comforting others, and sharing their food—behaviors that human beings definitely call moral behavior when we see it among ourselves. Morality had analogues in nonhuman creatures. So Darwin proposed that ancestral forms of man also had these social instincts, that these drives "served him at a very early period as a rude rule of right and wrong. But as man gradually advanced in intellectual power . . . so would the standard of his morality rise higher and higher."[38]

It is not difficult to imagine that the evolution of serial monogamy and clandestine adultery triggered the beginnings of selection for this moral wiring some four million years ago. What conflict this dual reproductive strategy produced. To form a pair-bond and also be adulterous required the skills of deceit and judgment and the ability to weigh the odds, to equilibrate, as Chance has said. Then, if what Fox has proposed is right, as human social life became more complex and our ancestors continued to jockey for sex and power, they acquired a conscience too.

Anthropologist Mary Maxwell dissects the evolution of conscience even further.[39] As men and women became engaged in larger and larger networks of social obligations, she proposes, individuals became more driven by the opposing values of reproductive self-interest and the necessity to cooperate within a larger group. Here was conflict. The Good Samaritan would die out as he overlooked his own sexual opportunities in order to obey the rules. So as individuals became adept at conniving for personal reproductive gain, moral precepts—along with the human predilection to evaluate the rightness and wrongness of an action, known as conscience—evolved to counteract this selfishness.

Biologist Richard Alexander adds one last stimulus to the evolution of moral rules and conscience: warfare. He proposes that our hunter-gatherer ancestors lived in high-density, rich environments where they experienced considerable trouble with neighbors. Bands needed to present a united front against these foes. Because each individual was ultimately self-centered, moral rules necessarily arose. These widespread, agreed-upon opinions—moral strictures—set standards. And as members of the group conformed, they acquired internal cohesion, peace, and a unified front against hostile neighbors.

Cheaters were also selected for, however—they could reap ancillary personal benefits from their indiscretions, as long as they were not caught. So as individuals began to weigh the costs and benefits of adhering to these mores, as opposed to cheating here and there, men and women developed the ability to distinguish between right and wrong. They also developed a conscience, "the still small voice," as Alexander puts it, "that tells us how far we can go in serving our own interests without incurring intolerable risks."[40]

"A society works best when people want to do what they have to do," said the American psychoanalyst Erich Fromm. He knew the power of the conscience as social glue.

What, then, of Cro-Magnon men and women? Carefree savages, free to wander, copulate, and desert their partners, these ancestors certainly were not. Undoubtedly the core of their moral spirit came directly out of nature and was present in some embryonic form by four million years ago when our first hominid forebears evolved the human reproductive strategy of monogamy, infidelity, and divorce. The Neanderthals, with modern brains but a society largely devoid of art, probably had feelings of right and wrong, a few moral rules, and a sense of duty to abide by group mores. Then, by the time Cro-Magnon people were painting symbols on cave walls beneath ancient France, our ancestors had become beleaguered by sexual codes, by peer pressure, by superstition, and by their conscience.

"The heart of man is made so as to reconcile contradictions," the eighteenth-century Scottish philosopher David Hume once said. I imagine more than one Cro-Magnon woman lay awake in her warm skin hut, tossing, listening to the sighing of the embers and the breathing of her husband as she debated whether to meet another man in a secluded glade early the next morning.

Such women would not be the last to struggle with the fickle passions of humanity.

~ 14 ~

Fickle Passion

Romance in Yesteryears

I am the family face;
Flesh perishes, I live on,
Projecting trait and trace
Through time to times anon,
And leaping from place to place
Over oblivion.
The years-heired feature that can
In curve and voice and eye
Despise the human span
Of durance—that is I;
The eternal thing in man,
That heeds no call to die.

—Thomas Hardy, "Heredity"

"Up the stream, past the overhanging rock, you'll see some small white pebbles on the trail that lead into the bush. Follow these. Not far along the animal path you'll come across water dripping from an overhanging rock. Above the rock is a piney overlook. Wait there. I'll come." He sat and listened, thinking of her laugh, her good directions, this secret spot. As he mused, he whittled a fist-sized ivory horse. He'd give her the present today, he thought.

How many million men and women have loved each other in all the seasons that preceded you and me? How many of their dreams have been fulfilled? How many nights did our ancestors beseech the stars for a change in their fortune or thank the gods for their tranquillity as they nestled in one another's arms? Sometimes I walk through the halls at the American Museum of Natural History and wonder about the great love stories that still live in the little ivory horses, the shell beads, the amber pendants, and the old tools and bones and stones that now rest in the museum cases.

How did our ancestors love?

We have one final clue to the nature of sexuality in yesteryear— the lives of traditional peoples around the world today. So I have picked two to write about, the !Kung of the Kalahari Desert and the Mehinaku of Amazonia, largely because anthropologists Marjorie Shostak and Thomas Gregor have so vividly described their sexual attitudes and behaviors.[1]

Neither culture represents life as it was 20,000 years ago when our Cro-Magnon ancestors had begun to moralize and worry, to worship and obey, to carve big-busted women and draw vaginas on the walls of dank caverns deep beneath the soil. But these contemporary traditional societies do have patterns of sexuality in common. These themes, these similarities, these basic patterns of romance, are also seen in other societies across the continents, so they must have evolved with the dawn of modern humankind—if not long before.

Sex on the Kalahari

Nisa's first sexual memories were of lying beside her parents in their tiny hut of brush and sticks, just large enough to lie in. If Nisa feigned sleep, she could watch her parents "do their work." Daddy would wet his hand with saliva, put this liquid on Mommy's genitals and move up and down on top of her. Sometimes during a trip into the bush to collect vegetables, her mother would set Nisa down beneath a tree and go off to copulate with another man. Once Nisa got so impatient that she screamed through the bush, "I'll tell Daddy he had sex with you!"

Nisa knew in infancy that sex was yet another thing that grown-ups did and that it had rules that were often broken.

After Nisa was weaned, she no longer accompanied her mother on her gathering expeditions. The !Kung say children walk too slowly, they are nothing but a nuisance. Instead, Nisa stayed in camp and played with friends. Regularly the gang of children left the circle of five or six huts, however, to build a "pretend village" some distance into the bush. Here they played at hunting, gathering, singing, "trancing," cooking, sharing—and "marrying."

"Marrying" consisted of pairing up, sharing their "pretend catch" of food with a "make-believe spouse," and playing with this partner—sexually. The boys would remove the leather aprons the girls were wearing, lie down on top of them, wet their genitals with saliva and poke around with a semi-erection as if they were having intercourse. At first Nisa was not an avid player, she told the anthropologist, but she liked to watch.

Boys and girls also sneaked into the bush to meet and play at sex with forbidden lovers. The boys normally initiated this pastime, saying, "We'll be your lovers because we already have wives in the other huts over there. We'll come and do what lovers do, then go back to them." "Being unfaithful" was another variation. Once again the boys began the game, saying to the girls, "People tell us that you like other men." The girls would deny it. But the boys would insist the girls had philandered, threatening to hit them so that they wouldn't take extra lovers any more. This way, as Nisa says, "they played and played."

!Kung parents do not approve of these sexual games, but they do nothing more than scold their children and tell them to "play nicely." With teenagers they use the common tactic of Americans and just look the other way.

Nisa's first teenage crush was on Tikay. She and her boyfriend built a little hut, and every day they played at sex, "doing everything but screw." But Nisa noted, "I still didn't understand about sexual pleasure—I just liked what Tikay did and I liked playing that play." Nisa did not want to share her lover either. She became fiercely jealous when Tikay decided to "take a second wife," playing one day with Nisa and the next day with the other girl.

Did our Cro-Magnon ancestors begin in childhood to play at marrying and being unfaithful, then start in teenage to have infatuations? Probably. American children play doctor, invent all sorts of other softly sexual pastimes, and begin a series of puppy loves in their early teens. These childhood games and teenage crushes are quite common around the world; they probably emerged long ago.

Nisa's sex life as an adult—her several marriages and numerous love affairs—strikes another familiar chord.

Around the age of sixteen or seventeen !Kung girls "begin the moon" or start to menstruate. Often they enter a marriage arranged by parents at this time, although many marry somewhat before puberty begins. Parents have definite opinions about a suitable match. They generally select a man several years older than their daughter. Because boys must go through secret initiation ordeals and also kill a large animal before they become eligible to wed, grooms are often as much as ten years older than their brides.[2] Parents also seek good hunters and responsible men who are unmarried, rather than a married man looking for a second wife.

Girls seem not to express opinions about whom they want to wed. Young men, however, say they want young, industrious, attractive, pleasant, fertile women. And when Shostak asked a man whether he would marry a woman who was smarter than himself, the man replied, "Of course. If I married her, she would teach me to be smart, too."

Nisa married before puberty. Her parents picked an older boy — but responsible he was not. As was customary, after the bargaining and the preliminary exchange of gifts, her wedding ceremony took place. At sunset friends led the couple to their new marriage hut built some distance from the camp. They carried Nisa over the threshold and laid her down inside while her new husband sat outside the door. Then Nisa's family and the relatives of the groom brought coals from their hearths to start a new fire in front of the marriage hut, and everyone sang and danced and joked until well after dark. The following morning both wife and husband were ceremonially rubbed with oil by their partner's mother — a normal celebration.

But Nisa had a bizarre wedding night — and a marriage that lasted only a few angry days. Nisa had not begun to menstruate, and as is normal among the !Kung, an older woman bedded with Nisa and the groom in their marriage hut to reassure the pubescent bride. But Nisa's chaperone had other ideas. She took the new husband as her own lover, bumping Nisa with her ardent copulating. Nisa couldn't sleep. When her parents heard of the goings-on two days later, they became incensed. After announcing that the marriage was finished, they stormed out of camp, taking Nisa with them.

Nisa's second marriage had other problems. Virginity is not a prerequisite for betrothal among the !Kung; in fact, Shostak could find no word for virginity in their language. But young girls often do not consummate their marriages on their wedding night. They are so much younger than their husbands that they act indifferent and reject the groom. This was Nisa's style. Her breasts were just beginning to develop; she was not ready to make love. And her refusal to copulate was so persistent that, after several months of waiting, her second husband, Tsaa, grew impatient and departed.

Then Nisa fell in love—with Kantla, a married man. Kantla and his wife encouraged Nisa to become a co-wife. But she refused. !Kung women do not like to share a husband; they say that the sexual jealousy, the subtle favoritism, and the quarrels outweigh the companionship and the help with domestic chores. Moreover, all three partners often share the same tiny bedroom hut, so none of them has any privacy. As a result of all these pressures, only about 5 percent of all !Kung men maintain a long-term relationship with two wives simultaneously. The other 95 percent amuse themselves endlessly, telling stories about the complications that arise in these ménages à trois.

Nisa liked her third husband; eventually she loved him—and made love to him. As she told Shostak, "We lived on and I loved him and he loved me. I loved him the way a young adult knows how to love; I just *loved* him. Whenever he went away and I stayed behind, I'd miss him. . . . I gave myself to him, gave and gave."

Nisa soon had secret lovers, though. Kantla, her teenage sweetheart, was the first of many. Sometimes she met a lover in the bush when her husband went traveling or hunting; sometimes she entertained in her hut when she was alone. If she visited relatives, she had lovers in other settlements as well.

These rendezvous were both thrilling and dangerous; often they were emotionally painful too. The !Kung believe that if you copulate with a lover while pregnant you will abort your child. Nisa did abort a fetus after a tryst with a lover. But she had more lovers anyway. And some caused her a lot of jealousy, as well as that sickening feeling of despair that jilted people suffer.

After her young husband died prematurely, Nisa became a single mother with small children. She got meat from her father and other relatives and seemed determined to raise her family without a spouse. The single parent is not a phenomenon unique to Western family life.

Then one of Nisa's three paramours, Besa, persevered, and she married for the fourth time. Nisa and Besa argued continually, usually about sex. As she said to anthropologist Shostak, he was "like a young man, almost a child, who lies with his wife day after day after day. Don't her genitals get sore after a while?" Nisa would exclaim. "You're just like a rooster," she shouted at Besa, ". . . At night, once is good; once is enough; . . . in one night you'd screw a woman to death!"[3] And the arguments would escalate from there.

But Nisa and Besa lived together for several years, and they both had extramarital affairs. Once Besa followed Nisa's tracks. Nisa had gone out to collect firewood, and her footprints joined those of a man. Soon Besa found his wife relaxing with her paramour beneath a tree. The lovers began to tremble when they saw Besa's face. And after a lot of bitter words an irate Besa ushered the couple back to camp where the headman ordered beatings for both Nisa and her boyfriend. Nisa refused hers, impudently offering to be shot with a bullet instead. Then she stalked off. Her partner took his punishment, four hard whacks.

Here, then, are patterns of human sexuality among the !Kung that are common in Western cultures too: childhood frolic, teenage crushes, youthful experiments at pairing up, then a lattice of marriages and affairs during reproductive years. All of these patterns were probably commonplace by the time our ancestors were painting murals of stampeding beasts in the dark caves of France and Spain some 20,000 years ago.

The !Kung also have all sorts of sexual codes, another fundamental element of the human mating game. Unlike the vast majority of traditional peoples, the !Kung have no fear of menstrual blood or other body fluids. They believe a woman must refrain from joining a hunt while she bleeds. Men and women also generally avoid intercourse during the height of menses. But spouses resume copulating during its final days if they want to have a child. Menstrual blood, they believe, combines with semen to make the infant.

And the !Kung love sex. "Sex is food," they say. They think that if a girl grows up without learning to enjoy coitus, her mind doesn't develop normally and she goes around eating grass. "Hunger for sex," they are convinced, "can make you die."

Women have specific complaints about men's genitals, however. They do not like a man's penis to be too big, since this hurts, or too full of semen, since this is messy. So women discuss among themselves the contents and the fit of their men's penises. And they demand orgasms. If a man has "finished his work," he must continue until a woman's work is finished too. Women should be sexually satisfied.

Men, of course, also have opinions about what constitutes good sex. One summed up a bad rendezvous this way: "She's so wide, she's like a Herero's mouth.[4] I just flounced around inside, but I couldn't feel anything. I don't know what it was like for her, but today my back hurts and I'm exhausted." Men also worry about their performance. When they are unable to get an erection, they take medicines.

The !Kung love to kiss each other on the mouth. But they do not perform cunnilingus. "A vagina would burn a man's lips and tongue," Nisa explains. Both women and men masturbate occasionally. Everybody jokes about sex too; an afternoon sometimes becomes a theater of witticisms, puns, and bawdy banter. Sexual dreams are considered good. And women talk endlessly about their lovers while they forage with close friends.

But some sexual etiquette is strict. Men and women always try to hide their love affairs from their spouses. They feel that these trysts tap into intense emotions—a "burning heart." Because spouses get jealous, it is wise to hide one's passion for fear of violence at home. So paramours try to meet in safe places—away from spying eyes and tattling tongues. They say their love for their spouses is a different matter. After the torrid sexual craving of early marriage has subsided, husband and wife often become good friends, almost parents to each other.

Nisa's fifth husband plays this role. She says, "We fight and we love each other; we argue and we love each other. That's how we live." And she still sneaks into the bushes with her first love, Kantla, as well as with other men.

Did our Cro-Magnon ancestors 20,000 years ago feel Nisa's zest for sex? Did they have childhood frolics and teenage beaux as they and their parents followed reindeer across the grasslands of France and Spain? Did they marry after gruesome puberty rituals in caverns deep below the ground? And, like Nisa, did they divorce and remarry when things went wrong, as well as meet other lovers in secret spots to dally through an occasional afternoon?

Probably, for the sexual escapades of traditional people living far from the arid bush of southern Africa are not too different from those of Nisa and her friends. Both cultures evidently reflect a world of sexuality and romance that evolved long before contemporary times.

Love in the Jungle

"Good fish get dull, but sex is always fun," explains Ketepe, a Mehinaku tribesman of central Brazil in the heart of Amazonia, to anthropologist Thomas Gregor. Ketepe has a wife he says is dear. He likes to take her and his children off on long fishing trips so that they can spend time by themselves. When he tries to copulate with her in his hammock after his children are asleep, someone nearby invariably gets up to stoke the fire or goes outdoors to relieve himself; home is not a private, sexy place. Moreover, Ketepe is often too busy to meet his wife in the family garden to make love in the afternoon. Village life, he says, is too hectic.

Ketepe is out of his hammock by dawn. Sometimes he and his wife go to the river to bathe together, stopping along the trail to chat with other couples. But on most days he joins a fishing party that leaves soon after the sun comes up. His wife stays home to feed their children and do other chores, women's work. By noon Ketepe returns, gives his fish to his spouse, and joins his friends in the village "men's house," which stands in the middle of the plaza.

The men's house is forbidden to women. None has ever entered—for here the sacred flutes reside, hidden in a corner. If a woman accidently sees these sacred objects, the men will waylay her in the forest and gang-rape her, a practice common among several Amazonian societies.

The men's clubhouse is a jovial place. Amid the teasing, lewd jokes, and chitchat, the men make baskets, work on their arrows, or decorate their bodies with paints in preparation for "wrestling time" in midafternoon. Then, after all the straining, grunting, dust, and cheers that the matches regularly provoke, the triumphant and the defeated all adjourn to their thatched homes which encircle the plaza playing field. Here Ketepe sits around the family fire with his wife, eats manioc bread heaped with a thick, spicy fish stew, and plays with his children until they all retire to their hammocks and drift off to sleep.

The Mehinaku are busy. Women work as much as seven to nine hours every day processing manioc flour, weaving hammocks, spinning cotton, making twine, fetching firewood, and carrying tubs of water from the nearby stream. Men do a good deal less. Fishing, trading, helping in the family garden plot, and taking part in their many local rituals take only about three and a half hours every day—except in the dry season, when men work hard to clear the land for the new manioc garden.

But the villagers also avidly engage in another time-consuming activity—sex. "Sex," they say, "is the pepper that gives life and verve." And sex liberally seasons daily life.

Soon after a Mehinaku child begins to walk, he or she joins other youngsters in play groups in the plaza. As the tots roll and tussle on the ground, adults tease them, saying, "Look, look, my boy is copulating with your daughter." Children soon learn the game. As they age, they, like !Kung children, begin to play a fantasy they call marrying.

Little boys and girls sling hammocks to the trees beyond the village, and while the girls stoke "pretend fires" or play at weaving cotton, boys gather big leaves. These "make-believe fish" they proudly present to their spouses to be cooked. (This, as you recall, is symbolic courtship feeding.) Then, after the couple eat together, they start another fantasy, "being jealous." Either the boy or girl sneaks into the bushes, followed closely by a suspicious "spouse." When he or she catches the other in a make-believe assignation, the cuckolded partner gets angry.

Older children have seen their parents copulating in the family garden, and they often abandon their innocent games for more-serious, grown-up sexual sports. If parents catch their young trying to couple, however, they taunt them unmercifully, so children learn early to be prudent.

The carefree days of childhood sex end abruptly around age eleven or twelve, when formal rules of sexual decorum demand that a boy enter up to three years of seclusion. His father builds a wall of palm wood staves and palm leaves at one end of the family house and hangs his son's hammock behind this barrier. Here the teenager spends much of his time, taking medicines that ensure that he will grow. The adolescent must speak softly, follow several dietary restrictions, and, above all, avoid any sexual encounters. Toward the end of his stay he begins to sneak out and have affairs, however.

Hearing of a tryst, his father then tears down the partition. The boy has become a man—equipped to go on long fishing trips alone, ready to cut a garden and have a wife.

Now young men are free to indulge in sexual adventures, dalliances that will become a normal part of adult life. Boys meet their girlfriends in the woods to copulate.[5] They take little time for foreplay.[6] If a couple find a spot where a thick log lies along the ground, they may make love on top of it in the missionary position, with the man on top. But comfortable logs are rare, the ground is often muddy, and insects bite. So lovers normally sit facing each other; she is on top, her legs wrapped around his hips.

In another common stance, he kneels and spreads his legs, holding her thighs, buttocks, and lower back above the ground while she braces her upper body with outstretched arms. Couples also like coitus in a pool of quiet water—chest high is best for leverage, they say. And if there is little time, lovers may copulate standing up; she wraps one leg around her sweetheart while he raises her slightly off her feet.

Sex is over after the man has ejaculated. Although the Mehinaku have no word for female orgasm, they are well aware that the clitoris swells during intercourse and is the seat of female pleasure. They liken the female genitals to a face; the clitoris is the nose; it "sniffs out sexual partners." But whether women have orgasms regularly is unknown to anthropologists.

Soon after ending coitus, lovers take different paths back home— but not without exchanging small gifts. Fish are currency for sex. After a fishing expedition, a man often stops just prior to entering the village, selects the oiliest of his catch, and sends it by a messenger to a lover. He gives her a fish when they meet too. And lovers regularly give one another other mementos, like a spindle of cotton, a basket, or some shell jewelry. This teenage sexuality is so common-place that when a girl walks into the central plaza smeared with her boyfriend's body paint, no one blinks; the Mehinaku see nothing wrong with premarital coitus in the woods.

But parents get exceedingly upset if their unmarried daughter gets pregnant. So soon after a girl emerges from her period of seclusion, which begins at her first menses and lasts a year or more, she weds. This is a special day. The new husband moves his hammock into his wife's home and presents her with an abundant catch of fish. She makes a particularly sweet batch of manioc bread. And over the course of several days friends and kin exchange more gifts and senti-ments.

The Mehinaku think a display of romantic love is silly, in poor taste, so newlyweds are supposed to be reserved. Excessive thoughts of a loved one, they believe, can attract deadly snakes, jaguars, and malevolent spirits. Yet newlyweds sleep in the same large hammock and spend their days together bathing, talking, and making love in the woods outside the village. Young married people get jealous, too, particularly if they catch a mate in an affair.

These outside dalliances generally begin soon after marriage. Cen-tral to the rendezvous is something the Mehinaku call alligatoring. A man who has established a liaison with a woman lies in wait for her in an "alligator place," either in the woods behind her house, along one of the trails that radiate from the village plaza, or near the gardens or bathing spots. As a paramour walks by, her would-be lover smacks his lips to beckon her, then propositions her as she draws near. She may oblige or make a later date. Men say women are "stingy with their genitals," although you might not agree. Tamalu, the most promiscuous woman in the village, has fourteen lovers. On average, Mehinaku men have four separate affairs at any given time.

These extramarital liaisons, Gregor reports, have a valuable social function: village cohesion. The Mehinaku think that semen makes a baby and that several copulations are needed to form a child. As men report, baby making is a "collective labor project," something like a fishing expedition. Thus every lover is convinced that a woman's forthcoming infant is partly his. Occasionally a man publicly recognizes the infant of a lover as his own and helps raise the child.[7] But spouses get jealous; as they say, they "prize each other's genitals." So the real father of an infant rarely reveals himself. This belief about baby making, however, silently links men and women in an elaborate web of kinship ties.

Probably as a result of all these veiled sexual connections, adulterers rarely get fined or beaten. In Mehinaku myths philanderers are hit, dismembered, even put to death. But in real life only newlyweds make a fuss or confront a spouse about infidelity—for an understandable reason. Villagers often jeer a jealous husband, calling him a kingfisher, because these birds flap about aimlessly, screeching and scolding. Rarely does a man put aside his dignity to invite this scorn.

This is not to say that men and women with roving spouses do not suffer; sexual tensions often lead to divorce. Marital discord is most easily measured by where a couple sleep. If spouses have strung their hammocks inches from one another, they probably are relatively happy. These couples tend to talk about the events of the day after their children are asleep, even copulate in one or the other's hammock. As their quarrels escalate they string their hammocks farther apart; sometimes they even sleep on opposite sides of the fireplace. And if a wife becomes enraged, she may take a machete and cut down her husband's bed. This often initiates divorce.

Although some single women with small children live in the village, the vast majority of adults remarry. As far as the Mehinaku are concerned, a man needs a wife to carry firewood, make manioc, and mend his hammock, as well as for companionship and sex. Like the !Kung and many other peoples, the Mehinaku regularly pursue the mixed human reproductive strategy of marriage, adultery, divorce, and remarriage.

Also like the !Kung, the Mehinaku love sex—a preoccupation that is evident in their myriad beliefs. Fish and manioc, their staples, both have sexual connotations. When women grate manioc tubers, something they do most of the day, villagers say they are having sex. Sex is the fabric of the daily litany of jokes. Men and women frequently tease each other sexually. Women paint their bodies, pluck their pubic hair, and wear a G-string through their vulvar lips and buttocks to accentuate their genitals. The Mehinaku's myths, their songs, their rituals, their politics, their dress, and their daily activities are all saturated with sexual symbolism.

Yet their sexuality has a macabre undercurrent of fear. Gregor thinks that Mehinaku men have rampant castration anxieties. In a study of Mehinaku dreams, he discovered that 35 percent of the men worried about the amputation or mangling of their genitals, a rate much higher than that among American men. The Mehinaku are also scared of impotence, for good reason. Gossip is endemic in this village of only eighty-five people, and the extent of a man's sexual prowess quickly becomes common knowledge. Hence dysfunction in the morning can turn into "performance anxiety" by night.

Men are also terrified of women's menstrual blood. This dark, "foul-smelling" secretion, they say, "races" into the water containers, the fish stew, the manioc drinks, and the bread the moment a woman begins to bleed. If this poison gets under a man's skin, they say, it turns into a foreign body that causes pain until a shaman magically removes it. So it is not unusual for a wife to throw a whole day's manioc flour into the jungle if one woman in the house begins to menstruate in late afternoon.

Sex, the Mehinaku believe, stunts growth, weakens a man, inhibits his wrestling and fishing ability, and attracts evil spirits. Even thinking about coitus while traveling may be dangerous to one's health.

A few men are cowed into abstention or impotence by these beliefs; many others try to moderate their trysts; and some cast caution to the wind and sow their seed whenever and wherever possible. But all the Mehinaku, Gregor thinks, are troubled; they believe that too much sex, sex at prohibited times, or sex with a partner in the wrong kin relationship can cause disease, injury, even death. "Anxious pleasures," as Gregor calls their dalliances, may be an understated description of these people's sexual escapades.

Blueprint of Human Sexuality

Are Ketepe's sojourns in the woods beside the Amazon any different from Nisa's rendezvous with Kantla on the Kalahari? Surely our Cro-Magnon forebears grew up with sex around them, played at coitus when they were children, went through ceremonies in teenage to announce their adult sexual status,[8] and then entered a labyrinth of marriages and affairs drenched with passion, rules, and superstition.

Cro-Magnon children almost certainly huddled in mammoth-bone huts on bear rugs in the middle of the night, listening to their parents' jostling and heavy breathing. In the morning they saw their parents smile at each other. Occasionally after their father had left camp to hunt, they saw mother vanish beyond the meadow with a man who admired her and gave her gifts. And like their counterparts in many other cultures, the more astute children knew what their parents were up to and could rattle off the clandestine lovers of most of the grown-ups in their band. They probably didn't tattle, though.

By age ten, Cro-Magnon youngsters must have begun their own journeys into sex and love.[9] Little girls may have slipped off to a river to bathe and play at "marrying" and "being jealous" with the boys. They probably roamed in gangs, and by early teenage some had started to play seriously at sex—long before puberty.[10] A few may have loved one boy and then another, while others had a constant "puppy love" for a single mate.

As teenagers they spent hours decorating themselves—as adolescents do in many cultures—plaiting their hair, donning garlands of flowers in order to smell sweet, wearing bracelets and pendants, and decorating their tunics and leggings with fur, feathers, beads, and red and yellow ocher. Then they strutted, preened, and showed off for one another around the fire's glow.

Sometime before puberty our Cro-Magnon forbears began the important rituals for adulthood that culminated in the caverns beneath the earth. Here they entered the spirit world and danced and sang in ceremonies designed to teach them to be brave and smart. And as girls matured, they wed older boys who had established their hunting skills.

When the reindeer started their annual migration in the spring, a "newly married" couple and their friends must have set brushfires that drove the giant beasts stampeding to their death in a steep ravine, then butchered these creatures and carted home great chunks of meat. Around a roaring blaze they reenacted the high points of the hunt. Then some vanished from the firelight to hug and nuzzle in the woods.

During the summer months a wife probably tanned the hide of a bear her husband had trapped; she roasted the fish he had caught in the teeming streams; and she came home from gathering expeditions to tell him where the horses were feeding and where the bees were making honey. Her husband showed his wife new nutting groves and fishing pools. Together they collected raspberries and blueberries. And together they lay in secret spots on lazy afternoons.

In autumn, they may have gone together on trading expeditions to where the waves pounded on the shore; here they exchanged fox hides for purple shells and golden stones and saw old friends and relatives. Then, as winter began to rage, they probably spent hours in the house, drilling beads, carving figurines, and telling tales.

Some men and women married more than once. Some had extra lovers. But they all had hopes and fears and sweethearts. For in their souls they carried an ancient script—a template for human bonding: "The family face," as Thomas Hardy called it, "the eternal thing in man that heeds no call to die."

This basic human nature would be sorely challenged by what happened next. By 10,000 years ago, the most recent Ice Age had passed into the present interglacial thaw. The land began to warm. Glaciers that had gripped the earth as far south as modern London retreated north, and the vast grasslands that stretched across Eurasia from Europe to the South China Sea turned into miles and miles of deep, thick woods. The woolly mammoth, the woolly rhino, and many other large mammals died out, replaced by red deer, roe deer, boar, and all the other modern creatures that still roam the European woods. Now men and women were forced to hunt smaller game, catch more fish, fell more birds, and collect lots of forest vegetables.[11]

Soon some would settle down, domesticate wild seeds and tame wild beasts. With this, the ancestors of Western men and women would change the face of marriage with two new ideas: honor thy husband; till death us do part.

~15~

"Till Death Us Do Part"
Birth of Western Double Standards

To have and to hold from this day forward,
for better for worse,
for richer for poorer,
in sickness and in health,
to love and to cherish,
till death us do part.

— Book of Common Prayer *(1549)*

Thwack, thwack, thwack. A giant willow crackled, swayed, then thundered down beside the lake. Trout, perch, pike, chub, and catfish sped below the lily pads and darted among the bulrushes that lined the lake with marsh. A forest boar dashed, stricken, from the underbrush. Ducks and geese and mud hens lifted, flapping, from the reeds. Two otters froze, listening, among the cattails. Someone new was in the woods.

By 5000 B.C. central Europe was strewn with ponds and lakes and streams, signatures of massive glaciers that had retreated north some five thousand years earlier. Surrounding these glacial footprints were deep, thick forests. First birches and pines had spread across the grass. Then oaks, elms, spruce, and fir trees appeared. And by 5000 B.C. beech trees, chestnut trees, ashes, and maples cloaked the river valleys. Where oak trees spread their limbs, light bathed the forest floor. Here thistles, stinging nettles, and other underbrush could thrive, providing luxuriant hotels for teeming forest life. But where beech trees took root, their thick leaves drank the sunlight, and only ferns, wild onions, garlic, and grasses grew.

No more did mammoths and mastodons trumpet in the morning air. Gone the open plains, the swaying grasses, low shrubs, and early-morning chill. Instead, the August light danced off crystal lakes and dew on leaves and bark. Solitary creatures like red deer, boars, elk, and badgers picked among the forest browse. Roe deer and brown bears hung along the rims of meadows where the hazel, raspberry, strawberry, and elderberry bushes grew. And wildcats stalked rabbits in fields of dandelions. The modern landscape and all the fauna that now live in Europe had appeared.[1]

New people lived here too: farmers.

Along the river valleys of Germany, Austria, Czechoslovakia, Poland, and the Low Countries, men and women had begun to fell the trees and till the soil. In some clearings only a single farmstead stood. Elsewhere tiny hamlets comprised four to ten squat, rugged wooden buildings. In small "kitchen gardens" just outside their doors, these first European cultivators grew peas, lentils, poppy plants, and flax. They housed domesticated cattle, pigs, sheep, and goats in barns attached to their homes. Dogs slept at their feet. And behind their houses lay scattered fields of planted wheat.

How the first farmers in southwestern Germany got along with the local hunter-gatherers we may never know. But archaeologist Susan Gregg has an hypothesis based on ingenious data.[2]

To reconstruct daily life along these riverbanks, she chose a hypothetical village consisting of six households, with thirty-four women, men, and children. Then, by meticulously studying the landscape, the artifacts of this period, and the life cycles of wheat, peas, pigs, and other plants and animals that lived here, Gregg pieced together these first farmers' work schedule, their cultivating and herding practices, and their estimated production and consumption of meat, milk, grains, and vegetables per individual per year.

Included in her calculations were the precise amount of time needed to plant each hectare of ancient wheat, the most suitable size for each field and garden plot, and the crop losses due to snails, mice, birds, and winter storage. To the equation she added the straw yield of each harvest and the amount of pastureland, forest browse, and winter fodder necessary to maintain the optimal number of cattle, sheep, goats, and pigs. She also weighed the life span of these species, the number of baby animals born each year, the abundance of wild berries, greens, and condiments, the time spent to cut wood, and many other factors in order to establish the most efficient way these farmers might have lived.

Her conclusion: they planted wheat in spring, and they employed the local foragers to help them seed their crop.

In exchange, she theorizes, the farmers gave these hired hands surplus meat—ewes, calves, and piglets that had expired just after birth in early spring, the leanest time of year for nomads. Then, in August when the wheat ripened, Gregg thinks, the farmers hired the local wanderers again to help cut the grain and carry straw to storage bins—this time in exchange for milk. They may also have bartered with the foragers for wild game, special flint and volcanic rocks for making axes. Most important, they got information—news of other farmers that these gypsies collected as they roamed.

The foragers, Gregg thinks, welcomed the farmers not only for their meat, milk, and grain but also for their abandoned fields. These clearings made gaps in the thick woods where new shrubs, herbs, and grasses took hold and attracted wild deer and forest swine. So around these fallow fields hunting may have been particularly good. More important, with farm produce at hand, the foragers could forgo some of their arduous long-distance fishing expeditions. They, too, could begin to settle down.

No doubt these early contacts between farmers and foragers were not all as friendly or as symbiotic as Gregg reports. Surely hunters and planters sometimes fought. But eventually the latter prevailed. These settlers would fundamentally alter ancient gender roles, initiating sexual codes and attitudes regarding women that have been passed down the centuries to us.

The Gentrification of Europe

How and why farming took root in Europe is avidly debated.[3] But Western agriculture had its origins on hillsides that stretch like a horseshoe from Jordan north through Israel, Lebanon, Syria, and Turkey, then south through Iraq and Iran—the Fertile Crescent. Here, by 10,000 B.C., in clearings among the pistachio and olive trees, the cedars, junipers, oaks, and pines, wild grasses grew and feral cattle, pigs, sheep, and goats all grazed.

Our nomadic ancestors had probably visited these meadows to hunt and collect grains for millennia. As the hot, dry summers got even hotter and drier, however, and as people clustered around the few remaining freshwater lakes, food supplies grew short. And with time these people began to store the grain they had collected and plant seeds in an effort to intensify their harvest of these wild cereals. The earliest farmers may have lived in the Jordan valley. But by 8000 B.C. many more hamlets had taken root and early villagers of the Fertile Crescent had begun to sow wild wheat, rye, and barley and herd sheep and goats.[4] The hearth of Western civilization had been laid.

Agriculture then spread north and west. And as the custom of planting grains and vegetables seeped into Europe along the riverbanks from Asia Minor, farming gradually became a way of life. For four million years our ancestors had meandered across the ancient world in a constant search for food. Now nomadism was becoming a thing of the past. As archaeologist Kent Flannery summed it up, "Where can you go with a metric ton of wheat?"

The Plow. There is probably no single tool in human history that wreaked such havoc between women and men or stimulated so many changes in human patterns of sex and love as the plow. Exactly when the plow appeared remains unknown. The first farmers used the hoe or digging stick. Then sometime before 3000 B.C. someone invented the "ard," a primitive plow with a stone blade and a handle like a plow's.

What a difference this made.

In cultures where people garden with a hoe, women do the bulk of the cultivating; in many of these societies women are relatively powerful as well.[5] But with the introduction of the plow—which required much more strength—much of the essential farm labor became men's work. Moreover, women lost their ancient honored roles as independent gatherers, providers of the evening meal. And soon after the plow became crucial to production, a sexual double standard emerged among farming folk. Women were judged inferior to men.

Honor Thy Husband

The first written evidence of women's subjugation in farming communities comes from law codes of ancient Mesopotamia dating from about 1100 B.C. when women were described as chattels, possessions.[6] One code indicated that a wife could be killed for fornication but her husband was permitted to copulate outside of wedlock—as long as he did not violate another man's property, his wife. Matrimony was primarily for procreation so abortion was forbidden.[7] And if a woman produced no children, she could be divorced.

The treatment of women as child-producing property, subservient beings, was not singular to people in the Middle East. These mores sprang up among many farming folk.[8]

In traditional agrarian India an honorable wife was supposed to throw herself on the burning funeral pyre of her husband—a custom known as suttee. In China an upper-class girl's toes (all but the big toe) were curled underneath her foot and tightly bound when she was about four, making it terribly painful to walk, impossible to run away from her husband's home. During the golden age of ancient Greece, upper-class girls were married off by the age of fourteen, ensuring they were chaste on their wedding day. Among the Germanic peoples who invaded classical Rome, women could be bought and sold.[9]

"Wives, be subject to your husbands, as is fitting in the Lord," the New Testament bid.[10] This credo was not just a Christian view. In ancient Sumeria, Babylonia, Assyria, Egypt, classical Greece and

Rome, across preindustrial Europe, in India, China, Japan, and the farming communities of North Africa, men became the priests, political leaders, warriors, traders, diplomats, and heads of household. A woman's sovereign was first her father and her brother, then her husband, then her son.

As the fifth-century B.C. Greek historian Xenophon encapsulated a wife's duties to her spouse, "Be therefore diligent, virtuous, and modest, and give your necessary attendance on me, your children, and your house, and your name shall be honorably esteemed even after your death."[11]

I do not wish to imply that the sexual double standard is unique to farmers. Among some gardeners of Amazonia (who use the digging stick rather than the plow) and some herding peoples of East Africa, women are definitely subservient to men in most arenas of social life. But a codified sexual and social double standard is not common to all peoples who herd, who garden with a hoe, or who hunt and gather for a living, whereas it does prevail in societies with the plow.[12]

I also do not wish to suggest that *all* women in farm societies experience the same degree of sexual restriction and social inferiority. Women's status changed from century to century. Class, age, and economic and social station affected women's position too.

Hatshepsut, for example, ruled Egypt in 1505 B.C., and she was only one of several powerful Egyptian queens. Unlike the cloistered housewives of classical Greece, courtesans were educated and highly independent. Some urban, upper-class Roman women of the first and second centuries A.D. became literary figures; others were politicians. During the Middle Ages a number of nuns were educated power brokers in the church; others wielded enormous influence in the marketplace. In the 1400s some Islamic women of the Ottoman Empire owned land and ships. And a sizable number of Renaissance women of England and the Continent were just as well read as any man.

Moreover, even where the sexual double standard is rigorously maintained, it does not always guarantee informal power, day-to-day influence. As we all know, the most insipid woman of a higher class or a more prestigious ethnic group can sometimes dominate a man from a lower social rung. Older women often control younger men. Young, sexy women can manipulate much more influential men. Sisters can rule brothers. And certainly wives can govern husbands. Even where the sexual double standard has been extreme, men have never universally dominated women—not in agricultural America, not in the little farmhouses that hugged the Danube several thousand years ago.

These exceptions notwithstanding, there is no question that during our long European farming ancestry female sexuality was seriously curbed; in almost all circumstances women became second-class citizens as well. Unlike women in nomadic foraging societies who left camp regularly to work and brought home precious goods and valuable information, who traveled freely to visit friends and relatives and ran their own love lives, a farming woman took her place in the garden or the house—her duty to raise children and serve a man.

With plow agriculture came general female subordination, setting in motion the entire panorama of Western sexual and social life.

Exactly how the plow and farm life led to changes in Western sexuality has been debated for at least a hundred years. I will propose that sedentary living, the need for lifelong monogamy, the rise of ranked societies, the escalation of warfare, and a peculiar property of testosterone, the male sex hormone, all played important roles. But before I present my scenario for the evolution of the sexual double standard in the European past, I would like to review some of the major modern theories on the subject. Interestingly, lifelong monogamy plays a part in each.

First, a reminder: *matriarchy* means political *rule* by women; *matriliny* means tracing one's descent through the female line.

The Mother Right

One of the first to offer a scenario for women's fall from power was Johann Jakob Bachofen, a German lawyer who wrote *Das Mutterrecht* (The mother right) in 1861. In this tome Bachofen proposed that humankind first lived in a state of sexual promiscuity in which women were every bit as powerful as men. With the invention of agriculture—by women—society then evolved its first form of social order, the matriarchy.

Because no one could be positive which man had sired any specific child, Bachofen reasoned, early agriculturalists reckoned descent through the female line—matriliny. Because women were the sole parents of the next generation, women were also honored; thus women ruled—matriarchy. Society overthrew the "mother right" for the "father right" during the Greek heroic age because of the adoption of *monogamy* and because of changing religious precepts. Bachofen based his theory for the fall of women on innumerable passages in classical literature, texts that referred to ancient myths in which women were once all-powerful.[13]

The concept of the primitive matriarchy swept through nineteenth-century intellectual circles. Soon the American anthropologist Lewis Henry Morgan marshaled evidence to "prove" Bachofen's scenario for the decline of women.

Because Morgan had lived among the Iroquois, who traced their descent through the female line, he hailed these Indians as a living relic of this primeval matriarchal stage of human social order. Like Bachofen, Morgan believed that primitive promiscuity evolved into matriarchal social life with the beginning of agriculture and that matriarchy was supplanted by patriarchy as agriculture advanced. Unlike Bachofen, he offered an economic explanation for the evolution of male rule.

Private property, Morgan thought, was at the root of the sexual double standard. So in his 1877 book *Ancient Society,* he proposed that as agrarian men increasingly gained private ownership of communal farmlands, they gained the power to overthrow matriarchal rule. Most interesting, basic to Morgan's theory on the rise of patriarchy was the origin of "exclusive pairing." Only as *permanent* monogamy evolved—assuring early farmers of paternity—could they seize power and begin to pass their property to their male heirs.

Friederich Engels elaborated on Morgan's scheme—and advanced his own economic formula for the decline of women's rights. In the earliest days of agriculture, Engels proposed, property was communally owned; women and men lived in matrilineal kin groups rather than in nuclear families headed by males; paternity was relatively unimportant; divorce and philandering were commonplace; women gathered at least as many subsistence foods as men did; and women ran the extended family home. Then, as men and women began to grow crops and herd animals, men's roles as farmers and shepherds became increasingly important. With time, men emerged as owners of the only valuable property—the soil and these beasts. Men then used their power as property owners to institute patriliny and patriarchy.

Like Bachofen and Morgan before him, Engels believed that monogamy—which he defined as strict female fidelity to a single *lifetime* partner—was central to the decline of women's power. Monogamy evolved to ensure paternity, he wrote. And as monogamy undermined a wife's ties and obligations to a wider kin group, monogamy ushered in slavery for women. He called this transition "the world historical defeat of the female sex."[14]

Paradise Lost? Scientists have now proven these early theories largely wrong—but somewhat right. Modern thinking started after the turn of the century, when anthropologists began to notice that no extant society was matriarchal; most were not even matrilineal.[15] Since then anthropologists have studied many more cultures and have still not found a single matriarchal culture. Moreover, there is no archaeological evidence that a primitive matriarchy ever existed anywhere on earth.

Some modern feminists do not agree. They argue that the female figurines on ancient pots and the feminine gods and other feminine motifs found in archaeological and traditional contemporary societies are evidence of primitive matriarchies.[16] But this reasoning is also undermined by data. Of the ninety-three societies surveyed by sociologist Martin Whyte in the 1970s, eighty-three had no folk beliefs that women were once all-powerful. And in those cultures where people did worship female gods and recount myths of female dominion, no female political supremacy existed.[17]

There is, however, some truth to the belief that women were once much more powerful. As was discussed in chapter 11, the vast majority of hunting-gathering peoples are (and probably always were) relatively egalitarian. No extant hunting-gathering, foraging, or gardening society has a rigid codified sexual double standard. And women have had inferior status in societies that use the plow for agriculture.[18] So, although there probably never were any primitive matriarchies, Bachofen, Morgan, and Engels were all partly correct: a *relative equality* between the sexes was probably the rule in many ancient, preagricultural societies, and this balance of power between the sexes indeed became *pronounced inequality* sometime soon after the plow was introduced.

In the 1970s the Marxist-feminist anthropologist Eleanor Leacock streamlined all of these ideas with yet another scenario. She wisely dropped the idea of the primitive matriarchy. But she marshaled data from around the world to prove that in prehistoric band societies men and women were, in fact, largely equals (see chapter 11). And she hypothesized that as farming men began to make trade goods, sell trade items, and monopolize trade networks, farmers' wives became subordinate to their husbands.[19] Like Bachofen, Morgan, and Engels before her, Leacock also proposed that the emergence of the monogamous nuclear family as the vital economic unit (in conjunction with sedentary living and the plow) was central to the deterioration of women's lives.

"Big Men"

"All thought is a feat of association," Robert Frost once said. So I wish to borrow from all these lines of reasoning, add a biological perspective, and propose a slightly fuller hypothesis for the fall of women.

To begin, then, with what we've got. The plow was heavy; it needed to be pulled by a large animal; it required the strength of men. As hunters, husbands had supplied the luxuries that made life thrilling as well as some of the daily fare; but as tillers of the soil, they became critical to survival. Women's vital role as gatherers, on the other hand, was undermined as our ancestors began to rely less on wild plants for food and more on domesticated crops. Long the providers of substantial daily fare, women now assumed the secondary tasks of weeding, picking, and preparing the evening meal. So anthropologists agree that as men's farm labor became essential to survival, the primary role in subsistence shifted from women to men.

This one ecological factor—the skewed division of labor between the sexes in subsistence and men's control of the vital resources of production—is sufficient to explain women's decline from social power. Those who own the purse strings rule the world. But other factors conjoined to create women's fall. With the advent of plow agriculture, neither husband nor wife could divorce. They worked the land together. Neither partner could dig up half the soil and depart. They had become tied to their mutual real estate and to one another—permanent monogamy.

How the plow and permanent monogamy contributed to the decline of women's worlds is best understood in conjunction with a third insidious phenomenon of farming peoples—rank. For millennia "big men" must have arisen among our nomadic ancestors during hunting, foraging, and trading expeditions. But hunter-gatherers have strong traditions of equality and sharing; for the vast majority of our human heritage, formal ranks did not exist. To organize the yearly farming harvest, however, and store grain and fodder, distribute surplus food, oversee long-distance, systematic trade, and speak for the community at regional gatherings, chiefs arose.

There is some evidence of rank in the European archaeological record as early as fifteen thousand years ago; some graves had much fancier goods than others. Village headmen had thus probably gained power with the rise of these first seasonal, nonagricultural communities. Moreover, along the Danube by 5000 B.C. one home in a hamlet was often larger than the rest, so social stratification had surely begun by then. Then with the subsequent spread of plow agriculture and village life, political organization grew more and more complex—and undoubtedly more hierarchial as well.[20]

So now we have sedentism, permanent monogamy, and rank.

Another factor that surely played a role in the decline of women's social and sexual rights was war. As villages proliferated and population density increased, people were obliged to defend their property, even extend their landholdings when they could. Warriors became invaluable to social life. And as anthropologist Robert Carneiro points out, everywhere in the world where fighting enemies is important to daily living, men come to increase their power over women.

Men's more-important economic roles as farmers, couples that were obliged to remain together on their mutual home range, villagers who needed chiefs to organize their work, and societies that needed warriors to defend their soil—what a volatile mixture. Here was a perfect opportunity for one sex to gain authority over the other.

Indeed, that's just what happened. Patriarchy sprang up across Eurasia and seeded deep into the soil.

But why patriarchy instead of matriarchy? Why didn't women seize the rule? The brute force necessary to drive the plow and the strength required in warfare both suffice to answer this question. But I think at least one more primary factor was involved in the florescence of patriarchy and the decline of women's worlds—biology.

In every single society where ranks are prevalent, men hold the majority of the authoritative roles. In fact, in 88 percent of ninety-three societies canvassed, *all* local and intermediate political leaders are men; in 84 percent of these cultures men hold *all* of the top leadership positions in the kin group too.[21] This is not because women are barred from these positions. In many of these cultures—such as the United States—women are permitted to seek influential positions in government. Today greater numbers of women are indeed running for office. But even now women do not seek political positions with anywhere near the regularity that men do.

To explain this enormous gender difference in who seeks and obtains political rank, sociologist Steven Goldberg has proposed that men are neuro-endocrinologically wired, by means of testosterone that sexes the fetal brain, for a greater drive to seek status; he calls this drive "male attainment." Thus, because of their biological drive to acquire rank, men more regularly give up time, pleasure, health, safety, affection, and relaxation to attain positions of rank, authority, and power.[22]

This is a dangerous idea. Most feminists will certainly reject it, as will anyone who dismisses the biological factors involved in human action. But as one who takes science seriously, I cannot ignore the possibility that biology plays a role in the acquisition of rank. In fact, several lines of reasoning support this conclusion.

The brain is indeed sexed before birth by fetal hormones. There is a clear link between testosterone and aggressive behavior in animals and people.[23] High rank is also associated with high levels of male hormones in men[24] and monkeys.[25] Last, women in many cultures assume more leadership positions after their childbearing years are over.[26] There certainly are cultural reasons for this. Released from the constant chores of rearing young, postmenopausal women are certainly liberated to pursue activities outside the home. But there may be a biological reason for their assertiveness as well. Levels of estrogen decline with menopause, unmasking levels of testosterone. Nature has concocted a chemical that possibly contributes to the drive for rank.

There may be another chemical in the cocktail too. Serotonin, another of the brain's molecules. The highest-ranking male vervet monkey in a troop, scientists have established, has consistently higher levels of serotonin in his blood. Male monkeys that rise in dominance exhibit a natural rise in levels of blood serotonin. And when a monkey's rank drops, his natural levels of serotonin decrease.[27] Even when male monkeys are artificially administered serotonin, their rank goes up; and male monkeys given drugs that inhibit the secretion of serotonin experience a drop in rank.[28]

Among human males the same correlations prevail. Officers in college student groups show higher levels of serotonin in their blood than do nonofficers, as do leaders of college sports teams.[29] These simple correlations seem not to be exhibited in women. And scientists preliminarily conclude that women and female nonhuman primates exhibit a more complex behavioral and physiological system of dominance.

Nevertheless, there seems to be a rather direct correlation between testosterone and rank—as well as some evidence that other brain substances contribute to the biology of hierarchy.

"Till Death Us Do Part"

So our European ancestors settled down to farm. They paired for
life. They plowed and warred and traded. And gradually men's new
jobs as plowmen and warriors became crucial to survival, while
women's vital roles as gatherers dwindled in importance. Then, as
ranks emerged and men scrambled for these positions, women's formal power vanished. For every farmer's foot was now sown into the
soil. A mixture of immobility, skewed economic roles, permanent
monogamy, an emerging ranked society, the burgeoning of warfare,
and, quite possibly, a peculiarity of testosterone and other physiological mechanisms set in motion systems of patriarchy seen in agrarian
societies. With patriarchy, women became possessions to be cov-
eted, guarded, and exploited—spawning vicious social precepts
known collectively as the sexual double standard. These credos were
then passed on to you and me.

The common belief that men have a higher sex drive than women,
the conviction that men are more adulterous, the tradition of feminine chastity at marriage, and the long-held assumption that women
are often weak, stupid, and dependent are rooted deep in the plow-
man's dirt. Of all the social changes that farm life produced, however, the most dramatic were our patterns of divorce.

Divorce rates were very low through much of our agrarian past. In
the ancient lands of Israel, for example, divorce was rare.[30] The
classical Greeks reveled in almost any sexual experiment, but they
prohibited sexual practices (like bringing a courtesan into the home)
that threatened the stability of the family.[31] Among the Greeks of
the Homeric age, divorce was permitted but uncommon. Marital
dissolution was low in Rome's early days, when the vast majority of
citizens were farmers; only as cities bloomed and some women became wealthy, independent—and urban—did divorce rates soar
among the upper classes.[32]

Early Christian fathers regarded marriage as a necessary remedy
for fornication; to them bachelors and spinsters, celibates and virgins

in honor of the Lord were far more pure. On the subject of divorce they were divided. "What therefore God has joined together, let no man put asunder," Jesus had advised.[33] Yet different passages of the Bible sent conflicting messages and some scholars think early Christian men had both the legal and religious right to divorce a wife for adultery or for being a nonbeliever. Regardless, divorce was never common among farming Christians, either before or after the decline of Rome.[34]

When Teutonic peoples overran Roman soil, they brought customs of their own. Divorce and polygyny were permitted among the ruling classes of prefeudal Germany. Pre-Christian Celtic and Anglo-Saxon peoples also allowed divorce and remarriage. Given the genetic payoffs of polygyny for men, it is no surprise that those with money took several wives. But what evidence is available suggests that the rate of divorce was low among European peasant farmers during the dark centuries following the fall of Rome.[35]

During the ninth century feudalism spread across Europe from its birthplace in France. As was customary in this system, feudal lords granted land to their vassals in exchange for allegiance and military duty. Each vassal then subgranted his lands to tenants in return for special services. Theoretically, vassals and tenants "held" these homesteads rather than owning them, but in actuality vassals and tenants passed these land grants—and the land—from generation to generation within their families. Under feudalism, therefore, marriage continued to be the only way most men and women could acquire soil and secure it for their heirs.

European couples could have a marriage annulled on grounds of adultery, impotence, leprosy, or consanguinity—which the rich and the well connected indeed did.[36] A spouse could also leave a mate if a properly constituted court pronounced a judicial separation that ordered partners to live apart. But this agreement carried a restriction: neither party was permitted to remarry.[37] In that case, who was to look after the goods, the lands, the animals, the house? Without a mate, a farmer could not make ends meet. In feudal Europe only the rich could afford to divorce a spouse.

Permanent monogamy. What nature and economics had prescribed for plowmen, Christian leaders sanctified. Augustine is generally thought to be the earliest church leader to regard marriage as a holy sacrament, but as the centuries passed, most Christian authorities came to agree with him. Divorce became impossible under any circumstances for members of the Roman Catholic church.[38] Although Catholic doctrine continued to make provisions for annulment and separation, lifelong marriage—a requisite of farm living—became a mandate straight from God.

With the rise of cities and trade in Europe in the tenth and eleventh centuries, women entered all sorts of occupations. In medieval London in the 1300s women were textile dealers, grocers, barber-surgeons, silk workers, bakers, beer makers, servants, embroiderers, shoemakers, jewelers, hatmakers, and craftsmen of many other kinds. Not surprisingly, some women like the Wife of Bath, Chaucer's bawdy entrepreneur, married five husbands in succession. But she was exceptional. A woman normally worked along with her spouse; she was socially subservient to him too. In fact, a woman's business debts were her husband's responsibility—a woman was not "a free and lawful person."[39] Predictably divorce was uncommon in medieval European cities.

This pattern of low divorce persisted. After the Reformation marriage became a civil contract, rather than a sacrament, for Protestants. So beginning in the 1600s women in non-Catholic countries could obtain a divorce from civil authorities.[40] In fact, divorce rates clearly fluctuated throughout the centuries following Christ's call for permanent monogamy. Where married men and women *could* leave each other, they did. But divorce rates remained notably low in Scandinavia and the British Isles, across the farmlands of Germany, France, the Low Countries, Spain, and Italy, through Hungary and the other eastern European cultures, in Russia, Japan, China, and India, and in Moslem farm societies of North Africa until the Industrial Revolution began to erode farm life.[41]

And when a spouse died (and where remarriage was permitted), a farmer took a new bride. Men who owned land often wed a few days after the mourning period ended. Remarriage by widows was widely discouraged in preindustrial European farming cultures, perhaps because this jeopardized the pattern of inheritance. But a great many women took a new husband anyway.

The realities of farm life required pairing.

Not all of our farming ancestors believed in God. Not all of these men and women were happily wed. Not all were excited about re-marriage either. But the vast majority of these people lived by the sun and by the soil. These farming men and women were tethered to their land and to one another—forever.

Not until factories emerged behind the barns of agricultural Europe and America did men and women start to regain their inde-pendence. Now patterns of sex and love and marriage begin to swing forward to the past.

~16~

Future Sex
Forward to the Past

And the end of all our exploring
Will be to arrive where we started
And know the place for the first time.

—*T. S. Eliot,* Four Quartets

"Thus the sum of things is ever being replenished and mortals live one and all by give and take. Some races wax and others wane, and in a short space the tribes of living things are changed, and like runners hand on the torch of life."[1] Lucretius, the Roman poet, spoke of the unbrokenness of human nature—those dispositions that emerged with our nativity and can be seen in men and women around the world today. Among them is our human reproductive strategy, the way we mate and reproduce.

Day by decade by century our ancestors fell in love, paired, philandered, abandoned each other, and paired again, then settled down as they got older or had more young—selecting for this blueprint of human romantic life. Not everyone conformed to this multipart sexual script. Individuals differed in the past as they do today and will two thousand years from now. But these natural patterns prevail around the world. Stomp as culture may, she will not wipe them out.

Culture can, however, change the incidence of adultery and divorce, the *number* of people who play out this ancient text. Farm living, for example, produced permanent monogamy in our elastic tribe. Will American divorce rates go up and up?[2] Will marriage survive? What kinds of families will we see? Where are we headed now?

As you know, all sorts of sociological, psychological, and demographic forces contribute to divorce rates. "Nomadism" is one. The vast majority of us have moved away from home; our parents live in different cities, often with new partners. So the wide network of family and community support that couples need when times are tough has vanished, increasing the likelihood of divorce. Those who choose partners with different habits, different values, different interests, and different leisure activities are more likely to divorce. Urbanism and secularism are associated with marital dissolution. The contemporary emphasis on individualism and self-fulfillment has also contributed to the rising incidence of divorce.

But of all the major factors that promote marital instability, perhaps the most powerful in America today can be summed up in two words: working women.[3] Divorce rates are high in marriages where the husband's income is markedly lower than the wife's.[4] Men in higher socioeconomic classes maintain more stable marriages because they tend to have more money than their spouses. And generally women with a good education and a high-paying job divorce more readily.[5]

Money spells freedom. Working women have more of it than those who mind the house. And demographers regularly cite this correlation between working women and high divorce rates.

This is not to blame working wives for the high American divorce rate. Although 60 percent of today's divorces are filed by women, demographers will never know who actually leaves whom. But where women work outside the home and bring back staples, luxuries, or money, people caught in difficult relationships can leave each other. And they do.

The Road to Modern Divorce

The Industrial Revolution launched this trend of more women in the workplace. Tracing this single phenomenon in the United States explains much about the pulse of modern family life.

As soon as hamlets of European settlers began to dot the Atlantic coast, American women began to make money outside the home by selling their surplus soap, their jars of raspberry preserves, their scented candles, and home-baked pies. A few spinsters set up shops to sell books or imported clothes. Some widows became innkeepers or land agents. But the vast majority of women kept a home.

By 1815, however, textile mills had begun to rise behind the cherry trees and chicken yards and some young women had begun to leave home for factory work. They sought regular pay and shorter work hours—time and money to spend thumbing through catalogs for store-bought clothes. Even married women began to take home piecework for extra cash. America was turning industrial. And around the middle of the nineteenth century the divorce rate started to rise.

Divorce rates have increased by fits and starts ever since. In the mid-1800s cheap labor—immigrant men—stole women's jobs. This vast new work force, the flight of American men from the farm into the factory, the belief that working women drive men's wages down, and the conviction that more children produce a larger tax base, a stronger military, a larger consumer market, and more bodies in church on Sunday then popularized the dictum "A woman's place is in the home."[6] By 1900 only about 20 percent of the women were in the labor force, most of them immigrants, youths, and singles. Nevertheless, more married women worked than in preceding decades—and divorce rates rose some more.

The twentieth century saw a periodic escalation of these social trends launched by the industrial age: more working women, more divorce.[7] With one exception. America's emergence as a superpower after World War II brought an era of marital stability some tend to think of as a golden age.

Actually the 1950s was the most unusual decade of our century. Millions of women left the labor market as war veterans returned home and claimed their jobs in industry. Tuition loans, cheap life insurance for servicemen, government-guaranteed morgages, tax advantages for married couples, and the expanding economy provided economic opportunities for postwar husbands. These young men and women had also grown up during the Great Depression, when family life was particularly turbulent. They valued a stable home.

So in the 1950s Americans settled down. Adlai Stevenson summed up the times in 1955, advising graduating women of Smith College to "influence man and boy" through the "humble role of housewife."[8]

America took Stevenson's advice. Homemaking became fashionable. Women's magazines warned brides of the dangers of mixing work with motherhood. Psychiatrists described women with careers as struggling with "penis envy." And social critics proclaimed that mothering and keeping house were women's natural roles. Anthropologist Ashley Montagu delivered the coup de grace, saying, "No woman with a husband and small children can hold a full-time job and be a good homemaker at one and the same time."[9]

Not surprisingly, men and women married younger in the 1950s than in any other twentieth-century decade; 20.2 was the median age for women and 22.6 for men.[10] The divorce rate remained unusually steady. Remarriage rates declined. And the birthrate rose to its twentieth-century high—the baby boom. In 1957 the bumper crop of infants peaked; the spreading suburbs became a cradle.

"Clap hands, clap hands until Daddy comes home, because Daddy's got money and Mommy's got none." This nursery rhyme became obsolete in the early 1960s, when historic trends sparked by the Industrial Revolution resumed: more working women, more divorce. The wide use of new kinds of contraceptives like "the pill," as well as several other forces, could have played a role.[11] But demographers point to young wives as a key factor in soaring rates of marital instability.

Many of these women, however, were not looking for careers.

They wanted pink-collar jobs, positions to supplement the family income or buy a dishwasher, a washing machine and dryer, an automobile, or a TV set. Their goal: the good life. And American employers embraced them. Here were women who spoke English, women who could read and write, women willing to take part-time, go-nowhere, dead-end, boring jobs. As anthropologist Marvin Harris wrote of the times, "With the generation of immigrant coolies fading from the scene, the dormant white American housewife was the service-and-information employer's sleeping beauty."[12]

You know what happened next; the women's movement erupted. More important to our story, America resumed its modern course: between 1960 and 1983 the number of working women doubled.[13] Between 1966 and 1976 the divorce rate doubled too.[14] And in 1981 remarriage rates hit a modern high.[15]

After many centuries of permanent monogamy among our farming forebears, the primitive human pattern of marriage, divorce, and remarriage had emerged again.

Will this spiraling divorce rate ever end? Demographer Richard Easterlin thinks the divorce rate is now stabilizing, although his critics disagree. Easterlin predicts that in the 1990s America will return to another era like the 1950s—marked by earlier marriage, more children, and less divorce.[16]

Easterlin points out that behind the baby boom came a baby bust generation, born in the late 1960s and 1970s. And he reasons that because there are fewer people in this bust cohort, its young men will get into their preferred colleges, land better jobs, and advance up the corporate ladder faster in the 1990s. Because these young men will secure good incomes, they will be able to afford to marry earlier and have more children. And because they will have financial security and larger families, they will divorce less readily. Hence Easterlin thinks that the trends of the 1950s will repeat themselves.

We will see. After a divorce peak in 1979 and 1981, divorce rates did decrease slightly, and they have remained relatively stable since 1986.[17] So Easterlin may be proven right. But he has based his predictions on the coming scarcity of young men. I would add that an inbred characteristic of human nature, in conjunction with a fluke of contemporary American demography, will also contribute to marital stability.

Risk of divorce is greatest among men and women in their twenties.[18] Because our newspapers and magazines regularly write about people who divorce in middle age, we tend to think that most people divorce while in their thirties, fourties, or fifties. Not so. As you recall from chapter 5, divorce is for the young. With advancing age, your chances of divorcing becomes less and less.

This simple fact of human nature takes on unusual significance when coupled with the reality that the boomers have come of age. A staggering seventy-six million babies were born in the United States between 1946 and 1964. The bulge. These baby boomers are traveling through American society like a pig moving through a python— visibly changing our culture as they get older. When the boomers were young, advertisers invented baby-proof bottles for medicine shelves. When they were teenagers, rock 'n' roll music became the rage. When they entered their twenties, the sexual revolution (and the drug revolution) occurred. And now that the boomers are in their thirties and early forties, day care, working women, and abortion are major issues in the news.

So what the boomers do, America seems to do. And next the boomers will settle down. Why? Because these boomers are way past the age of highest divorce risk. Many are having children too— further reducing their likelihood of parting. As Margaret Mead once said, "The first relationship is for sex; the second is for children; the third is for companionship." The boomers seem to be entering this final state, searching for a soul mate. Most will marry or remarry and remain together. It's in their genes.

And as tiny aging boomer families seed across America, these couples may help usher in about two decades of relative marital stability.

Through the Looking Glass of Prehistory

"If you can look into the seeds of time and say, which grain will grow, and which will not, speak then to me," Shakespeare wrote. Predicting the future is dangerous. But the human animal has been built by evolution to do certain things more easily than others. Using our prehistory as a guide, I will venture a few more guesses about the future of male/female relationships. What can the past say about tomorrow?

Women will continue to work.

Sociologist Eli Ginzberg recently hailed the entry of women into the work force as "the single most outstanding event of our century."[19] But are working women really so astonishing? Female chimpanzees work. Female gorillas, orangutans, and baboons work. For millennia, hunting-gathering women worked. On the farm women worked. The housewife is more an invention of privileged people in ranked societies than a natural role of the human animal. The double-income family is part of our human heritage.

So if the nineties woman retreats to keeping house, as some predict, she will, I suspect, be no more than another blip on demographic charts—as she was in the 1950s. From the anthropological perspective, working women are here to stay, tomorrow and a thousand years from now.

What more can yesterday say about tomorrow?

I do. I do. I do. "Marriage," Voltaire said, "is the only adventure open to the cowardly." Indeed, Americans participate with gusto. Today over 90 percent of all American men and women eventually wed. And although our newspapers tell us that fewer men and women are willing to take the plunge, marriage rates have changed very little through our history. In fact, the percentage of "never married" people was almost the same in 1989 as in 1890, almost a hundred years ago.[20]

Americans aren't even marrying any later—as we are often told.[21] In 1990 the median age at which a bride wed was 23.9 and her groom's age was 26.1; in 1890 a woman married at the median age of 22.0 and a man wed at 26.1.[22] Because Americans tend to compare present marriage patterns with those of the 1950s, when men and women did indeed wed much earlier, we think the current marriage age is a new phenomenon. It is not. Furthermore, despite claims that marriage is passé, marriage is a badge of *Homo sapiens.*

To bond is human. This drive evolved some four million years ago—and if we survive as a species, it should be with us four million years from now.

Women will continue to have fewer children too—another hall-mark of our past. Large families are contrary to human nature. !Kung women and mothers in other traditional societies bear about four or five babies each, but only about two offspring live to adulthood. Thus families were small during our long nomadic ancestry. On the farm, however, infants were cheap to raise, and little hands were needed in the gardens, fields, and barns. So in the early 1800s American women bore, on average, seven to eight infants. Only with industrial-ization did birthrates begin to slide as urban parents began to see children as more expensive.[24]

Today American women bear an average of 1.8 infants that live to maturity.[25] Thus, as children have became unnecessary as farm-hands, women are reverting to a more natural breeding pattern—small families.

Why should this pattern change?

Women have begun to space their children farther apart as well.[26] As you know, in societies where women gather or garden for a living, they tend to bear their young about every four years. This gives the mother uninterrupted time with her infant before she bears a second child. Today this trait, wide birth spacing, is returning.

Bravo. Several studies indicate that children in smaller families achieve higher test scores in school. They advance farther up the education pyramid. And they get more attention from their parents as they mature.[27] Wider birth spacing is healthy for parents too. Men and women were not built by evolution to cope with two in-fants simultaneously. Having fewer children at greater intervals should not only increase their educational potential but reduce the incidence of child abuse among parents who cannot deal with the problems of rearing more than one youngster at a time.

To review, then. Knowing what we do of human nature and the forces of modern culture, we may plausibly propose that, as the twenty-first century begins, our ancient human reproductive script will remain basically unaltered: young couples will fall in love and form pair-bonds; many will then leave each other and find new mates. The older people get, the more children they produce, and the longer they remain together, the more likely spouses will be to mate for life. Women and men will continue to marry later than in the 1950s and have fewer children, more widely spaced apart. Women will continue to work outside the home, keeping divorce rates relatively high. Serving to counterbalance this trend will be all the couples who marry later and all the boomers who settle down. Hence relative marital stability should reign.

This is not to suggest that the boomers or any of the rest of us will return to the life of TV's Ozzie and Harriet, the consummate 1950s couple. On the contrary, in 1987 only 10 percent of all American families were of the traditional agrarian type, in which the father brought home all of the income and the mother stayed home to rear the children. Today mothers go to work. And some observers say we are entering an age of new kinds of partnerships.

We are not. Take hypergamy, for example. This practice of "marrying up" is indeed dying out. On the farm a girl's primary goal was to marry well; marriage was her only source of economic and social gain. But today a woman's career path is marked by her education and her job. Women still tend to marry men with higher salaries, because men still generally make more money. But women no longer *need* to marry up to get ahead. They can choose partners for companionship and not for financial and social gain.

Is this so very new? Throughout our hunting-gathering past, women and men undoubtedly also wanted to marry well. And certainly spouses were somewhat dependent on each other to make ends meet. But a woman's partner was not her entire economic and social future; she had her kin, her friends, her own productive and socially valuable livelihood. So in our ancient past, women in most societies were able to chose their partners without worrying about upward mobility—just as more and more women have begun to do again today.

Perhaps as hypergamy declines, we will see more older wives with younger husbands and growing numbers of men and women marrying into different ethnic, religious, economic, or social groups.

Commuter marriages are not altogether new either. Today it is common to know a woman working in New York who is married to a man who lives in Boston or Chicago. These relationships have both perquisites and drawbacks. Some aging boomers with high-power jobs find commuter marriages a relief—at first. Partners can ease into the commitment. Neither spouse's career is threatened. No property needs to be melded. And some boomers say that commuting keeps the marriage fresh.

From an anthropological perspective, they are partly correct. The human animal is not built to live with a mate cheek by jowl around the clock. Among many traditional peoples, spouses often do not even interact until they retire to share their thoughts before they sleep. Moreover, men go off hunting for days, whereas women leave home to visit relatives for weeks. These geographic barriers can enliven a relationship. They also help modern couples separate work from pleasure—creating "dating time," unencumbered hours when spouses can leave their office troubles on the desk and court.

But commuting does run contrary to other natural human tendencies. Young couples need to spend time together to establish their roles, their jokes, their intimacies, their goals. Commuter marriages inhibit this bonding process. Older people suffer the consequences of commuting too. As a friend in his mid-fifties said to me, "In the get-ahead years you are always thinking about tomorrow. But as you age, you become more interested in today. You want to come home at night and share your thoughts with your sweetheart this evening, not next weekend." Another problem with commuting is the likelihood of philandering; the human animal has a taste for infidelity that commuter marriages facilitate.

In the jazz age of the 1920s, "advanced" social theorists suggested that men and women engage in "visiting marriages"—that couples should maintain separate households and meet by appointment only.[28] A few did. So commuter marriages are not new. They were around in the 1920s and they were probably prevalent a million years ago.

"Living in Sin"

In her famous *Redbook* article of July 1966, Margaret Mead proposed that Americans should forge another seemingly unconventional wedding pattern: marriage "in two steps."[29]

Mead suggested that a young couple with no immediate plans to reproduce should first make an "individual marriage," a legal tie that excluded bearing children, did not imply a lifelong commitment, and had no economic consequences should the couple part. Mead recommended that when this couple decided to produce young, they enter a "parental marriage," a legal relationship that confirmed a long-term bond and made formal provisions for their children should they divorce.

In the 1960s, Mead's proposal was considered avant-garde. But a version of the first part of this two-step marriage erupted like a fumarole in the 1970s—"living together." Numbers more than tripled between 1970 and 1981; what had been scandalous became routine. Interestingly, 60 percent of these relationships eventually lead to the altar.[30] It is difficult to judge the effect of trial marriages on divorce, however, because the available data conflict. In some studies these live-in partnerships are associated with more divorce; in others the reverse is true.[31] It is entirely possible that premarital living arrangements are not an important factor in the incidence of divorce.

Sociologists know little about these live-in partnerships except that they show no signs of ceasing. I am not surprised. Trial marriages are probably as old as humanity itself.

An essential ingredient of Mead's marriage plan has been forgotten, though: American couples who go on to the second step often make no provisions for their forthcoming children in case of divorce. We do not like prenuptial agreements. And here we are at loggerheads with our prehistory.

Long before their wedding day, spouses in many traditional societies know exactly what rights they have to the house, the land, the children. A Navajo child, for example, is born into his or her mother's clan, so everybody knows who "owns" the infant should the couple part. Land and goods are not negotiable either. Navajo women own their own property; men own theirs. As a result, despite all the traumas of divorce, there are no squabbles over who owns what.

Not so among most Americans. At marriage we generally merge

our goods. And we are so caught up with romantic emotions that we refuse to anticipate separation or make the most cursory agreements about the future of our children should the marriage fail.

This cocktail of sentimentality and impracticality becomes flammable at the time of divorce. Judges, bailiffs, lawyers, detectives, mediators, property assessors, realtors, artists that airbrush faces out of family albums—the individuals entangled in an American divorce can be legion. From greeting cards to therapists to tax experts, an indefatigable "divorce industry" thrives in America. Anthropologist Paul Bohannan thinks we should convert this immense enterprise into a "well-family industry."[32] Starting at the altar with a prenuptial agreement, Mead might add.

The "remarriage industry" is also booming.[33] Our health, sports, travel, and singles clubs, support groups, therapists and counselors, self-improvement books, women's magazines, dating services, and want ads are all tied to our search for "him" or "her." Despite some stabilizing of marriage in the 1990s, some 50 percent of all Americans who marry will probably divorce. So these divorce and remarriage industries should flourish. The old custom of matchmaking may even spring back into vogue.

Prisoners of the Present Tense

So today women work. They have fewer children, more widely spaced apart. Women no longer consider marriage a career. Some engage in trial marriages. Some spouses commute between two homes. And all these patterns have antecedents in early stages of human evolution. But what about our single parents and "blended" families? Are these really new, or are we yet again prisoners of the present tense?

In 1987 some 20 percent of all American families with children were headed by single parents; some 90 percent of these were run by mothers and almost 10 percent by fathers. The number of these single-parent households has doubled since the early 1970s—not only because of soaring divorce rates but also because more women are having children out of wedlock.[34] One out of every four boys and girls spends some time in a single-parent home. Is this unusual?

Yes and no. Less than a century ago single mothers customarily gave up their young to orphanages or relatives; as recently as 1940 one in ten American children lived with *neither* parent. These days only one in thirty-seven youngsters lives in a foster home. One parent should be an improvement over none. Moreover, many single-parent families are not permanent. The vast majority of divorced parents remarry; about half do so within three years of their divorce.[35] So the average length of time a child of divorced parents spends in a single-parent home is about four years.[36] These single-parent households, then, are generally temporary arrangements.

Moreover, single parenting is nothing new. Given that divorce rates were probably quite high among our hunting-gathering forebears, as they are in many traditional societies today, single parents are almost certainly another throwback to the past.

So are all of our blended families. Over one in six American children live in a family with a stepparent; many live with stepbrothers and stepsisters as well. And here history speaks loud and clear. Because more men and women died younger in the past, nuclear families actually remained intact for *shorter* periods.[37] Thus remarriage, blended families, and stepparents were all quite common a hundred years ago.

Is the family an endangered species? Absolutely not. These remarriage links, these trellises of marriage ties, were not new in the nineteenth century; they were not new among our forebears who first kindled flame in the caves of Africa over a million years ago. Divorce, single parents, remarriage, stepparents, and blended families are as old as the human animal—creations of a distant prehistoric age. As Paul Bohannan summed it up, "The family is the most adaptable of all human institutions, changing with every social demand. The family does not break in a storm as oak or pine trees do, but bends before the wind like the bamboo tree in Oriental tales and springs up again."[38]

New Kin

So what is genuinely new? From an anthropological perspective the only remarkably novel phenomenon of contemporary family life is the prevalence of single and divorced people, and of widows and widowers living by themselves. "Soup for one" could be the motto of the day.

Actually, the number of single American adults has not changed in the past one hundred years. Some 41 percent of all Americans over age fifteen are single today; 46 percent of all people over age fifteen were single in 1900.[39] But in our American past and in *all* traditional societies, single parents, young singles, and single widows and widowers lived with relatives; they did not live alone. Yet, in 1990, nearly twenty-three million Americans lived by themselves. (Interestingly, the median length of time that men and women spend living by themselves is 4.8 years.)

This is new. Moreover, this modern habit is generating what might be a truly modern family type: the association. Associations, anthropologists say, are composed of unrelated friends.[40] Members talk to one another regularly and share their triumphs and their troubles. They assemble for minor holidays like birthdays and Labor Day. And they help care for one another when one is sick. These people have a network of friends that they consider family. This network often breaks down, however, during major festivals like Christmas when people join their genetic relatives. No wonder holidays can be so stressful. Displaced from their daily family world, people find themselves out of touch, out of place.

So for the first time in human history some Americans and other industrialized peoples have begun to pick their relatives—forging a brand-new web of kin based on friendship instead of blood. These associations may eventually spawn new kinship terms, new types of insurance policies, new paragraphs in health plans, new rent agreements, new types of housing developments, and many other legal and social plans.

What else is really new?

Well, we are seeing a revolution in psychiatry that could change the face of love. The brain has been a mystery for centuries; scientists still call it the black box. But now we have begun to unravel the mechanisms of the mind. As was discussed earlier in the book, psychiatrists Michael Liebowitz, Hector Sabelli, and others think infatuation is associated with natural amphetamines that pool in the emotional centers of the brain, while attachment is linked to morphine-like substances, the endorphins. And a few psychiatrists have begun to treat lovesick men and women with drugs that act as antidotes to some of these brain chemicals.

Could we cure the "playboy syndrome" with pills? Could new elixirs eventually help "attachment junkies" break unsatisfactory partnerships? Perhaps scientists will refine their understanding of attraction and attachment during the coming century and bottle love potions or temporary cures. If so, you can be sure that would-be lovers and jilted, pining sweethearts will buy these concoctions by the jug—either to fuel obsession or snuff passion out.

"Love magic" sold a thousand years ago; it will sell a thousand years from now.

Etienne-Emile Baulieu, the French physician, has sparked a revolution in birth control with his development of the drug RU-486. At last, we may have a safe, efficient abortion pill—an antidote to unwanted childbearing that would reinforce several of the aforementioned modern social trends.

But RU-486 is not legal or available in America. Largely because of widespread opposition by prolife groups, it may take several years before RU-486 becomes widely available—at your doctor's office. But when have Americans ever waited for legal drugs? If RU-486 is not legalized, some version of it will almost certainly be a black-market item in the United States by the year 2000.

If so, teenagers will buy it like a balloon ride off a burning building. Our teens have been duped by evolution. In prehistoric times, puberty occurred around age sixteen or seventeen for girls—followed by at least two years of irregular ovulation, a phase known as adolescent subfertility. So throughout our long hunting-gathering past, teenagers could copulate for several years without the risk and costs of pregnancy. Today, however, our fatty diet and sedentary life-style have raised the critical body weight and tricked the body into early puberty. Hence the median age at menarche in many Western cultures is around thirteen now, as opposed to sixteen in 1900.[41]

No wonder our young get pregnant long before they should. They are designed by nature to experiment with sex and love, yet their natural mechanisms for birth control are gone. If RU-486 becomes a black-market drug, however, American teenagers may risk solving their problem of pregnancy by themselves—no matter what America's abortion laws maintain. And this reproductive option should fuel trends toward more working women, fewer children, more divorce, and more remarriage.

Rise of the Entrepreneur

The United States is at the confluence of several business trends that should affect women, men, and love. Foremost, many of the baby boomers are going into business for themselves. These men and women joined the work force in their twenties, and now many feel stuck in middle management. They have the training, the experience, the networks, and the wish to break away from conventional employment. Corporate America would like to see them go. Businesses are suffering from a bloated middle management. Three million American executives lost their jobs in the 1980s, and corporate "down scaling" is likely to continue.[42]

And as corporations push the boomers out, the service industries are sucking the boomers in. Our senior citizens, working women, all of the singles, even the large corporations buy a host of services. Not just day care and take-out restaurants but masseuses, decorators, and the like; some harried careerists even employ specialists to clean and organize their closets.

So as the futurist Marvin Cetron sees it, "By the turn of the century, most of our middle-sized institutions will have vanished but thousands of tiny companies will be flourishing beneath the feet of giants."[43] And facilitating the growth of all these small businesses are a host of new technological innovations, such as home computers and fax machines. The timing is perfect; Alvin Toffler's vision of the "electronic cottage" has come of age.

Globalization is a second major shift in business. Companies are spreading their offices around the world. These businesses need "culture brokers," individuals who can move effectively between different societies with different manners and different languages.

How will these trends, entrepreneurism and globalization, affect romance?

They favor women.

As you recall from chapter 10, women are, on the average, more verbal than men. They are also better at picking up all sorts of nonverbal cues. And they are outstanding at networking. Before the computer, before the knitting needle, even before the bow and arrow, women also developed another business tool—arbitration. Remember Big Mama, the queen of the chimpanzee colony at the Arnhem Zoo? Mama was the group arbiter; she regularly broke up fights and soothed hurt feelings after the incessant political skirmishes that plagued this chimp community. For millennia ancestral women must have played a similar role, manipulating their peers with their wits and tongues, rather than their fists. Negotiating is a female skill.

A last strength of the twenty-first-century woman will be her age. In traditional societies women become more assertive and self-assured as they get older; they generally become more powerful in political, religious, and social life as well. Undoubtedly this is because they are less tied to the chores of raising children. But as I have mentioned, biology may play a role. With menopause, levels of estrogen decline and the body's dosage of testosterone becomes unmasked—and testosterone is often found in the company of authority and rank.

"There is no greater power in the world," Margaret Mead once said, "than the zest of a post-menopausal woman." With words, with nonverbal acuity, with networking and negotiating skills—and also with unleashed testosterone—women will probably become increasingly visible in modern national and international business life.

And powerful working women will almost certainly sustain the long-term trends initiated by the Industrial Revolution: later marriage, fewer children, more divorce, and more remarriage.

Our problems with sex in the office will probably get worse, for here we are once again at loggerheads with our prehistory. For millennia, men and women did separate tasks. As a result, it is sometimes awkward for the sexes to work in close proximity; we tend to flirt. No wonder the workplace has long been a bog of sexual harassment. Some of this tomfoolery is useful, of course; a few office affairs turn into happy marriages. But I am referring to the sexual overtures that are not welcome.

Mead suggested an antidote to office lechery; she proposed we institute taboos. Periodic consciousness-raising sessions are a good beginning. At these meetings the staff and management assemble to learn about the four-part flirt, how not to smile, the power of the gaze, the subtle messages people cast with touch, gait, body posture, vocal tone, clothing, and use of space—and all the other components of sexual harassment. Despite all the jokes about the meeting, some standards will have been set.

Office mediators, trained specialists employed to hear sexual complaints and empowered to recommend specific actions, may also become commonplace. These policemen do not always deter predators or save the prey. But at the very least, each peacekeeper will stress the policy of the company and be a beacon flashing: "Warning! Management does not condone unfair play." Another deterrent probably will be fear. As more and more cases of sexual harassment hit the newspapers, as more politicians, CEOs, and well-known personalities are publicly admonished, and as laws become enacted and enforced, sexual harassment might be contained.

I doubt that it will disappear, however; the genders were built to court—even when it leads to trouble. The only really new development may be that more of the offenders will be women.

Hundreds of other forces will affect our marriages. More flexible work hours, part-time employment, job sharing, and parenting leave for new mothers and fathers should vary our romantic lives. Working wives will certainly not be the kinds of companions that homemakers have been. Conversations will be different. Styles of arguing may change. Who pays for dinner may shift. But I doubt that many wives will be able to enlist their husbands into doing more household chores. As I mentioned earlier, around the world women do the vast majority of housework, in cultures where they are economically powerful and in those where they are not.

I suspect that spouses will continue to allot household duties according to their personal rules. And the rise of economically powerful women will not dramatically alter these arrangements.

Forward to the Past

So we are creatures living in a sea of currents that pull and stretch our family lives. Upon the ancient blueprint for serial monogamy and clandestine adultery, our culture casts its own design. The fact that America is getting older will tend to stabilize divorce rates. That we are marrying later than we did in the 1950s is another factor that makes for stable divorce rates. However, working women and commuter marriages should counter these stabilizing influences, keeping divorce rates relatively high. And other phenomena such as trial marriages, single mothers, smaller families, and blended families should be commonplace in the decades of tomorrow.

But none of these modern social trends are new. Instead, they have come across the centuries, up from primitives who wandered onto the plains of Africa at least four million years ago.

Of all the social changes that are occurring, however, the most interesting to me is the following. We are shedding the agricultural tradition and, in some respects, returning to our nomadic roots.

Few of us still live in the house where we grew up. Rather, many of us have several places we call home—our parent's house, the office, our own residence, and perhaps a vacation spot. We migrate between them. We no longer grow our own food. We now hunt and gather in the grocery store and then carry home our catch—as Twiggy and *Homo erectus* did over a million years ago. (I am not surprised that we like fast foods either, or eat between meals here and there as we move through the day; our ancestors certainly ate as they marched along.) We commute to work again. And we have a loose network of friends and relatives, many of whom live far away.

These are habits from our past.

We are shedding the sexual attitudes of farm life too. In preindustrial Europe, a wedding often marked a merger of property and an alliance between families. So marriages had to be stable and permanent. This necessity is gone. A woman's job was to bear her husband's seed and raise his young; hence our agrarian forerunners required virginity at marriage. This custom is gone. Many of our farming ancestors carefully arranged their marriages. This practice is largely gone. They banned divorce. This is gone. They had a double standard for adultery. This has changed. And they celebrated two marital mottoes: "Honor thy husband" and "Till death us do part." These, too, are disappearing.

For the past several thousand years, most farm women had only three basic options: to be uneducated, subservient housewives; to be cloistered nuns; to be courtesans, prostitutes, or concubines. Men, on the other hand, held the sole responsibility for the family income and welfare of the young.

Now vast numbers of women work outside the home. We have double-income families. We are more nomadic. And we have a growing equality between the sexes. In these respects, we are returning to traditions of love and marriage that are compatible with our ancient human spirit.

Notes

The citation numbers in each chapter refer to specific sources, groups of sources or footnotes that appear in the endnotes. To find the complete bibliographical reference for any source turn from the endnotes to the bibliography. If you would like to know the source for data not referenced, please contact me at the American Museum of Natural History, New York City.

1 Courting: *Games People Play*

1. ETHOLOGY: The word *ethology* comes from the Greek *ethos,* meaning "manner" or "behavior" (see Gould 1982). Ethology is generally considered to be the observation and analysis of animal behavior in the natural environment. It is based on the premise that characteristic behavior patterns of a species evolved in the same way that physical traits evolved, through selection and evolution. Darwin laid the groundwork for the science of ethology with his examination of motor patterns, such as snarling and other facial gestures, in different species (see Darwin [1872] 1965).

2. For cross-species similarities in body language and facial expressions, see Givens 1986, 1983; Goodall 1986; Van Hooff 1971; Darwin [1872] (1965).

3. Eibl-Eibesfeldt 1989; Hess 1975.

4. De Waal 1987.

5. Smuts 1985, 1987.

6. Ekman 1985.

7. Darwin [1872] 1965.

8. Ekman, Sorenson, and Friesen 1969; Ekman 1980, 1985; Goleman 1981. CARTOGRAPHY OF THE FACE: Using anatomy texts, cameras, and a mirror, psychologist Paul Ekman and his colleagues learned to contract their individual facial muscles at will. When they were unsure which muscles they were using, they inserted specially wired needles into specific muscles to

isolate the activity of each. Ekman reports that the human "open smile" is among the least complicated facial expressions. It takes only the "lip corner puller," the "dimpler," and the "cheek raiser" to make our wide, inviting grin. The ninety-six major variations of anger use several hundred different muscle combinations, depending on their intensity. See Ekman 1985; Goleman 1981.

9. Field et al. 1982; Trevathan 1987.

10. Givens 1983; Perper 1985.

11. HUMAN SPATIAL TERRITORIES: People divide space into four distinct types. For Americans "intimate space" is generally about eighteen inches around the head. You permit only intimate companions and pets into this private territory for any length of time. "Personal space" is the two to four feet surrounding you; you allow friends to enter here. "Social space," about four to eight feet away, you use when you interact with others during work or social gatherings. "Public spaces" are all the areas beyond nine to ten feet from you. Different societies measure the territory around the body differently, but they all have a code for proximity. See Hall 1966.

12. CONVERSATIONAL COURTING TACTICS: As a couple begin to talk, they search for common interests and try to establish compatibility. They may test each other by disagreeing, then watch how the other handles this adversity. The goal is trust. One may reveal a weakness, yet wrap it in a positive self-image. And early in the courtship they may ask a minor favor—another test. Vital to these interactions are three subtle undercurrents. People strive to "make a good impression," they seek the attention of the other, and they revert to cooing and other babylike behaviors. All the while they try to convey a panoply of assets, including stability, self-control, intelligence, kindness, caring, acceptance, competence, reliability, bravery, humor, and, most important, availability. See Eibl-Eibesfeldt 1989.

13. TOUCH: Our ancestors were held constantly as babies and slept next to their mother's breast, so human beings are designed to live in skin contact with others. In some cultures, infants are held so continually that they never crawl; their first solo exploration of the world comes when they try to walk. As a result, we naturally like to touch and be touched unless we are trained otherwise. See Hall 1959; Montagu 1971; Morris 1971; Henley 1977.

14. Givens 1983.

15. Eibl-Eibesfeldt 1989.

16. Hall 1976.

17. Douglas 1987.

18. Whyte 1978.

19. Yerkes and Elder 1936.
20. Daly and Wilson 1983.
21. COURTSHIP FEEDING: It is possible that this courtship feeding mimics feeding between mother and infant, triggering feelings of caring and protection by the man and childlike acceptance by the woman that enhance the bonding process. See Eibl-Eibesfeldt 1989.
22. Goodall 1986; Teleki 1973a.
23. Ford and Beach 1951.
24. Ibid.
25. Jespersen [1922] 1950.

2 Infatuation: *Why Him? Why Her?*

1. Hunt 1959, 45.
2. Tennov 1979.
3. Stendhal [1822] 1975.
4. Ackerman 1990; Russell 1976; Hopson 1979.
5. PHEROMONES: The term *pheromone,* coined in 1959, can be applied to any chemical substance that a creature excretes as a signal that elicits a specific, unlearned response in other creatures. Although creatures give off pheromones as repellants and for other uses, the term *pheromone* is generally used to describe sex attractants. See Shorey 1976.
6. Hopson 1979; Ackerman 1990.
7. Gregersen 1982.
8. Cutler et al. 1986; HUMAN MALE PHEROMONES: These data on human male pheromones are speculative at present (see Wilson 1988). But the presence of a male does stimulate estrus of other species. Scientists at the Monell Cemical Senses Center suggest that "male essence" may eventually be useful in correcting certain kinds of infertility, regulating the menstrual cycle, improving the rhythm method of birth control, and alleviating some of the symptoms of menopause.
9. Forsyth 1985.
10. McClintock 1971. Those who question these data include Graham and McGrew 1980; Quadagno et al. 1981.
11. Preti et al. 1986.
12. Eibl-Eibesfeldt 1989.
13. Givens 1983.
14. Money 1986.
15. Ibid. 19.

16. SEXUAL PERVERSIONS: John Money (1986) proposes that paraphilias, or sexual perversions, begin in childhood when traumatic events curtail the normal development of erotic, sexual, and loving feeling and the child's sexual impulses are redirected toward deviant patterns of attraction and arousal. By adolescence the individual has developed an eccentric love map. These people are unable to find a partner whose love map complements theirs, so they begin to seek inappropriate partners to fulfill their drive for sexual arousal. The link between love and lust has been severed, blocked, or distorted, and the individual starts to indulge in sexual perversions. For a discussion of human sexual perversions and their etiology, see Money 1986.

17. Feinman and Gill 1978.

18. Bower 1990.

19. Ford and Beach 1951; Frayser 1985.

20. Buss 1989.

21. Shepher 1971; Spiro 1958.

22. Tennov 1979.

23. Capellanus 1959.

24. Jankowiak 1992.

25. Ibid.

26. Jankowiak and Fischer 1992.

27. Givens 1983.

28. Fehrenbacker 1988.

29. Liebowitz 1983.

30. Sabelli et al. 1990.

31. Sabelli 1991.

32. THE ROLE OF LHRH IN INFATUATION: Several other neurochemicals are probably also associated with infatuation. Among them is LHRH, or luteinizing hormone-releasing hormone. The hypothalamus produces LHRH, which then travels to the nearby pituitary. Here it triggers the production of hormones that regulate the production of estrogen and progesterone in the ovaries and androgens in the testes. In some animals LHRH also travels directly from the hypothalamus to the emotional and thinking parts of the brain, informing them when to court and copulate. The association between hypopituitarism and lack of erotic/sexual arousal suggests that this hormonal feedback loop plays a role in infatuation. See Money 1980.

33. Money and Ehrhardt 1972.

34. Money 1980, 65.

35. Liebowitz 1983, 200; Bowlby 1969.

36. OXYTOCIN AND SEXUAL AROUSAL: Undoubtedly other neurotransmitters in the brain, as well as hormones secreted by the brain, will be discovered that contribute to our human system of attachment—and detachment. Oxytocin, for example, is a peptide synthesized primarily by the hypothalamus, which lies at the base of the brain and forms part of the limbic system; it is known for its role in stimulating uterine contractions during childbirth and the production of human breast milk. Scientists now think oxytocin may also play a role in stimulating the sex drive, the drive to nuzzle and protect infants, and feelings of pleasure and satisfaction during body contact, sexual arousal, and sexual fulfillment. One study of men found that levels of oxytocin in the blood became three to five times more abundant during orgasm (Angier 1991).

3 Of Human Bonding: *Is Monogamy Natural?*

1. Daly 1978.

2. Van Valen 1973.

3. Hamilton 1980; Hamilton et al. 1981.

4. Dougherty 1955.

5. Parker, Baker, and Smith 1972.

6. ORIGIN OF TWO SEXES: There are several theories for why *two* sexes evolved. Some primitive blue-green algae have two mating types, designated + and − because the gender of neither is distinguishable. One theory holds that these algae evolved two mating types to avoid inbreeding (see Daly and Wilson 1983). The "genetic repair" theory proposes that with sexual reproduction new combinations could repair the mutational damage to DNA material that had occurred during preceding cell divisions (see Michod 1989). Another theory is known as the parasitism hypothesis. The sexes arose in the same fashion that modern viruses parasitize host cells: the virus incorporates its own DNA into the host cell; then, as the host cell reproduces itself, it replicates the DNA of the virus too. Thus the precursors of males were tiny gametes that parasitized larger female gametes. For an overview of the advantages of asexual and sexual reproduction, the costs of sexual reproduction, and theories on the origin of sexual reproduction, see Daly and Wilson 1983; Williams 1975; Maynard Smith 1978; Low 1979; Daly 1978; Michod and Levin 1987.

7. Hamilton 1964.

8. "INCLUSIVE FITNESS" AND ALTRUISM: The theory of inclusive fitness was first suggested by Darwin (1859) when he noted that natural selection may operate on the level of the family rather than on that of the individual. Inclusive fitness was anticipated again in the 1930s by the British geneticist

J. B. S. Haldane. But the theory was formally proposed in 1964 by the British population geneticist William D. Hamilton, to explain the evolution of altruism: if an ancestral man sacrificed himself to save his drowning brother, he was actually saving half of his own DNA and, thereby, some of his altruistic nature. Hence one's fitness is measured by the number of one's own genes and those of one's relatives who survive. With Hamilton's concept of inclusive fitness many other social behaviors became explicable: creatures defend a common territory; animals share and cooperate; people are nationalistic because when they help their relatives they further their own DNA (see Wilson 1975). Today inclusive fitness and the related concept of kin selection are standard means for explaining some patterns of animal behavior. See ibid.; Barish 1977; Hamilton 1964.

9. REPRODUCTIVE STRATEGIES: This adaptation of terms has been incomplete; the two variants of monogamy—monogyny and monandry—are not used to describe human marriage systems. As a result, the *separate* reproductive tactics of men and women are largely overlooked. For example, we are told that the Afikpo Ibo of eastern Nigeria are "polygynous." Some Afikpo Ibo men have several wives. But Afikpo Ibo women marry only one man at a time, monandry. So two marriage patterns occur, polygyny and monandry, depending on whether you are describing men or women. When social scientists describe a society as polygynous, they ignore the reproductive tactics of women.

10. Wittenberger and Tilson 1980, 198.

11. See Trivers 1985; Mock and Fujioka 1990; Westneat, Sherman, and Morton 1990; Hiatt 1989; Wilson and Daly, in press.

12. Bray, Kennelly, and Guarino 1975.

13. Gibbs et al. 1990.

14. Lampe 1987; Wolfe 1981.

15. DEFINITIONS OF MARRIAGE: Many anthropologists have defined marriage. Suzanne Frayser's version is a good one: "Marriage is a relationship within which a group socially approves and encourages sexual intercourse and the birth of children" (Frayser 1985, 248). Anthropologist Ward Goodenough's similar one defines the three essential components of marriage as the jural or legal dimension, the priority of sexual access, and the eligibility to reproduce (Goodenough 1970, 12).

16. Cherlin 1981.

17. Fisher 1989.

18. Murdock 1967; van den Berghe 1979; Betzig 1986.

19. Betzig 1982, 1986.

20. TIWI MARRIAGES AND THE ROLE OF WOMEN: Tiwi women are not pawns in the marriage wars of men. On the contrary, women play crucial roles in

negotiating marriages. Every son-in-law must cater to the needs of the woman who will bear his brides, and a mother-in-law can break this contract if his gifts and work are paltry. So Tiwi women are powerful nodes in the marriage system, as well as being powerful in other aspects of society. See Goodale 1971; Hart and Pilling 1960; Rohrlick-Leavitt, Sykes, and Weatherford 1975; Berndt 1981.

21. Verner and Willson 1966; Orians 1969; Borgerhoff Mulder 1990.

22. POLYGYNY AND WOMEN: Women living with co-wives are generally less fertile than women in monogamous marriages (Daly and Wilson 1978). However, among women living with polygynous husbands, the first wife often bears more children then junior co-wives do, probably because she does less strenuous work and has access to more food (Isaac and Feinberg 1982).

23. Bohannan 1985; Mealey 1985.

24. FORMS OF POLYGYNY: Males in the animal community acquire harems in at least four ways; each has parallels in humankind (Flinn and Low 1986). Polygyny is frequently found in species where the food supply, hiding places, nesting spots, or mating grounds are located in clusters. Females tend to gather at these places to feed or breed, and if a male can succeed in becoming the sole proprietor of one of these rich locations, he may acquire a harem simply by driving off other males and waiting for the females to arrive. This tactic is known as RESOURCE-DEFENSE POLYGYNY (Emlen and Oring 1977). Among the Kipsigis of Kenya, women regularly choose to marry polygynous men with large pieces of real estate (Borgerhoff Mulder 1990).

Males of some species round up a group of females and then forcibly prevent other males from courting them; this is known as FEMALE-DEFENSE POLYGYNY. If a Tiwi husband of Australia suspected a young wife of adultery, he sometimes beat her or complained to the girl's natal family. If a boy eloped with an adolescent married woman and refused to repent, an irate husband might kill the thief (Goodale 1971). This guarding behavior is reminiscent of female-defense polygyny seen in other species (Flinn and Low 1986).

Another strategy is known as MALE-DOMINANCE POLYGYNY. Male sage grouse maneuver among themselves to acquire "mating stations" on a lek (see chapter 1), from which they can be easily seen by passing females. Females then walk among them and rest in their mating stations to mate. Older, more vigorous males tend to attract most of the passing females (De Vos 1983). Among the !Kung San of the Kalahari Desert of southern Africa some men are charismatic, strong, and healthy, and they occasionally acquire two wives not with resources but with their personalities (Shostak 1981). Orangutans, moose, and bumblebees persistently seek out receptive females, mate, and move on; this is known as SEARCH POLYGYNY. A variation of this form of harem building is characteristic of truck drivers, traveling salesmen, international businessmen, and sailors who have "a wife in every port." See Flinn and Low 1986; Dickemann 1979.

25. Frayser 1985; van den Berghe 1979; Murdock and White 1969.

26. Murdock 1949, 27–28.

27. Murdock 1967; van den Berghe 1979.

28. Klein 1980.

29. Alexander 1974; Finn and Low 1986; Goldizen 1987; Jenni 1974.

30. Lancaster and Lancaster 1983.

31. NAYAR MARRIAGE CUSTOMS: The Nayar of India's Malabar Coast in Kerala have a marriage form that defies classification. These people live in households consisting of siblings and mother. The head of household is a man. A woman's first marriage is a brief ceremony; after this ritual, she does not need to socialize or even have sex with her husband. If a wife wishes to take other lovers, she is free to do so. Her husband and lovers call on her only at night; thus they are called visiting husbands. Women have anywhere from three to twelve lovers at any one time. A marriage ends when a husband no longer gives his wife gifts at annual festivals. It is essential that one or more men of the proper social group claim paternity when a "wife" becomes pregnant, although the biological father often does little more than observe the incest taboo in later life—if he knows the child is his. For the Nayar, marriage provides nothing but legitimacy for children. See Gough 1968; Fuller 1976.

32. "FREE LOVE" COMMUNES: Studies of six American communes indicate that their members do not actually practice "free love"; instead, rules about copulation are rigid and sexual and social roles are hierarchical and highly structured. See Wagner 1982; Stoehr 1979; Constantine and Constantine 1973.

33. See van den Berghe 1979.

34. Bohannan 1985.

35. POLYGYNY AND POLYANDRY—SECONDARY HUMAN REPRODUCTIVE STRATEGIES: Because polygyny provides males with genetic advantages and polyandry provides females with extra resources, some anthropologists argue that these reproductive strategies are primary reproductive tactics of humankind, that men and women endure monogamy only because men are unable to gain the resources they need to acquire harems and that women endure monogamy only because they are unable to entice several males to provide resources. Supporting this view is the ample evidence for polygyny among powerful men (Betzig 1986). But the *variant* reproductive strategy of monogamy in conjunction with adultery provides similar reproductive advantages; males have the opportunity to inseminate multiple

partners; females can garner extra resources. Moreover, *most* human beings exhibit monogamy in conjunction with adultery. So I think this is the
primary reproductive strategy of *Homo sapiens,* while polygyny and polyandry are *opportunistic, secondary* reproductive tactics.

36. Whyte 1978, 74; Frayser 1985, 269.
37. Mace and Mace 1959.

4 Why Adultery?: *The Nature of Philandering*

1. Diana, n.d.
2. Carneiro 1958.
3. WORLD PATTERNS OF ADULTERY: In 72 percent of 56 societies surveyed,
   female adultery is moderate to common (van den Berghe 1979). Of 139
   societies surveyed in the 1940s, 39 percent permitted men and women to
   have extramarital affairs either during certain holidays or festivals, with
   particular kinfolk, such as one's wife's sister or husband's brother, or under
   other special circumstances. Extramarital relations were extremely common
   in 17 of the remaining 85 cultures, and offenders were rarely punished (see
   Ford and Beach 1951). In a different study anthropologist George Murdock
   surveyed 148 societies, past and resent, and found that 120 had taboos
   against adultery, 5 freely allowed adultery, 19 allowed philandering under
   some conditions, and 4 disapproved of but did not strictly forbid sex outside
   of marriage (Murdock 1949). In all cases, however, Murdock was measuring
   adultery as sexual activity with distantly related or unrelated people. This
   distinction is important. He confirms Ford and Beach's (1951) finding that
   a substantial majority of societies allow extramarital relations with individuals in certain kin relationships. Suzanne Frayser (1985) confirms the widespread taboo against adultery with unrelated individuals too: she reports
   that 74 percent of 58 cultures forbid adultery either for the woman or for
   both sexes. She notes that punishments for adultery vary. In 83 percent of
   48 societies, both partners receive penalties for adultery; in 40 percent of
   them men and women get the same degree of chastisement; in 31 percent
   of them the man's punishment is more severe than that of his female lover.
   No society tolerates a female's dalliances while punishing males; and significantly more cultures have restrictions on women than on men. Societies
   with few prohibitions against extramarital liaisons of any kind and with a
   high degree of extramarital sexual behavior for both sexes include the Dieri
   of Australia, the Gilyak of Northeast Asia, the Hidatsa Indians of North
   Dakota, the Lesu of New Ireland, the Masai of East Africa, the Toda of
   India, the Kaingang of Brazil, and the Yapese of the Pacific (Ford and
   Beach 1951). Stephens (1963) reports that even in those cultures where
   adultery is condoned, men and women suffer from jealousy.
4. Schneider 1971.

5. Gove 1989.

6. Westermarck 1922.

7. *People* magazine 1986.

8. Bullough 1976.

9. Ibid.

10. Lampe 1987.

11. Lampe 1987; Bullough 1976.

12. Bullough 1976.

13. Song of Solomon 3:16.

14. Lawrence 1989; Foucault 1985.

15. Lampe 1987; Bullough 1976.

16. ORIGIN OF SEXUAL TERMS: By the fourth century A.D. adultery was so commonplace in Rome that officials began to fine offenders. The revenue from this taxation was apparently so great that the state built a temple to Venus with it (Bardis 1963). The terms *cunnilingus, fellatio, masturbation,* and *prostitute* all come from ancient Roman vernacular (Bullough 1976).

17. Bullough 1976; Lawrence 1989.

18. See Bullough 1976; Lawrence 1989; Brown 1988; Pagels 1988.

19. Bullough 1976, 192.

20. Lampe 1987, 26; Lawrence 1989, 125; Pagels 1988.

21. Burns 1990.

22. Lawrence 1989, 169.

23. Kinsey, Pomeroy, and Martin 1948; Kinsey et al. 1953.

24. Hunt 1974, 263.

25. Tavris and Sadd 1977.

26. Wolfe 1981.

27. Hite 1981.

28. Lawson 1988; Lampe 1987.

29. *Marriage and Divorce Today* 1987.

30. Blumstein and Schwartz 1983.

31. TIMING AND DURATION OF EXTRAMARITAL RELATIONSHIPS: The duration of extramarital relationships is difficult to establish from the literature. In one study of 200 couples, husbands maintained their extramarital affairs for an average of twenty-nine months, whereas wives sustained theirs for an average of twenty-one months (Hall 1987). Kinsey (1953) noted that about 42 percent of his sample of women engaged in extramarital coitus for a year or less, 23 percent for two to three years, and 35 percent for four years or more. But he did not say how long each affair lasted, only how long these women engaged in extramarital coitus.

A study of about 600 British men and women found that men married in the 1970s had their first extramarital relationship 5 years after wedding and that women remained faithful 4.5 years after wedding. Men married in the 1960s waited an average of 7 years; women waited an average of 8 years before they had an affair. Among those married prior to 1960, men took an extra lover an average of 11 years after wedding, whereas women waited 14.5 years (Lawson 1988).

32. Kinsey et al. 1953, 409.
33. See Bateman 1948; Trivers 1972; Symons 1979.
34. Symons 1979, v, 291.
35. Ruse 1988.
36. Kinsey, Pomeroy, and Martin 1948; Kinsey et al. 1953.
37. Kinsey, Pomeroy, and Martin 1948.
38. Shostak 1981, 271.
39. Hrdy 1981, 1986.
40. Ford and Beach 1951, 118.
41. Kinsey et al. 1953, 415.
42. Werner 1984; Bullough and Bullough 1987.
43. Gregor 1985.
44. Reichard 1950.
45. Bullough and Bullough 1987.
46. Nimuendaju 1946.
47. Beals 1946.
48. Nadel 1942.
49. Symons and Ellis 1989.
50. See Lampe 1987, 178ff.; Brown 1987; Hall 1987; Lawson 1988; Pittman 1989; Atwater 1987; Wolfe 1981, Hite 1981; Hunt 1974; Tavris and Sadd 1977; Kinsey, Pomeroy, and Martin 1948; Kinsey et al. 1953.
51. Botwin 1988.
52. Shostak 1981.
53. Lampe 1987, 199.

5 Blueprint for Divorce: *The Four-Year Itch*

1. Abu-Lughod 1987, 24.
2. Abu-Lughod 1986.
3. Farah 1984.
4. Ibid.
5. Ibid. 26.
6. Ibid. 20.

7. Murdock 1965.

8. Weisman 1988.

9. Murdock 1965; Betzig 1989.

10. MALE/FEMALE RIGHTS TO DIVORCE: In thirty of forty traditional societies surveyed by George Peter Murdock in 1950, men and women had equal rights in initiating divorce; in 10 percent of these cultures women had superior privileges regarding divorce. He concluded that divorce was generally equally accessible to both sexes (Murdock 1965). In a study of ninety-three societies Whyte confirmed this, concluding, "We find equal divorce rights by far the most common pattern" (Whyte 1978). Suzanne Frayser reported that, of forty-five societies she surveyed, 38 percent allowed both husband and wife to obtain a divorce; one or both partners had a difficult time securing a divorce in 62 percent of these cultures. In many insular Pacific societies divorce was easy to obtain for both men and women. In circum-Mediterranean societies it was more difficult for women to obtain a divorce, but in many African societies it was generally harder for men to do so. See Frayser 1985.

11. Murdock 1965, 319.

12. Betzig 1989.

13. MARRIAGE AS A REPRODUCTIVE STRATEGY: Murdock (1949) argued that because sex and reproduction could be obtained outside of marriage, economic cooperation and the division of labor between the sexes were the primary reasons for marriage. But in the forty traditional societies he surveyed in 1950, he noted that reproductive issues were prominent reasons for divorce (Murdock 1965). A survey by Frayser confirms the important role that reproduction plays in divorce—and thus in marriage. In a sample of fifty-six cultures, men divorced their wives first for reproductive problems, second for incompatibility, third for illicit sex on the wife's part. In a sample of forty-eight cultures, women abandoned their husbands most frequently because of incompatibility; second, because of failure to meet economic and domestic responsibilities; third, because of physical violence. See Frayser 1985.

14. REMARRIAGE: A survey of thirty-seven traditional peoples found that remarriage was openly allowed in 78 percent of these societies; where remarriage was difficult to obtain (in 22 percent of these cultures), it was generally harder for the woman to remarry than for the man (Frayser 1985). Remarriage occurred in preindustrial western European societies, but it was regularly associated with the death of a spouse, rather than divorce, since divorce was banned by the Roman Catholic church. Common to several of these peoples was the *charivari tradition,* the belief that it was unethical for widows to remarry. Underlying this precept were the complex property transactions and mechanics of inheritance that widow re-

marriage threatened (Dupâquier et al. 1981). The disapproval of remarriage by widows (and sometimes widowers) among the European peasantry of past centuries notwithstanding, remarriage was both frequent and widespread (Dupâquier et al. 1981; Goody 1983). Remarriage by widows was difficult in preindustrial India, China, Japan, and other agrarian peoples as well (Dupâquier et al. 1981; Goody 1983, 40). *In all societies for which records are available, however, remarriage rates were highest for women of reproductive age.* See Dupâquier et al. 1981; Furstenberg and Spanier 1984; also see chapter 16 of this book.

15. Cherlin 1981.

16. Howell 1979; Shostak 1981.

17. Howell 1979.

18. FEMALE AUTONOMY AND HIGH DIVORCE RATES: Cultures that have a high degree of female autonomy and high divorce rates include those of the Semang of the Malay peninsula (Sanday 1981; Murdock 1965; Textor 1967); several Caribbean populations (Flinn and Low 1986); the Dobu, who live on an island off the eastern tip of New Guinea (Fortune 1963); the Fort Jameson Ngoni, the Yao, and the Lozi of southern Africa (Barnes 1967); the Turu of Tanzania (Schneider 1971); the Samoans of Oceania (Textor 1967); the Gururumba of New Guinea (Friedl 1975); the Trobriand Islanders of Papua, New Guinea (Weiner 1976); the natives of Mangaia, Polynesia (Suggs and Marshall 1971); the Tlingit of southern Alaska (Laura Klein, Dept. of Anthropology, Pacific Lutheran Univ., personal communication); the Kaingang of southern Brazil, the Crow of Montana and the Iroquois of New York (Murdock 1965).

19. Lloyd 1968, 79.

20. Friedl 1975.

21. Brenda Kay Manuelito, Dept. of Anthropology, Univ. of New Mexico, personal communication.

22. Van den Berghe 1979.

23. Le Clercq 1910, 262.

24. Dupâquier et al. 1981.

25. Mark 10:11–12; Lawrence 1989, 63.

26. Fisher 1987, 1989.

27. Cherlin 1981; Levitan, Belous, and Gallo 1988; Glick 1975; Espenshade 1985; Whyte 1990.

28. THE RISING AUTONOMY OF ROMAN WOMEN: Historians do not agree on the reasons or the timing for the increased emancipation and self-assertion of women in ancient Rome. Some point to the defeat of Hannibal in 202 B.C.; others, to the defeat of Macedonia in 168 B.C.; still others, to the

distruction of Carthage in 146 B.C. As a result of a series of historical developments, however, Rome experienced rising opulence in the centuries preceding Christ, a concomitant rise in women's economic, political, and social power and a rise in rates of divorce. See Balsdon 1973; Carcopino 1973; Rawson 1986; Hunt 1959.

29. Burgess and Cottrell 1939; Ackerman 1963; Lewis and Spanier 1979; Bohannan 1985; London and Wilson 1988.

30. Whyte 1990, 201.

31. Cohen 1971.

32. Levinger 1968.

33. Bernard 1964.

34. Guttentag and Secord 1983.

35. Paul Morgan, Department of Sociology, Univ. of Pennsylvania, personal communication.

36. Levitan, Belous, and Gallo 1988.

37. Fisher 1989.

38. DIVORCE DATA IN THE HUMAN RELATIONS AREA FILE: Cross-cultural data on divorce can be found in the Human Relations Area File. This file, known as the HRAF, was started in the 1950s by George Peter Murdock, who collected "ethnographies" (anthropological descriptions of specific cultures) and then cross-indexed these books and articles. Today over 850 cultures are cataloged. But the divorce data in this file present several problems. As Charles Ackerman (1963) reports, "For the most part, ethnographers have stated only that divorce is 'low,' 'common,' 'infrequent,' etc. Rarely has any ethnographer justified his assessment of the rate by any statement of the actual incidence of divorce." Ackerman also notes that HRAF data make it impossible to judge divorce rates *between* societies; one cannot tell whether a "low" divorce rate in one culture is equivalent to a "low" divorce rate in the next. In addition, the researcher does not know whether the "low" divorce rate of one community represents divorce rates in neighboring villages or in the same community in other decades. Synchronic and diachronic data on divorce are lacking. Moreover, different ethnographers of the same culture report different frequencies of divorce, and data in some of the entries conflict with reports by social scientists in other books and articles (Textor 1967). Last, few ethnographers tabulate the duration of the marriage that ends in divorce, the age at divorce, the number of children per divorce, and other data that could be used to make comparisons with Western peoples.

39. Ackerman 1963; Murdock 1965; Friedl 1975.

40. Cohen 1971.

41. Avery 1989, 31.

42. Barnes 1967; Murdock 1965; Textor 1967; Friedl 1975.

43. Fisher 1989, 1991, in preparation.

44. THE SEVEN-YEAR ITCH: The American concept of the seven-year itch stems from the demographic use of the *median* to establish marriage duration. The median is the middle number of a group of numbers; 50 percent of the incidents occur before the median and 50 percent after the median. In the United States between 1960 and 1982 the *median* duration of marriage that ended in divorce ranged between 7.2 and 6.5; thus 50 percent of all marriages had terminated by about seven years (U.S. Bureau of the Census 1986, chart 124). But I am interested in establishing what *most* people do, the divorce *peak* or *mode*. Across the United Nations sample, an average of 48 percent of all divorces occur within seven years of marriage—the median—but divorces cluster around a four-year *peak* (Fisher 1989).

45. Andrew Cherlin, Department of Sociology, Johns Hopkins Univ., personal communication.

46. Bullough 1976, 217.

47. Fisher 1989.

48. *Vital Statistics of the United States* 1981.

49. Ibid. 1964, 1974, 1984, 1985, 1987, 1990.

50. Cherlin 1981.

51. Bohannan 1985, 147.

52. PROCEDURAL MATTERS THAT SKEW THE UN DATA: The time from the petition of divorce to the granting of the decree generally ranges in the United Nations sample from a few weeks to about a year (United Nations 1958, 1984). Several other technicalities tend to skew these divorce statistics: some countries include annulments, which decrease the duration of marriage; some include legal separations, which increase the duration of marriage; some include certain grounds for divorce, such as "separation for two years," that extend the divorce process; some base their statistics on "petitions for divorce" rather than on final divorce decrees; and so on. Procedural problems such as the overloading of court cases and the hearing of cases near the end of the calendar year also skew the data. Fortunately the incidences of annulments and legal separations are few. (See United Nations 1984, table 37.) Because of the imprecision of these data on the legal duration of marriage, I would prefer to examine the duration of human pair-bonds—measured from the moment a man and women begin to court and behave like a couple to the moment they decide to end the tie. But these numbers are not available.

53. United Nations 1955, 1984; Fisher 1989.

54. Johnson 1983, 1.

55. Fisher 1989, 1991, in preparation.

56. Ibid.

57. DIVORCE RISK BY NUMBER OF DEPENDENT CHILDREN—AN IMPORTANT PROBLEM: To establish the *risk* of divorcing with any specific number of children in the family, one needs data not available in the yearbooks of the United Nations. For example, to establish the *risk* of divorcing with one dependent child, one must divide the number of couples who divorce with one dependent child by the number of couples who remain married with one dependent child. I have been unable to find the appropriate correlating census data to establish the divorce risk by number of dependent young for any year in any foreign country or for any year in the United States. Thus these above data on divorce with dependent children *suggest* that the presence of "issue" stabilizes a marriage—but they do not prove it.

58. London and Wilson 1988.

59. Glick 1975.

60. Levitan, Belous, and Gallo 1988.

61. Cherlin 1981.

62. United Nations 1984.

63. RELATIONSHIP BETWEEN THESE DIVORCE PROFILES: Because these data from the demographic yearbooks of the United Nations on the duration of marriage that ends in divorce, on the age at divorce, and on divorce with dependent children are not available in multivariate form, they cannot show the relationships between these three divorce profiles. The divorce peak among couples with one or no children, for example, may be an artifact of the divorce peak during and around the fourth year of marriage.

64. Chute 1949.

65. Chagnon 1982.

66. Barnes 1967.

67. Murdock 1965.

68. Betzig 1989.

69. Beardsley et al. 1959.

70. Radcliffe-Brown 1922.

71. East 1939.

72. WORLD PATTERNS OF CHILD CUSTODY AND PROPERTY DIVISION FOLLOWING DIVORCE: The most common constraints on divorce stem from decisions about the custody of children and about the allocation of property and other resources. A survey of forty-one cultures showed that 44 percent granted the custody of children according to the circumstances that precipitated the separation or according to the wishes or ages of the "issue." In 22 percent of forty-one societies surveyed, children were placed in the

custody of the husband; in 20 percent of them they became the property of the wife. The circumstances of the divorce governed property allocation in 41 percent of thirty-nine societies. In 29 percent of thirty-nine cultures, economic resources were divided equitably between spouses; in 23 percent of them the wife incurred greater financial loss, and the husband and his relatives saw greater economic devastation in 15 percent of them (Frayser 1985).

73. Henry 1941.

74. Cohen 1971, 135.

75. Howell 1979.

6 "When Wild in Woods the Noble Savage Ran"
Life Among Our Ancestors in the Trees

1. The fauna and flora mentioned here and in subsequent sections of the book are ancient varieties of ancient species and families that are now extinct.

2. Chesters 1957; Andrews and Van Couvering 1975; Bonnefille 1985; Van Couvering 1980.

3. Corruccini, Ciochon, and McHenry 1976; Rose 1983.

4. Sibley and Ahlquist 1984; Simons 1985.

5. Corruccini, Ciochon, and McHenry 1976; Rose 1983.

6. Andrews 1981.

7. Smuts 1985, 16.

8. Nadler 1988.

9. Goodall 1986; Fossey 1983; Galdikas 1979.

10. Tutin and McGinnis 1981; Fossey 1979; Veit 1982; Galdikas 1979.

11. PYGMY CHIMPANZEE SEXUAL BEHAVIOR: Pygmy chimps, also known as bonobos, have sex lives quite different from those of the other apes. They engage in a great deal of homosexuality, and although homosexual activities peak during estrus, these contacts occur during other parts of the menstrual cycle (De Waal 1987; Thompson-Handler, Malenky, and Badrian 1984). Bonobo heterosexual activities also occur throughout most of the menstrual cycle (ibid.). And female bonobos resume sexual behavior within a year of parturition (Badrian and Badrian 1984). Because pygmy chimps exhibit these extremes of primate sexuality and because biochemical data suggest that pygmy chimps emerged as recently as two million years ago (Zihlman et al. 1987), I do not feel they make a suitable model for life as it was among hominoids twenty million years ago.

12. Hrdy 1981; Goodall 1986; De Waal 1982.

13. Conoway and Koford 1964; Goodall 1986; Rowell 1972; Harcourt 1979; Veit 1982; Fossey 1983.

14. Goodall 1986; MacKinnon 1979.

15. Fossey 1983.

16. Veit 1982; Fossey 1983; De Waal 1982, 1987.

17. RAPE IN OTHER SPECIES: During several free-access tests (FATs) a single female common chimp, gorilla, or orangutan was housed with a single male of the same species in a common cage; each animal had continual access to the other. In some cases in all three species the male dominated the female and forced copulation—regardless of the female's sexual status or her preference (Nadler 1988). The most frequent and conspicuous examples of rape were offered by male orangutans. Rape occurred every day a couple were housed together, regardless of the stage of the female's estrus cycle or her interest in sex. In a second test a doorway was installed that divided the cage in half and was so designed that the female could pass freely to join the male but the male could not pass freely to join the female. Under these conditions, females of all three species sought copulations only during a restricted period associated with midcycle estrus (ibid.). Hence when females were able to control mating, sex was markedly periodic (ibid.).

Rape does occur among free-ranging apes. Two incidences of forced copulation have been reported among chimpanzees (Tutin and McGinnis 1981). In both cases a male trapped a female in a tree and forced copulation. On a few occasions a male gorilla was observed expressing aggressive gestures toward a female during courtship, but in no instance was copulation forced (Harcourt 1979). Rape may be among the primary reproductive strategies of subadult male orangutans. Dominant, fully adult males establish a consortship with a female during her period of receptivity; they do not coerce a female into copulation (Galdikas 1979). But subadults often accost a female and try to copulate by force (MacKinnon 1979). This "sneak rape" behavior is now considered a "stable alternative strategy" for reproduction among orangutans (Rodman 1988). Rape has also been observed in other species such as ducks, gulls, herons, albatrosses, and bank swallows. In monogamous, colonially nesting bank swallows, for example, a male mated to one female will attempt to knock another mated females out of the sky and force copulation (see Daly and Wilson 1983).

18. Van Couvering 1980.

19. Berggren and Hollister 1977.

20. Van Couvering and Van Couvering 1975; Berggren and Hollister 1977; Thomas 1985.

21. Axelrod and Raven 1977.

22. Andrews and Van Couvering 1975, 65.

23. Van Couvering 1980; Axelrod and Raven 1977.

24. Andrews and Van Couvering 1975.

25. A savanna is a "well-drained grassy vegetation with 10% to 40% cover by trees" (Retallack, Dugas, and Bestland 1990).

26. Andrews and Van Couvering 1975; Van Couvering 1980; Retallack, Dugas, and Bestland 1990.

27. Andrews and Van Couvering 1975; Van Couvering 1980; Axelrod and Raven 1977; Maglio 1978; Bernor 1985; Vrba 1985.

28. Kay 1981; Pilbeam 1985.

29. Greenfield 1980, 1983; Andrews and Cronin 1982; Conroy et al. 1990.

30. Wolpoff 1982; Ciochon and Fleagle 1987.

31. DATING THE DIVERGENCE OF HUMANKIND: Data from DNA and other biochemical, anatomical, and genetic analyses of differences between humankind and the African apes suggest somewhat different dates for the divergence of the human line. Estimates range from 10 to 4 my BP (million years before present). See Sarich and Wilson 1967a, 1967b; Cronin 1983; Sibley and Ahlquist 1984; Andrews and Cronin 1982. New data suggest that human beings are most closely related to chimpanzees and that gorillas diverged earlier (Miyamoto, Slightom, and Goodman 1987). Some of this research is in question however (Lewin 1987b).

32. Veit 1982.

33. Nadler 1975.

34. Veit 1982.

35. Fossey 1983.

36. Darwin 1871; Freud 1918; Engels [1884] 1954.

37. Lucretius 1965, 162–63.

38. Kano 1979; Kano and Mulavwa 1984.

39. Kano 1979; Badrian and Malenky 1984.

40. De Waal 1987; Thompson-Handler, Malenky, and Badrian 1984; Kano and Mulavwa 1984.

41. Kuroda 1984; De Waal 1987; Savage-Rumbaugh and Wilkerson 1978.

42. De Waal 1987.

43. Ford and Beach 1951.

44. De Waal 1987.

45. Kano 1980.

46. FACE-TO-FACE COITUS IN NATURE: Several animals copulate face-to-face on some occasions, including gorillas (Nadler 1975), orangutans (Galdikas 1979), siamangs (Chivers 1978), and whales and porpoises (Harrison 1969).

47. Coolidge 1933; Zihlman et al. 1987; Zihlman 1979; Susman 1984.
48. Ellen Ingmanson, anthropologist, personal communication.
49. McGinnis 1979; Goodall 1986.
50. Tutin 1979; McGinnis 1979; McGrew 1981; Goodall 1986.
51. McGrew 1981; Goodall 1986; De Waal 1982; McGinnis 1979.
52. McGinnis 1979; Tutin 1979; Goodall 1986; McGrew 1981.
53. Pusey 1980.
54. McGinnis 1979; Tutin 1979; Goodall 1986.
55. Tutin and McGinnis 1981.
56. Bygott 1979; Goodall et al. 1979; Wrangham 1979b; Goodall 1986.
57. Goodall et al. 1979.
58. Bygott 1974, 1979; Goodall et al. 1979; Goodall 1986.
59. Teleki 1973a, 1973b; Goodall 1986.
60. Teleki 1973a; McGrew 1981.
61. Plooij 1978.
62. Goodall 1968, 1970, 1986; McGrew 1981.
63. De Waal 1989.
64. McGrew 1979, 1981; also see Boesch and Boesch 1984.
65. Goodall 1970, 1986; McGrew 1974, 1981.
66. Goodall 1986.
67. Fouts 1983.
68. Moss 1988
69. Tanner 1981; McGrew 1981; Fisher 1982; Mansperger 1990; Foley and Lee 1989.

7 Out of Eden: *A Theory on the Origin of Monogamy and Desertion*

1. Hay and Leakey 1982.
2. THE TERMS HOMINOID AND HOMINID: Traditionally anthropologists used the term *hominoid* to designate the ancestors of the great apes and humankind. The term *hominid* they used to designate the ancestors of human beings only. Since then the science of cladistics has matured. This school of thought maintains that species should be grouped according to the recency of their common ancestry, and because of the distant biochemical relationship between humans and orangutans and the close biochemical similarities between humans, chimpanzees, and gorillas, some of these scientists would like to change these terms accordingly. I use the traditional term, *hominoid*, to designate all ancestors of the apes and people and *hominid* to signify the ancestors of humanity only (see Marks 1989).

3. Leakey and Hay 1979; Hay and Leakey 1982.

4. Leakey et al. 1976; White 1977, 1980.

5. Johanson and Edey 1981; Johnston 1982; Lewin 1983a.

6. Johanson and White 1979; see Johnston 1982; Susman, Stern, and Jungers 1985; Jungers 1988; McHenry 1986.

7. Johanson and White 1979; White 1985; Tuttle 1990.

8. Van Couvering 1980.

9. Ibid.; Vrba 1985; Axelrod and Raven 1977; Bernor 1985.

10. Pilbeam 1985.

11. Binford 1981, 1985; Blumenschine 1986, 1987, 1989; Shipman 1986; Potts 1988; Sinclair, Leakey, and Norton-Griffiths 1986; Lewin 1987b.

12. Tunnell 1990; Schaller and Lowther 1969; Blumenschine 1986.

13. SCAVENGING AMONG NONHUMAN PRIMATES: Goodall reported scavenging among the chimps at the Gombe Stream Reserve, Tanzania, on ten occasions. On most of them, a chimp returned to eat meat left behind after a group of chimps had made a kill earlier in the day. In one case, a chimp stole the limp body of a monkey as Goodall was photographing it. Gombe chimps ignored the fresh meat of a dead bushbuck fawn and guinea fowl. But on four occasions chimps in the nearby research site at the Mahale Mountains scavenged the carcasses of blue duikers or bushbucks (Goodall 1986). Savannah baboons also scavenge (Strum 1990; Cavallo and Blumenschine 1989).

14. Cavallo 1990; Cavallo and Blumenschine 1989.

15. McHenry 1986; Ryan and Johanson 1989.

16. Gaulin and Konner 1977.

17. MODERN HUNTING-GATHERING PEOPLES AS MODELS FOR HOMINID EVOLUTION: In the 1960s it became fashionable among anthropologists to use the !Kung as a model to reconstruct life as it may have been during our hunting-gathering past (Lee 1968). Today this has become unstylish. Wilmsen (1989) argues that the !Kung have been in contact with surrounding pastoralist peoples for several centuries and that their appearance as foragers is a function of recent historical events (ibid.). Thus the !Kung do not represent the pristine hunting-gathering society anthropologists once thought they did; nor do they provide a suitable model for understanding life in the past.

    Recently anthropologists have begun to analyze the hunting and gathering activities of traditional peoples in terms of "OPTIMAL FORAGING STRATEGIES." This line of investigation contends that a society will vary its daily quest for food, depending on the ease of acquisition and processing, on the dependability, quantity, and quality of the food source, and on several other factors, so as to maximize its intake of nutrients while minimizing its expenditure of energy, time, and risk (Hawkes et al. 1982; Torrence 1989). Hence because we do not know the specific micro-environment of East Africa in past millennia, we cannot be sure that modern hunter-gatherers are reasonable models for a reconstructing of past populations.

   With these caveats, it remains fair to say that the traditional !Kung lived in an environment basically similar to that of early hominids and that they displayed a social organization remarkably uncontaminated by outside influences. So I shall continue to use the !Kung as a model in the attempt to understand our past. (See Schrire 1984; Solway and Lee 1990; Wilmsen and Denbow 1990.)

18. Sahlins 1972.

19. Darwin 1871, 434.

20. Tanner and Zihlman 1976; Zihlman and Tanner 1978; Zihlman 1981; Tanner 1981.

21. Potts 1988; Watanabe 1985.

22. FATHERHOOD ACROSS SPECIES: Males of many species exhibit parental behavior, although most are not monogamous. Male parental investment occurs in two forms: *(a)* direct care, such as feeding young, carrying infants, baby-sitting, sleeping in contact with young, grooming young, retrieving, and/or playing with young; *(b)* indirect care, such as defending resources, stockpiling food for infants, building shelters for young, helping pregnant or nursing females, marking and/or maintaining a territory, defending and patrolling borders of a range, expelling intruders, and/or calling to drive competitors away (Kleiman and Malcolm 1981; also see Hewlett 1992).

23. Wittenberger and Tilson 1980; Kleiman 1977; Orians 1969; Lack 1968; Mock and Fujioka 1990.

24. MONOGAMY IN CROSS-SPECIES PERSPECTIVE: Several circumstances operate together to produce monogamy, and researchers provide alternative explanations for the evolution of monogamy in different creatures. I am particularly influenced by the work of Devra Kleiman—specifically by her contention that monogamy occurs "whenever more than a single individual (the female) is needed to rear the young" (Kleiman 1977, 51). This was said differently by Ember and Ember (1979): "Heterosexual partnerships develop wherever the need of the mother to obtain her nutrition interferes with the care of the young. The duration of this bond is dependent upon the parental care time." I think this factor was critical to the evolution of monogamy in *Homo sapiens.* For discussions of monogamy in birds and mammals, see Kleiman 1977; Wittenberger and Tilson 1980; Lack 1968; Orians 1969; Rutberg 1983; Peck and Feldman 1988; Mock and Fujioka 1990.

25. PRECOCIAL YOUNG: Creatures that deliver their young in a state of relative maturity, as opposed to immaturity, are said to deliver "precocial" young. Horses provide a good example; a foal can see and walk a few hours after birth.

26. Kleiman 1977; Henry 1985; Lloyd 1980; Zimen 1980; Gage 1979; Rue 1969.

27. Trivers 1972; Emlen and Oring 1977.

28. Henry 1985; Lloyd 1980; Zimen 1980; Gage 1979; Rue 1969.

29. Orians 1969; Mock and Fujioka 1990.

30. Eugene Morton, Dept. of Ornithology, Smithsonian Institution, personal communication.

31. SEXUAL DIMORPHISM, POLYGYNY, AND MONOGAMY: In many polygynous species, males battle for the privilege of becoming harem master, the weak and small are driven off, and the large males breed—selecting for large males. Because the bones unearthed at Hadar and Laetoli were of different sizes, some anthropologists suggest that these individuals had a polygynous breeding system. This argument has several problems. *(a)* The correlation between large males, small females, and polygyny is not a regularity of nature. The exceptions are so extensive that anthropologists now postulate that there is no necessary connection between degree of sexual dimorphism and mating strategy (Frayer and Wolpoff 1985; Mock and Fujioka 1990). *(b)* Very few fossil bones are found at Hadar and Laetoli and small sample sizes often say nothing about whole populations (Gaulin and Boster 1985). *(c)* The size differences in these bones can be explained by other ecological forces. Scavenging and hunting (as well as serial monogamy) may have selected for large males whereas Lucy's diminutive frame may have been a compensation for the demands of bearing young. Because of pregnancy and lactation, female mammals need extra calories; they must eat for two and then nurse a child, so the smaller Lucy was, the less she needed to feed herself. For more data on sexual dimorphisms, see Hall 1982.

32. Cohen 1980; Hassan 1980; Lee 1980; Short 1976, 1984; Konner and Worthman 1980; Simpson-Hebert and Huffman 1981; Lancaster and Lancaster 1983; Frisch 1978.

33. Birdsell 1979.

34. Galdikas and Wood 1990.

35. Raymond Hames, Dept. of Anthropology, Univ. of Nebraska, personal communication.

36. Briggs 1970.

37. Gorer 1938.

38. Heider 1976.

39. Lancaster and Lancaster 1983.

40. FOUR-YEAR HUMAN BIRTHING CYCLE — MODERN VARIATIONS, APE ORIGINS: Modern living has changed this general four-year human birthing cycle. Even continually breast-feeding women in India, Bangladesh, the United States, and Scotland begin to ovulate about five to eighteen months after delivering a child (Simpson-Hebert and Huffman 1981; Short 1984). Thus modern birth spacing can be as short as two years or even less. This is, at present, explained by the "CRITICAL FATNESS" HYPOTHESIS. In the 1970s Rose Frisch and colleagues proposed that a woman needs adequate stores of body fat to trigger ovulation (Frisch and Revelle 1970; Frisch 1978, 1989). Because of the modern diet high in calories, lack of exercise, and limited nursing frequency, women often ovulate and get pregnant a few months after childbirth.

Modern patterns of birth spacing do not conform to traditional patterns, however. When our ancestors walked miles to collect dinner, when they ate fruit and lean meat, and women nursed their infants continually, fat stores were lower and women probably bore their young about four years apart (Lancaster and Lancaster 1983). Data on birth spacing among the apes support the antiquity of this reproductive pattern. Among chimpanzees and gorillas, birth spacing is in general approximately four to five years, whereas birth intervals among orangutans are often about eight years (Allen et al. 1982; Galdikas and Wood 1990).

41. Tanner 1981; McGrew 1981; Fisher 1982; Foley and Lee 1989; Mansperger 1990.

42. Strum 1990; Smuts 1985, 1992.

43. EARLY HOMINID GROUP SIZE: Birdsell (1968) proposed that early hominid bands were composed of about twenty-five individuals, half of whom were adults. I think this standard model is a reasonable one for early hominid social groups. (Also see Foley and Lee 1989.)

44. Laura Betzig, Evolution and Human Behavior Program, University of Michigan, personal communication.

45. ADAPTIVE REASONS FOR MALES TO "REMARRY": Among apes males tend to seek copulation with older, more mature females rather than with adolescents — presumably because females with young have a good reproductive track record. This raises the question, Why would ancestral hominid males seek to form pair-bonds with young females rather than with more mature ones? The answer, I think, lies in the ecology of monogamy. In monogamous species the male will invest time and energy rearing his offspring himself. Hence the values of youth — such as fresh eggs, a supple body, a resilient personality, and a long reproductive future — may be more important to a male than the female's reproductive track record.

46. ADAPTIVE REASONS FOR FEMALES TO "REMARRY": Psychologist David Buss (Dept. of Psychology, Univ. of Michigan, personal communication)

argues that once a woman produced a child, her reproductive value went down, making her less attractive to prime males. Hence as a woman aged, her subsequent pair-bonds were with men of lower reproductive worth. Thus serial monogamy was not an adaptive strategy for ancestral females. This argument is logical. But several practical variables must be considered. *(a)* Band size and infrequency of interband contact may have reduced opportunities for a female to acquire a prime mate on her first mateship, providing her with the opportunity to "marry up" on her second try. *(b)* The female's first mate's reproductive value might go down dramatically as a result of injury; hence although her second mate might not be prime, he would be of higher reproductive value than the first. *(c)* A young male was probably strong and quick but inexperienced at hunting and protecting, whereas an older male was undoubtedly more experienced at hunting, scavenging, and fathering (as well as economically burdened by previous wives and children). The reproductive value of males thus probably varied enormously with factors other than age. *(d)* A female's reproductive value may have gone up with age if she became a more proficient provider and remained fertile, thereby attracting more prime males in subsequent mateships. I suspect the reproductive value of each male and female rose or fell according to several variables; the vicissitudes of the environment added more variables as well. Hence a reproductive strategy of flexible *"opportunistic"* serial monogamy would have been adaptive for females.

47. Bertram 1975; Schaller 1972; Hausfater and Hrdy 1984.
48. Daly and Wilson 1988.
49. Tylor 1889, 267–68.
50. Friedl 1975.

8 Eros: *Emergence of the Sexual Emotions*

1. Liebowitz 1983.
2. Tennov 1979; Money 1980.
3. Shostak 1981, 268.
4. Jankowiak and Fischer 1992.
5. Liebowitz 1983, 90.
6. Bischof 1975; Wickler 1976.
7. SITES OF ATTACHMENT: Ethologists note that animals attach (seek and maintain proximity) to several different things: an object, such as a tree or fence; a site, such as a field or patch of beach; or an individual or group of conspecifics, such as an infant, a mate, or a congregation of cohorts. People attach to all of the above-mentioned phenomena: to a home, to certain

pieces of land, and to children, relatives, and friends. Several scientists have confirmed that the motivation to attach is instinctual. See Wickler 1976; Bowlby 1969.

8. ATTACHMENT IN ANIMALS: Infant puppies, baby monkeys, chicks, and guinea pigs cry when their mother goes away—even if they are warm, comfortable, and satiated. Their heart races, their blood pressure increases, and their body temperature rises as "separation anxiety" escalates into panic. When they are administered endorphins or other natural opiates, however, these infants calm down. The locus ceruleus, an area in the brain stem, and other loci in the brain also play a role in episodic panic and anxiety attacks. See Liebowitz 1983.

9. Michael Trupp, New York City psychiatrist, personal communication.

10. Bowlby 1969.

11. Bieber et al. 1962; Ruse 1988.

12. Bell and Weinberg 1978.

13. Ruse 1988.

14. Merry Ratliff Muraskin, New York therapist and anthropologist, personal communication.

15. Kinsey, Pomeroy, and Martin, 1948; Kinsey et al. 1953; Silverstein 1981; Ruse 1988.

16. Adams 1980.

17. Daly and Wilson 1988.

18. Stephens 1963.

19. Hiatt 1989.

20. Goodall 1986.

21. Hiatt 1989.

22. David Buss, Dept. of Psychology, Univ. of Michigan, personal communication.

23. Weiss 1975.

24. Zuckerman, Buchsbaum, and Murphy 1980; Zuckerman 1971; Weiss 1987.

25. Sostek and Wyatt 1981; Weiss 1987.

26. Kagan, Reznick, and Snidman 1988.

27. Donaldson 1971.

28. Mellen 1981; Donaldson 1971.

29. Darwin [1872] 1965.

9 The Siren's Web: *Evolution of Human Sexual Anatomy*

1. NATURAL SELECTION VERSUS SEXUAL SELECTION: In terms of the transmission of genes, there is no difference between natural selection and sexual

selection. The distinction lies in the type of selection and the type of adaptive results. *Sexual selection* is defined as selection for characteristics that are specifically concerned with increasing one's success at attracting and obtaining mates. The results are the evolution of traits useful to sex and reproduction rather than adaptations to the general environment. Following Darwin, it is customary to distinguish two kinds of sexual selection: *(a)* INTRASEXUAL SELECTION is selection for traits that enable one to compete with members of the same sex for mates of the opposite sex; *(b)* INTERSEXUAL SELECTION is selection for characteristics that make one attractive to the opposite sex. See Darwin 1871; Campbell 1972; Gould and Gould 1989.

2. Eberhard 1987, 1990.

3. Smith 1984; Eberhard 1985, 1990.

4. Daly and Wilson 1983.

5. Smith 1984.

6. Short 1977; Moller 1988; Lewin 1988d.

7. Smith 1984.

8. Darwin 1871; Bateman 1948; Trivers 1972.

9. Morris 1967.

10. Gallup 1982.

11. Lancaster 1986.

12. Low, Alexander, and Noonan 1987.

13. Mascia-Lees, Relethford, and Sorger 1986.

14. Darwin 1871, 907.

15. Ibid. 881.

16. Alexander 1990.

17. Ford and Beach 1951.

18. NEOTENY: Ashley Montagu (1981) proposes that the human female downward-tilted vaginal canal and face-to-face coitus evolved as a by-product of "neoteny," or "growing young." Neoteny, meaning the extention of childlike characteristics into adulthood, is a remarkable phenomenon; we have several neotenous traits, including flat faces, rounded skulls, playfulness, curiosity, and other emotional and physical traits that nonhuman primates display in infancy but lose as they mature. The downward-tilted vagina occurs in the embryo of all mammals, but after birth the vaginal canal rotates backward and lies parallel with the spine. Women retain this embryonic, vaginal orientation into old age. Montagu (1981) hypothesizes that the immature position of the human vagina (and all other neotenous human traits) evolved as a package when evolution favored the growth of the brain millennia ago. The expanding fetal brain required the mother to deliver infants at an earlier stage of development. Along with immature

delivery, Montagu reasons, humans evolved slower maturation, a longer childhood, and the retention of many childlike traits into adulthood— including a tipped vagina. New data argue against Montagu's theory. Several neotenous features of the hominid skull may have evolved at different times, indicating that each was subject to direct selection (Lewin 1985).

19. Symons 1979.

20. Rancourt-Laferriere 1983.

21. ORGASM AS A MEANS OF STIMULATING PHYSIOLOGICAL SENSATIONS OF ATTACHMENT: Oxytocin, a peptide secreted by the pituitary gland in the brain, is secreted (at least in men) during orgasm and serves to produce feelings of pleasure and sexual fulfillment (Angier 1991). This suggests that orgasm could produce chemical responses that increase feelings of attachment.

22. Smith 1984; Alcock 1987.

23. Burton 1971; De Waal 1982; Whitten 1982; Lancaster 1979; Hrdy 1981; Savage-Rumbaugh and Wilkerson 1978.

24. THE FICKLENESS OF HUMAN FEMALE ORGASM: From data on how people learn, it is now established that partial or irregular reinforcement drives them to more persistent trials than does a 100 percent reward. So some suggest that sexual frustration caused by the irregular female orgasmic response served to drive ancestral females to seek renewed sexual intercourse (Diamond 1980).

25. SEX OUTSIDE OF ESTRUS IN OTHER ANIMALS: Female pygmy chimps engage in sexual behavior with other females on a daily basis. Heterosexual copulations also occur throughout most of the menstrual cycle, although not all of it (Thompson-Handler, Malenky, and Badrian 1984). Female dolphins reportedly masturbate and copulate regularly, with few signs of periodicity (Diamond 1980). Females of several primate species exhibit sexual behavior at times other than midcycle estrus, such as during troop upheaval, during captivity, or during pregnancy. One can cite many exceptions, but generally speaking, the vast majority of heterosexual interactions among female primates occur during midcycle estrus. See Fedigan 1982; Lancaster 1979; Hrdy 1981.

26. Kinsey et al. 1953; Ford and Beach 1951; Wolfe 1981.

27. Ford and Beach 1951.

28. MENOPAUSE: The complex programmed cessation of ovulation known as menopause, which occurs in all middle-aged women, does not appear to occur in other primates or other mammals, although elephants, pilot whales, and some primates exhibit some signs of menopause in advanced age (Alexander 1990, Pavelka and Fedigan 1991). Some scientists cur-

rently think menopause evolved in ancestral hominids as an adaptive strategy to aid existing offspring and other genetic relatives, in lieu of producing new ones that would require many years of investment. Hence the post-menopausal mother could be GRANDMOTHER and BABY-SITTER to grandchildren. Menopause could also be the by-product of the increased human life span or a pleiotropic effect (Pavelka and Fedigan 1991). Perhaps the hominid female's high postmenopausal *libido* evolved to enable them to maintain their pair-bonds (and the political-social coalitions these accrued), as well as enabling them to continue to garner extra resources from "extramarital" copulations. See Alexander 1990; Dawkins 1976; Pavelka and Fedigan 1991.

29. Strassman 1981; Alexander and Noonan 1979; Turke 1984; Fisher 1975, 1982; Lovejoy 1981; Burley 1979; Small 1988; Gray and Wolfe 1983; Benshoof and Thornhill 1979; Daniels 1983; Burleson and Trevathan 1990; Hrdy 1983.

30. Teleki 1973a; Goodall 1986.

31. Fisher 1975, 1982.

32. Rosenblum 1976.

33. NATURAL PEAKS IN THE HUMAN FEMALE SEX DRIVE: Studies suggest that the peak of a woman's sexual activity occurs at midcycle (Hrdy 1981). Married women given a variety of contraceptive devices exhibited a rise in female-initiated sex drive during ovulation under most conditions; this was suppressed by the use of oral contraceptives (Adams, Gold, and Burt 1978). Intercourse peaked among a sample of American women soon after the end of menstruation, however (Udry and Morris 1977). Other studies indicate that American wives (as well as women in other cultures) experience a peak of excitability immediately before or after menstruation (Ford and Beach 1951; Kinsey et al. 1953). These data lead me to propose that women have two natural peaks in sex drive: one during and around ovulation and another just before or during menstruation. The peak during ovulation may be a holdover from estrus. The peak during menstruation may have evolved with bipedalism; blood pools naturally in the pelvic area prior to menstruation, and bipedalism may act to heighten tension on genital tissues at this time.

34. Daniels 1983.

10 Why Can't a Man Be More like a Woman?
Development of the Human Sexual Brain

1. Gould 1981; Russett 1989.

2. Mead 1935, 280.

3. CULTURAL DETERMINISM: The sharp swing toward "cultural determinism" in the 1920s and 1930s did not focus on gender differences alone but was part of an intellectual reaction to the eugenics movement at the time and emphasized racial and ethnic commonalities too. For a history of the nature/nurture debate and the events of the early twentieth century that influenced this controversy, see Degler 1991.

4. Jost 1972; Otten 1985.

5. Maccoby and Jacklin 1974; McGuinness 1976, 1979, 1985.

6. Benderly 1987, 1989.

7. Sherman 1978.

8. Benderly 1987.

9. McGuinness 1985, 89.

10. Kimura 1989; Weiss 1988.

11. Fennema and Leder 1990.

12. Maccoby and Jacklin 1974; McGuinness 1979; Fennema and Leder 1990.

13. Benbow and Stanley 1980, 1983.

14. Leder 1990; Benderly 1987.

15. Kimura 1989; Moir and Jessel 1989.

16. Silverman and Beals 1990.

17. Fennema and Leder 1990; Sherman 1978; Benderly 1987; Bower 1986.

18. Darwin 1871.

19. McGuinness 1979; McGuinness and Pribram 1979; Hall et al. 1978, 1977; Zuckerman et al. 1976; Hall 1984.

20. De Lacoste-Utamsing and Holloway, 1982.

21. Kimura 1983; McGuinness 1985.

22. Geschwind 1974; Springer and Deutsch 1985.

23. ORIGIN OF WOMEN'S INTUITION—AN ALTERNATIVE VIEW: Donald Symons (1979) suggests that women evolved the superior ability to pick up nonverbal cues because early hominid females needed to choose the appropriate mate to help raise their children. Those females who could accurately "read" personality survived disproportionately (Symons 1979). Sociologists point out that individuals of low status are keener observers of high-status individuals than the reverse. And it can be argued that women's intuition stems from their long historical role as second-class citizens in patriarchal societies instead. Cultural factors certainly play a part in one's ability to detect nonverbal cues. But I suspect that women's ancestral roles as caretakers provided the *primary* selective pressure for female intuitive skills.

24. Kimura 1989.

25. McGuinness 1979, 1985; McGuinness and Pribram 1979.

26. Whiting and Whiting 1975.

27. Konner 1982.

28. Miller 1983.

29. Rossi 1984; Frayser 1985.

30. McGuinness 1979, 1985; McGuinness and Pribram 1979.

31. Otten 1985; Moir and Jessel 1989; Money and Ehrhardt 1972.

32. McGrew 1981.

33. McGuinness 1979.

34. Leakey 1971.

35. Behrensmeyer and Hill 1980; Brain 1981.

36. Bunn and Kroll 1986.

37. Cavallo 1990; Cavallo and Blumenschine 1989.

38. MORE ON SCAVENGING: There is a great deal of controversy about the role of scavenging in the early hominid diet. Pat Shipman, for example, suggests that our ancestors scavenged in a group, rather than hunting, and that they probably collected predominantly skin and tendons. Thus "animal carcasses . . . were not systematically cut up and transported for sharing at base camps." See Shipman 1984, 27; Shipman 1987; Binford 1985.

39. Potts 1984, 1988.

40. Zihlman 1981.

41. Lewin 1987b; McHenry 1986.

42. Brod 1987; Goleman 1986.

43. Gilligan 1982a.

44. Ellis and Symons 1990.

45. Bower 1988a; Susman 1989, 1990.

46. Johanson and Shreeve 1989.

47. Tobias 1991.

48. WHO MADE THE TOOLS AND BUTCHERED THE MEAT AT OLDUVAI? Although recent data suggests that robust australopithecines could have made and used tools and that these creatures had a bulge in Broca's area in the brain, several lines of evidence suggest that *Homo habilis* individuals made and stored these tools, as well as devised the system of cache sites to butcher meat at Olduvai two million years ago. *(a)* The reduced cheek teeth of *Homo habilis* suggest that these creatures relied on meat (McHenry and O'Brien 1986). *(b)* The increased cranial capacity of this species may even have required the consumption of energy-rich foods such as meat (Ambrose 1986). *(c)* The bones of *Homo habilis* lie in spacial patterns consistent with those of the stone tools found at Olduvai, and

these patterns at Olduvai Gorge fit well with patterns of fossils and tools left at Koobi Fora. *(d)* Several anatomical details of these fossil bones suggest that *Homo habilis* is in the direct line toward humankind.

11 Women, Men, and Power: *The Nature of Sexual Politics*

1. Van Allen 1976.
2. Ibid.
3. Van Allen 1976; Okonjo 1976.
4. DISCUSSIONS OF UNIVERSAL MALE DOMINANCE: Anthropologists have proposed several reasons why men universally dominate women. Some have pointed to biology: men are naturally stronger and more aggressive; hence men have always dominated women (Sacks 1979). Some have proposed a psychological explanation: men dominate women to reject the powerful women in their lives (Whiting 1965). Universal male dominance, others say, stems from female reproductive functions. Because women bear children, they are tied to the natural rather than the cultural world (Ortner and Whitehead 1981) or to the private rather than the public sector (Rosaldo 1974). For anthropological discussions of universal male dominance and theories of why gender relations vary cross-culturally, see Dahlberg 1981; Reiter 1975; Etienne and Leacock 1980; Leacock 1981; Friedl 1975; Harris 1977; Sanday 1981; Sacks 1979; Ortner and Whitehead 1981; Rosaldo and Lamphiere 1974; Collier 1988.
5. Elkin 1939; Hart and Pilling 1960; Rohrlich-Leavitt, Sykes, and Weatherford 1975; Berndt 1981.
6. Montagu 1937, 23.
7. Kaberry 1939; Goodale 1971; Berndt 1981; Bell 1980.
8. Reiter 1975; Slocum 1975.
9. Whyte 1978.
10. TRADITIONAL SOCIETIES WITH POWERFUL WOMEN: Pygymy women of the Congo, Navajo women of the American Southwest, Iroquois women of New York, Tlingit women of southern Alaska, Algonkian women of the American Northeast, Balinese women, Semang women of the tropical forests of the Malay Peninsula, women in Polynesia, women in parts of the Andes, Africa, Southeast Asia, and the Caribbean, Trobriand Islanders of the Pacific, and women in many other societies traditionally wielded substantial economic and social power. See Sanday 1981; Etienne and Leacock 1980; Dahlberg 1981; Reiter 1975; Sacks 1979; Weiner 1976.
11. Leacock 1980, 28.
12. Sanday 1981, 135.

13. TYPES OF POWER: Power in traditional societies comes in several forms. Sociologist Robert Alford divides power into three distinct varieties, however: *(a)* the ability to influence or persuade; *(b)* authority or formal institutionalized command; *(c)* what sociologists sometimes call hegemony, which is almost identical to one meaning of *culture* because it refers to the unquestioned, accepted mores of a culture that bestow power on one gender or individual rather than on another (Alford and Friedland 1985). See chapter 15 of this book for a discussion of the evolution of rank and authority.

14. Friedl 1975; Sacks 1971; Sanday 1974; Whyte 1978.

15. Friedl 1975.

16. Shostak 1981, 243.

17. Rogers 1975.

18. THE HUMAN RELATIONS AREA FILE: Many anthropologists regard this file as highly uneven and flawed because the data on each culture are taken by a different ethnographer. Each ethnographer has asked different questions in different ways, recorded his or her perceptions under different circumstances, and had his or her own subjective perspectives. The data in this file were then distilled by Whyte and his colleagues—further reducing the likelihood of accuracy. I use Whyte's analysis here because I do not wish to overlook an available source and because my experience with the ethnographic literature suggests that Whyte's conclusions on this topic represent some general cross-cultural truths.

19. Whyte 1978.

20. Belkin 1989; Hochschild 1989.

21. Sanday 1981.

22. De Waal 1982, 1989.

23. De Waal 1982, 187.

24. Hrdy 1981; Fedigan 1982.

12 Almost Human: *Genesis of Kinship and the Teenager*

1. USE OF FIRE—A DEBATE: Several anthropologists currently propose that the fire at the Swartkrans cave and other fires at sites in Africa, the Near East, Asia, and Europe dating between 1.8 million and 120,000 years ago occurred naturally—the result of brushfires, volcanic eruptions, lightning, spontaneous combustion, or burning branches that fell through cracks in cave ceilings (James 1989; Binford 1981, 1985, 1987). But there is a great deal of circumstantial evidence that humankind living in this period did make and use fire. *(a)* Bits of charcoal, burned bone, charred stones, baked

clay, reddened earth, and other indications of fire prior to 120,000 years ago have been found at thirty-four sites in Africa, the Near East, Asia, and Europe (James 1989). *(b)* Small brushfires occurred annually during the dry season, so humans had regular opportunities to experiment with fire— as well as the intelligence to control fire. *(c)* Caves are damp, cool, still places; they do not provide ideal conditions for lightning or the spontane- ous combustion of decaying dung. *(d)* Lightning rarely causes extensive grass fires on the plains; in fact, mankind may have created the grasslands of East Africa *with fire;* when modern people leave an area, savannas rapidly return to a more natural landscape of grasslands scattered with brush and trees. *(e)* In numerous caves across Africa and Eurasia are found the bones of ancestral hominids dating from this time range; could they have lived in freezing caves without controlling flame? These data have led several anthropologists to conclude that it is highly likely that mankind living at this time made campfires. See James 1989; Straus 1989.

2. Brain and Sillen 1988.

3. Brown et al. 1985.

4. HOMO ERECTUS AND SEXUAL DIMORPHISM: *Homo erectus* fossils show a reduction in sexual dimorphism in body size over earlier hominid forms. In the endnotes to chapter 7, however, I maintain that sexual dimorphisms in the size of male and female bones can tell us nothing about ancient repro- ductive strategies; hence I do not discuss the evolution of this trait here.

5. Brink 1957.

6. Behrensmeyer 1984.

7. Gibbons 1990b.

8. Montagu 1961; Gould 1977; Fisher 1975, 1982; Trevathan 1987.

9. HUMAN SECONDARY ALTRICIALITY: Human newborns are not uniformly altricial; instead, they display a mosaic of features, some of which exhibit more altriciality than others (Gibson 1981). Scientists at present debate whether the "secondary altriciality" of some neonatal traits evolved in response to cephalo-pelvic disproportion (Lindburg 1982). I use the stan- dard explanation that secondary altriciality *is* a response to cephalo-pelvic disproportion. See Montagu 1961; Gould 1977; Bromage 1987; Trevathan 1987.

10. Montagu 1961, 156.

11. Martin 1982; Lewin 1982.

12. Trevathan 1987; Bromage 1987.

13. Fisher 1975, 1982.

14. Trevathan 1987.

15. Bromage 1987; Smith 1986.

16. Lancaster and Lancaster, 1983; Lancaster in preparation.

17. Ackerman 1989.

18. EVOLUTION OF HUNTING—A DEBATE: Some anthropologists doubt that *Homo erectus* hunted large animals; they contend that *Homo erectus* subsisted primarily as a scavenger (Binford 1981, 1985, 1987). I think *Homo erectus* was a hunter of big game for several reasons: *(a)* Today there are over 130,000 pounds of big game in one square mile of Uganda's Albert National Park and archaeological data suggest that wild game was prevalent a million years ago. *(b) Homo erectus* individuals made stone tools that were efficient for butchering game, and these tools have been found along watercourses where large beasts gather. *(c)* Hawks hunt; sharks hunt; wolves hunt in coordinated packs; chimpanzees hunt large animals relative to their size and leave no archaeological record of their kills; one hardly needs a modern human brain to kill and eat meat. I think *Homo erectus* hunted, killed, and shared meat a million years ago.

19. Jia and Weiwen 1990.

20. ARCHIAC HOMO SAPIENS: Several anthropologists think that archaic *Homo sapiens,* rather than *Homo erectus,* is the species represented at these later sites (Wolpoff 1984). Moreover, some think that *Homo erectus* was a single species that changed gradually over time (ibid.); others think that these bones represent different varieties or even separate species and that only one strain led to modern *Homo sapiens* (Lewin 1989).

13 The First Affluent Society: *A Flowering of Conscience*

1. Conkey 1984.

2. Service 1978; Pfeiffer 1982.

3. Gargett 1989; Chase and Dibble 1987.

4. For a review of the arguments surrounding the evolution of *Homo sapiens neanderthalensis,* see Delson 1985; Mellars 1989.

5. Holloway 1985.

6. Arensburg 1989.

7. Lieberman 1984; Laitman 1984; Laitman, Heimbuch, and Crelin 1979.

8. Leroi-Gourhan 1975; Solecki 1971, 1989.

9. Gargett 1989; Chase and Dibble 1987.

10. Mellars 1989.

11. ORIGIN OF HOMO SAPIENS SAPIENS—THEORIES: Some anthropologists think *Homo erectus* spread out of Africa about a million years ago and then gradually evolved into modern peoples along parallel lines in different regions of Africa and Eurasia—the "candelabra" model. Others think a

single population of modern peoples originated in Africa more than 100,000 years ago and dispersed through the rest of the Old World, replacing more-primitive existing human populations (including the Neanderthals) as they spread—the "Noah's ark" or "out of Africa" hypothesis. African and Middle Eastern sites dating to over 70,000 years B.P. show evidence of fully modern peoples. By 30,000 years ago the skeletal remains of fully modern peoples are also found in Southeast Asia, Australia, New Guinea, and the New World.

12. For alternative hypotheses regarding the origins of Upper Paleolithic art, culture, and political organization, see Conkey 1983; Price and Brown 1985; Johnson and Earle 1987; Cohen 1977.

13. Gladkih, Kornieta, and Soffer 1984.

14. White 1986.

15. Ibid.; Mellars 1989.

16. White 1989a, 1989b.

17. EARLY CERAMICS—A RITUAL PURPOSE? Archaeological remains from Czechoslovakia suggest that these figurines were used in ceremonies. On the lower slopes of the Pavlov Hills, in what is today modern Moravia, these ancestors built their homes overlooking the confluence of two meandering rivers some 26,000 years ago. Eighty meters above their village on the rocky slope, they made a circular depression domed on two sides, one of several kilns found in this area. In it were thousands of shattered fragments of hard, durable ceramic figurines made of mammoth fat mixed with bone ash, local loess, and a bit of clay. Only one sculpture from these sites in Moravia remains intact, a wolverine the size of your fist. Either our ancestors were dreadful potters, or they intended to blow up their art in order to divine or for some other ritual purpose (Vandiver et al. 1989).

18. Fox 1972, 1980; Bischof 1975b; Frayser 1985.

19. Cohen 1964; Fox 1980; Malinowski 1965.

20. Tylor 1889.

21. EXOGAMY AS A PREFERRED BREEDING STRATEGY: Anthropologists are careful to distinguish between sexual rules, such as the incest taboo, and marriage regulations. These phenomena are closely connected, however, and the distinct political advantages of breeding outside of the immediate family may well have stimulated the common human marriage rule of *exogamy,* marrying outside of the community. In a study of cross-cultural marriage patterns in sixty-two societies, Suzanne Frayser (1985) reports that in 35 percent of them it is prescribed behavior to marry *outside* of the community; in 42 percent of them one is supposed to marry *within* one's community; in the balance, no preference is specified.

22. INBREEDING: It often takes many generations of extremely close inbreeding before harmful genes become selected and dreaded diseases emerge in

a family line. In fact, a certain amount of inbreeding is necessary to accentuate positive traits; this is why people breed dogs for temperament or endurance, for example. For good genetic health, a species needs enough inbreeding to fix positive traits and enough outbreeding to mask deleterious recessive genes and enrich the genome with vital fresh genetic material. So although the incest taboo (mating with nuclear-family members) is universal, marriages between first cousins are obligatory or preferred in many societies (Bischof 1975; Daly and Wilson 1983).

23. Westermarck 1934.
24. Spiro 1958.
25. Shepher 1971, 1983.
26. Bischof 1975b; De Waal 1989.
27. Sade 1968; Bischof 1975b.
28. Bischof 1975b; De Waal 1989; Daly and Wilson 1983.
29. Frayser 1985, 182.
30. Frazer [1922] 1963, 702.
31. Darwin 1871, 47.
32. Chance 1962.
33. Fox 1972, 292.
34. Ibid. 287.
35. Eibl-Eibesfeldt 1989.
36. Damon 1988; Kohlberg 1969.
37. Kohlberg 1969; Gilligan and Wiggins 1988; Damon 1988; Kagan and Lamb 1987.
38. Darwin 1871, 493.
39. Maxwell 1984.
40. Alexander 1987, 102.

14 Fickle Passion: *Romance in Yesteryears*

1. Shostak 1981; Gregor 1985.
2. AGE DIFFERENCE BETWEEN BRIDE AND GROOM: It is standard in cultures around the world that the groom is several years older than his bride (Daly and Wilson 1983).
3. Shostak 1981, 226.
4. The Herero are cattle-tending peoples who settled in the area of the Dobe !Kung in the mid-1920s.
5. PRIVATE SEX: Around the world people seek privacy for coitus. Chimpanzees, baboons, and other primates occasionally usher a partner behind a bush to copulate, but normally primates have coitus within view of con-

specifics. The human drive to seek private, uninterrupted, concealed sex is probably another trait born on the African veldt as our ancient forebears began to pair millennia ago.

6. FOREPLAY: The people of Ponape and the Trobriand Islanders of the insular Pacific spend hours at foreplay, whereas the Lepcha of Sikkim do almost no precopulatory caressing. The amount of foreplay varies from one society to the next. From a survey of worldwide studies of foreplay, Goldstein (1976a) lists types of precoital contact in descending order of worldwide prevalence. General body fondling is most important; we seem instinctively to hug, pat, and stroke before making love. "Simple kissing," mouth-to-mouth contact, is so nearly universal that it is probably basic to our human sexual repertoire as well, despite the few cultures that find kissing disgusting (Ford and Beach 1951). Tongue kissing is very common too. Fondling the woman's breasts comes next in descending order of worldwide habits of precopulatory sex, then touching the woman's genitals, oral stimulation of her breasts, caressing the man's genitals, fellatio, cunnilingus, anilingus, and, last, painful stimulations of body parts (Goldstein 1976a). Other species also engage in foreplay. Birds tap their bills together. Dogs lick. Whales stroke each other with their flippers. Most birds and mammals engage in some sort of precopulatory fondling.

7. COUVADE: Several societies in the world have an institution known as the couvade, from the French *couver*, "to incubate or hatch." This custom dictates that the father imitate some of his wife's behavior during and around pregnancy and birth. In some cultures the man acts out the physical pain of childbirth; in others he may simply observe certain dietary taboos. The Mehinaku demand only some dietary restrictions. Occasionally the father (who is not the woman's husband) will follow the restrictions of the couvade; more often he forgoes these traditions, lest he reveal his relationship with the newborn's mother.

8. PUBERTY RITUALS: Most cultures mark puberty with ceremonies for both boys and girls, so it is likely that in our ancestry both genders underwent puberty rituals prior to wedding. Because arranged marriages are also common around the world, it is probable that among our ancestors, parents regularly selected the first spouse for an adolescent child. See Frayser 1985.

9. PREMARITAL SEX: In most cultures of the insular Pacific and in many parts of sub-Saharan Africa and Eurasia, people tolerate premarital sex. In many places around the Mediterranean, premarital sex is strictly forbidden. In 82 percent of sixty-one cultures recorded, the same limitations (or lack of restrictions) apply to both genders equally; in these societies there is no double standard in regard to premarital sex. In those cultures where there is a double standard, the boy sometimes gets harsher punishment than his girlfriend; many of these societies are in sub-Saharan Africa (Frayser 1985, 205).

10. AGE AT MENARCHE: Today the median age at menarche for American white girls is 12.8; for American black girls it is 12.5. Early puberty is also common in contemporary European populations. Age at menarche has slowly declined over the last 150 years in American and European cultures, however. In 1840 the average age at menarche was 16.5–17.5 in several European peoples. This is not to suggest that menarche has been getting progressively earlier throughout human evolution. Among the classical Greeks and Romans, girls may have reached menarche as early as age 13 or 14 (Eveleth 1986). As you recall, among hunting-gathering peoples girls generally reach menarche between ages 16 and 17, suggesting that menarche occurred during late teenage in ancestral populations and that late menarche is typical of the human condition (Lancaster and Lancaster 1983).

11. Clark 1980; Cohen 1989.

15 "Till Death Us Do Part": *Birth of Western Double Standards*

1. Gregg 1988.
2. Ibid.
3. It is currently being debated whether domestication of plants and animals in Europe was introduced by immigrants or whether these practices spread as new ideas that were adopted by local foragers (Howell 1987).
4. Nissen 1988; Clark 1980; Lewin 1988a; McCorriston and Hole 1991; Blumler and Byrne 1991.
5. Whyte 1978.
6. Bullough 1976, 53.
7. ABORTION was not always illegal in Western history. The ancient Greeks, for example, believed in small families and approved of abortion. Abortion laws have varied dramatically in Western history, according to varying social circumstances.
8. Whyte 1978.
9. Lacey 1973; Gies and Gies 1978; Lampe 1987.
10. Colossians 3:18.
11. Hunt 1959, 22.
12. Whyte 1978.
13. Leacock 1972.
14. Ibid. 120.
15. Whyte 1978.
16. PRIMITIVE MATRIARCHY: Despite insufficient evidence for the absence *or* presence of a primitive matriarchy, several contemporary academics de-

fend the concept (see Fluehr-Lobban 1979; Davis 1971; Gimbutas 1989).
On the basis of the survival of female Greek and Roman deities, mysteri-
ous female figures in European folklore and fairy tales, and drawings of
goddess-like figures on ancient pottery and in frescoes, Gimbutas maintains that matriarchal societies existed in Europe seven thousand years ago
and that these peoples were then overrun by marauders from the steppes of
Russia who brought with them customs of patrilineal descent and patriarchal rule.

17. Whyte 1978.

18. SOCIAL SUBORDINATION OF WOMEN IN AGRARIAN CULTURES: A survey of
ninety-three preindustrial societies shows that women in peasant farming
communities have less domestic authority, less ritual solidarity with other
women, and less control over property than do women in gardening and
hunting-gathering cultures. Farming women resort more often to informal
means of influence. Men express more ritualized fear of women in these
cultures. Women's work is less valued, and less importance is placed on
women's lives (Whyte 1978).

19. Leacock 1972; Etienne and Leacock 1980.

20. EVOLUTION OF CHIEFDOMS: Johnson and Earle (1987) argue that European political organization characterized by permanent "big men," or
chiefs, arose in the Upper Paleolithic between 35,000 and 12,000 B.P.
because of large-scale hunting and territorial defense in highly populated
areas of Europe, but that chiefs became commonplace in Europe with the
introduction of agriculture. For a discussion of the evolution of human
political organization, see Carneiro 1991, 1987, 1981; Nissen 1988; Johnson and Earle 1987.

21. Whyte 1978, 169.

22. Goldberg 1973.

23. Davis 1964.

24. Eibl-Eibesfeldt 1989, 267; Sapolsky 1983.

25. Velle 1982; Sapolsky 1983; Rose, Holaday, and Bernstein 1971; Rose et al.
1974.

26. Brown 1988; this trend is widely seen in the anthropological literature.

27. McGuire, Raleigh, and Brammer 1982.

28. Raleigh et al., in press; Tiger 1992.

29. Frank 1985.

30. Goody 1983, 211; Queen and Habenstein 1974.

31. Bullough 1976; Lacey 1973.

32. Hunt 1959, 63; Carcopino 1973, 60; Phillips 1988.

33. Matthew 19:3–9.

34. Phillips 1988.
35. Gies and Gies 1978; Bell 1973; Bullough 1978; Hunt 1959; Phillips 1988.
36. Gies and Gies 1978, 33.
37. Queen and Habenstein 1974, 265.
38. Gies and Gies 1978, 18; Dupâquier et al. 1981.
39. Bell 1973; Power 1973; Abrams 1973.
40. Phillips 1988.
41. Goody 1983, 211; Dupâquier et al. 1981; Phillips 1988; Stone 1990.

16 Future Sex: *Forward to the Past*

1. Lucretius 1965.
2. DIVORCE RATE: The divorce rate is much more difficult to estimate than is generally thought. In 1989 the annual American divorce rate was 4.7 per 1,000 persons—which means that about 5 out of every 1,000 people divorced during that year. This tells us nothing about your chances of divorcing during the course of your life. To compute this, demographers use the "life table approach." They examine the lifetime divorce experience of adults in several successive age groups and establish all the factors that contributed to the frequency of divorce over time among the individuals in these cohorts. Then they evaluate the present force of all these factors, anticipate new factors that could contribute to divorce, and use all these data to estimate how many people will divorce this year and in coming decades. PRESENT ESTIMATES, projected from divorce trends in this century via this "life table approach," are that 47.4 percent of all Americans who married in 1974 will eventually divorce—if divorce and death rates prevailing in 1975 continue (Cherlin 1981, 25). Another estimate: 54 percent of all first marriages by women in the age category twenty-five to twenty-nine in 1987 will end in divorce (Levitan, Belous, and Gallo 1988, 1). For a comprehensive breakdown of the percentage of divorces by age, number of children, and previous marital status, see London and Foley Wilson 1988.
3. Cherlin 1981, 53; Levitan, Belous, and Gallo 1988, 32, 99; Glick 1975, 8; Espenshade 1985.
4. Cherlin 1978.
5. Glick 1975.
6. Harris 1981; Levitan, Belous, and Gallo 1988.
7. Evans 1987; Harris 1981; Cherlin 1981; Levitan, Belous, and Gallo 1988.
8. Cherlin 1981, 35.
9. Harris 1981.

10. Glick 1975; Levitan, Belous, and Gallo 1988.

11. BIRTH CONTROL AND DIVORCE: Some scientists argue that the introduction of the birth control pill, the intrauterine device, and surgical sterilization all played significant roles in the declining birthrate in the 1960s and subsequent decades. But the birthrate was low during the Great Depression, when couples in economic crisis wanted to postpone family life and these modern means of birth control were not available (Cherlin 1981, 57). Birthrates also fell in the early 1960s, before these contraceptive methods became widely available (Harris 1981). In fact, birthrates have been declining over the last hundred years, long before technological changes in contraception occurred (Goldin 1990). These new forms of birth control may have affected demographic trends in other ways, however. By using these devices, more unmarried women can avoid pregnancy; thus fewer women marry very young—probably increasing the average age at first marriage and enabling more women to enter the job market sooner. Demographer Andrew Cherlin (1981) concludes, however, that these new forms of contraception were not major forces in the 1960s trend toward later marriage, fewer children, and more divorce.

12. Harris 1981, 93.

13. Evans 1987.

14. Cherlin 1981.

15. Ibid.; Levitan, Belous, and Gallo 1988.

16. Easterlin 1980; also see Cherlin 1981; Espenshade 1985; Levitan, Belous, and Gallo 1988.

17. Levitan, Belous, and Gallo 1988; Barringer 1989b; Cherlin 1987.

18. Fisher 1989.

19. Levitan, Belous, and Gallo 1988, 77.

20. Norman Goodman, Department of Sociology, SUNY, Stony Brook, personal communication.

21. AGE AT MARRIAGE AND AGE DIFFERENCE BETWEEN HUSBAND AND WIFE: Late marriage is not the norm in traditional societies. In 69 percent of forty-five traditional cultures surveyed, girls married when they were less than 18; the age category with the highest frequency of brides was 12–15 (Frayser 1985, 208). In 74 percent of forty-two cultures, boys were at least 18 or older when they wed; the largest age category in which men wed was 18–21 (ibid.). Even in the United States about 25 percent of all women marry by age 19, and this figure has remained constant since 1910 (Cherlin 1981, 10). In agrarian cultures the dowry system often delayed marriage for a woman well into her twenties. Late marriage in America today is largely a result of women's completing college and entering the work force instead (Glick 1975). Around the world husbands tend to be two to six

years older than their wives. In the United States the age difference between husband and wife increases with the age of the groom because men who divorce tend to remarry younger women (London and Foley Wilson 1988).

22. Barringer 1991; Levitan, Belous, and Gallo 1988.

23. Lancaster and Lancaster 1983.

24. Harris 1981.

25. Levitan, Belous, and Gallo 1988.

26. Ibid.

27. Ibid.; Blake 1989a, 1989b.

28. Hunt 1959.

29. Mead 1966; Kirkendall and Gravatt 1984.

30. Krier 1988.

31. Cherlin 1981; White 1987; Barringer 1989b; Stone 1990.

32. AMERICAN AND EUROPEAN DIVORCE LAWS: For an overview of the history of divorce laws and practices in the United States and Western Europe, see Phillips 1988; Stone 1990; Bohannan 1985; Dupâquier et al. 1981.

33. PERCENTAGE OF DIVORCED PEOPLE WHO REMARRY AND TIMING OF RE-MARRIAGE: The Census Bureau reports that 76.3 percent of the women who divorce before age thirty eventually remarry; 56.2 percent of those who divorce in their thirties remarry; and 32.4 percent of those who divorce in their forties remarry (Levitan, Belous, and Gallo 1988). About 75 percent of the women and 80 percent of the men who divorce will remarry (Glick 1975; Cherlin 1981; Levitan, Belous, and Gallo 1988). One-third of all young adults today can expect to find themselves in a remarriage (Cherlin 1981, 69). One-half of all remarriages take place within three years of the divorce (Cherlin 1981; Furstenberg and Spanier 1984).

The median NUMBER OF YEARS BETWEEN DIVORCE AND REMARRIAGE is 2.9 for American women under the age of thirty with no children, about 3.0 years for women with one to two children, and about 4.4 years for women with three to five children (Levitan, Belous, and Gallo 1988). Other data conclude that women typically remarry 4 years after divorcing, whereas men typically remarry 3 years after divorcing (London and Foley Wilson 1988). Demographer Paul Glick (1975) reports that the average number of years between divorce and remarriage is 3 years. The average and median number of years a child spends in a single-parent home is 3.98 years (Marriage and Divorce Today 1986).

REMARRIAGE RATES have steadily increased since the 1930s with the exception of the 1950s (Levitan, Belous, and Gallo 1988, 33). Slightly more DIVORCES occur among REMARRIED couples than among first-married pairs (Cherlin 1981; Furstenberg and Spanier 1984). Very few men and women marry more than twice (Levitan 1988). Glick reports that women who divorce and REMARRY a never-married man end up with 3.1 children and that men and women who marry only once end up with 3.2 CHILDREN. In remarriages between two divorced persons, men and women end up with slightly fewer children—a total of 2.9 offspring (Glick 1975).

34. Levitan, Belous, and Gallo 1988; Espenshade 1985; Cherlin 1987.

35. Cherlin 1981; Furstenberg and Spanier 1984.

36. *Marriage and Divorce Today* 1986.

37. Bohannan 1985; Levitan, Belous, and Gallo 1988.

38. Bohannan 1985.

39. Krier 1988.

40. MORE ON ASSOCIATIONS: There is every reason to think that individuals in kin-based societies formed family connections with nonblood peers. But it is unlikely that these associations played the same role they do in modern societies where kinship ties do not define daily life (Leith Mullings, Department of Anthropology, CUNY Graduate Center, personal communication). Moreover, associations undoubtedly will not form in all American populations. For example, I would expect to see them occur more frequently in urban than in rural settings and more commonly in some ethnic groups that in others.

41. Eveleth 1986; Goldstein 1976.

42. Cetron and Davies 1989.

43. Ibid.

Appendix
Divorce charts

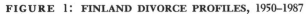

FIGURE 1: FINLAND DIVORCE PROFILES, 1950–1987

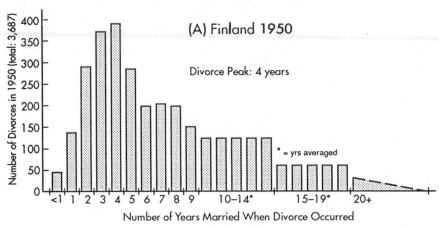

(A) Finland 1950

Divorce Peak: 4 years

* = yrs averaged

Number of Divorces in 1950 (total: 3,687)

Number of Years Married When Divorce Occurred

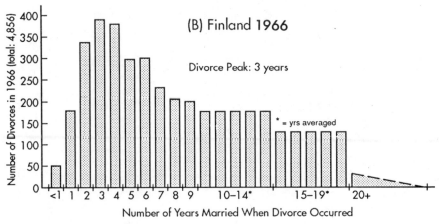

(B) Finland 1966

Divorce Peak: 3 years

* = yrs averaged

Number of Divorces in 1966 (total: 4,856)

Number of Years Married When Divorce Occurred

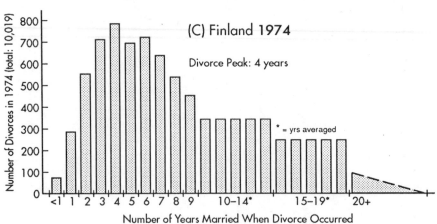

(C) Finland 1974

Divorce Peak: 4 years

* = yrs averaged

Number of Divorces in 1974 (total: 10,019)

Number of Years Married When Divorce Occurred

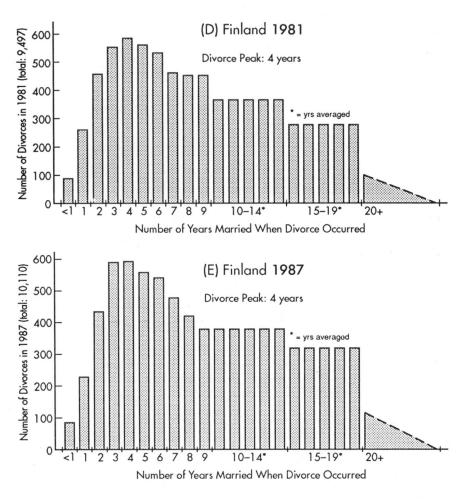

Figures A–E show the divorce profiles for Finland in five years for which data are available in the demographic yearbooks of the United Nations. In 1987, for example, 84 couples divorced in less than a year of marriage, 228 couples divorced after one year of marriage, 432 couples divorced after two years of marriage, and so forth. Most divorces occurred between the fourth and fifth years of marriage. Data on divorces occurring between 10 and 14 years of marriage and between 15 and 19 years of marriage were averaged because the raw data lumped them together. Divorces in the 20+ category were designated 20–40 years married and averaged as well. In actuality, divorces steadily declined with increasing number of years married. As can be seen in these histograms, divorces regularly cluster around a four-year peak, and this pattern shows little change despite steadily increasing divorce *rates* during these decades.

FIGURE 2: THE FOUR-YEAR ITCH: Divorce Peaks, 62 Societies,
All Available Years, 1947–1989 (188 Cases)

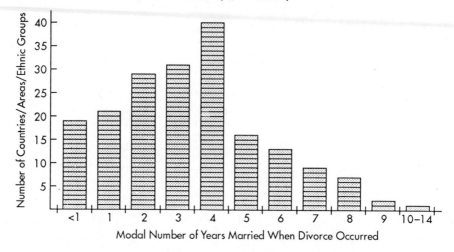

Figure 2 shows the divorce profiles for 62 countries, areas and ethnic groups
in specific years between 1947 and 1989 were drawn (188 cases). Then the
divorce peak (the mode) for each of these histograms was marked as a box on
this master chart. Finland 1987, for example, is represented as one box in the
column marked four. Thus human beings in a variety of societies tend to
divorce between the second and fourth years of marriage, with a divorce peak
during the fourth year.

FIGURE 3: EGYPT 1978 DIVORCE PROFILE

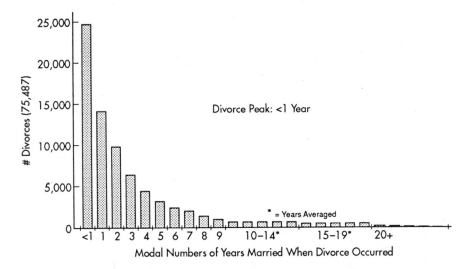

Figure 3 shows in Egypt 1978, as well as in almost all other Muslim countries for which the United Nations has data between 1947 and 1989, most divorces occurred during less than one year of marriage, and the longer a couple remained married the more likley they were to stay together. Explanations for this variation are given in chapter 5.

FIGURE 4: THE UNITED STATES 1986 DIVORCE PROFILE

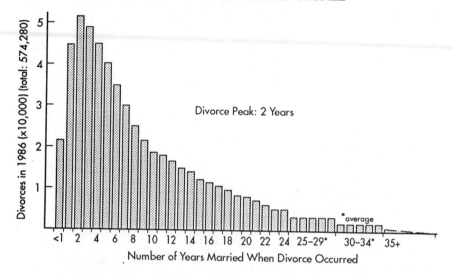

Figure 4 shows the divorce profile for the United States in 1986 as taken from the *Vital Statistics of the United States.* Data on divorces occurring between 25 and 29 years of marriage, between 30 and 34 years of marriage, and in the 35 + years category were averaged because the raw data lumped them together. Most divorces occurred between the second and third year of marriage—as in all other years I examined between 1960 and 1989. An explanation for this consistant divorce peak appears in chapter 5.

Bibliography

Abrams, A. 1973. Medieval women and trade. In *Women: From the Greeks to the French Revolution*, ed. S. G. Bell. Stanford: Stanford Univ. Press.

Abu-Lughod, L. 1986. *Veiled Sentiments: Honor and Poetry in a Bedouin Society*. Berkeley: Univ. of California Press.

—. 1987. Bedouin blues. *Natural History*, July, 24–34.

Ackerman, C. 1963. Affiliations: Structural determinants of differential divorce rates. *American Journal of Sociology* 69:13–20.

Ackerman, D. 1990. *The Natural History of the Senses*. New York: Random House.

Ackerman, S. 1989. European history gets even older. *Science* 246:28–29.

Adams, D. B., A. R. Gold, and A. D. Burt. 1978. Rise in female-initiated sexual activity at ovulation and its suppression by oral contraceptives. *New England Journal of Medicine* 299:1145–50.

Adams, V. 1980. Getting at the heart of jealous love. *Psychology Today*, May, 38–48.

Alcock, J. 1987. Ardent adaptationism. *Natural History*, April, 4.

Alexander, R. D. 1974. The evolution of social behavior. *Annual Review of Ecology and Systematics* 5:325–83.

—. 1987. *The Biology of Moral Systems*. New York: Aldine de Gruyter.

—. 1990. *How Did Humans Evolve?* Museum of Zoology, University of Michigan, Special Publication no. 1.

Alexander, R. D., and K. M. Noonan. 1979. Concealment of ovulation, parental care and human social evolution. In *Evolutionary Biology and Human Social Behavior*, ed. N. A. Chagnon and W. Irons. North Scituate, Mass.: Duxbury Press.

Alford, R. R., and R. Friedland. 1985. *Powers of Theory: Capitalism, the State, and Democracy.* New York: Cambridge Univ. Press.

Allen, L. L., P. S. Bridges, D. L. Evon, K. R. Rosenberg, M. D. Russell, L. A. Schepartz, V. J. Vitzthum, and M. H. Wolpoff. 1982. Demography and human origins. *American Anthropologist* 84:888–96.

Allen, M. 1981. Individual copulatory preference and the "Strange female effect" in a captive group-living male chimpanzee *(Pan troglodytes). Primates* 22:221–36.

Altschuler, M. 1971. Cayapa personality and sexual motivation. In *Human Sexual Behavior,* ed. D. S. Marshall and R. C. Suggs. Englewood Cliffs, N.J.: Prentice-Hall.

Ambrose, S. H. 1986. Comment on: H. T. Bunn and E. M. Kroll, Systematic butchery by Plio/Pleistocene hominids at Olduvai Gorge, Tanzania. *Current Anthropology* 27:431–53.

Andrews, P. 1981. Species diversity and diet in monkeys and apes during the Miocene. In *Aspects of Human Evolution,* ed. C. B. Stringer. London: Taylor & Francis.

Andrews, P. and J. E. Cronin. 1982. The relationships of *Sivapithecus* and *Ramapithecus* and the evolution of the orang-utan. *Nature* 297:541–46.

Andrews, P. and J. A. H. Van Couvering. 1975. Palaeoenvironments in the East African Miocene. In *Approaches to Primate Paleobiology,* ed. F. S. Szalay. Basel: S. Karger.

Angier, N. 1990. Mating for life? It's not for the birds or the bees. *New York Times,* Aug. 21.

——. 1991. A potent peptide promotes an urge to cuddle. *New York Times,* Jan. 22.

Arensburg, B., A. M. Tillier, B. Vandermeersch, A. Duday, L. A. Schepartz, and Y. Rak. 1989. A middle paleolithic human hyoid bone. *Nature* 338:758–60.

Atwater, L. 1987. College students extramarital involvement. *Sexuality Today,* Nov. 30, p. 2.

Avery, C. S. 1989. How do you build intimacy in an age of divorce? *Psychology Today,* May, 27–31.

Axelrod, D. I., and P. H. Raven. 1977. Late Cretaceous and tertiary vegetation history in Africa. In *Biogeography and Ecology of Southern Africa,* ed. M. J. A. Werger. The Hague: Junk.

Badrian, N. and R. K. Malenky. 1984. Feeding ecology of *Pan paniscus* in the Lomako Forest, Zaire. In *The Pygmy Chimpanzee,* ed. R. L. Susman. New York: Plenum Press.

Badrian, A., and N. Badrian. 1984. Social organization of *Pan paniscus* in the Lomako Forest, Zaire. In *The Pygmy Chimpanzee,* ed. R. L. Susman. New York: Plenum Press.

Balsdon, J. P. V. D. 1973. Roman women: Their history and habits. In *Women: From the Greeks to the French Revolution,* ed. S. G. Bell. Stanford: Stanford Univ. Press.

Barash, D. P. 1977. *Sociology and Behavior.* New York: Elsevier.

Bardis, P. 1963. Main features of the ancient Roman family. *Social Science* 38 (Oct.): 225–40.

Barnes, J. 1967. The frequency of divorce. In *The Craft of Social Anthropology,* ed. A. L. Epstein. London: Tavistock.

Barrett, N. 1987. Women and the economy. In *The American Woman, 1987– 88,* ed. Sara E. Rix. New York: W. W. Norton.

Barringer, F. 1989a. U.S. birth level nears 4 million mark. *New York Times,* Oct. 31.

—. 1989b. Divorce data stir doubt on trial marriage. *New York Times,* June 9.

—. 1991. Changes in U.S. households: Single parents amid solitude. *New York Times,* June 7.

Bateman, A. J. 1948. Intra-sexual selection in drosophila. *Heredity* 2:349–68.

Beals, R. L. 1946. *Cherán: A Sierra Tarascan village.* Smithsonian Institution, Institute of Social Anthropology, Publication no. 2. Washington, D.C.: Government Printing Office.

Beardsley, R. K., J. W. Hall, and R. E. Ward. 1959. *Village Japan.* Chicago: Univ. of Chicago Press.

Behrensmeyer, K. 1984. Taphonomy and the fossil record. *American Scientist* 72:558–66.

Behrensmeyer, K., and A. P. Hill. 1980. *Fossils in the Making.* Chicago: Univ. of Chicago Press.

Belkin, L. 1989. Bars to equality of sexes seen as eroding, slowly. *New York Times* Aug. 20.

Bell, A. P., and S. Weinberg. 1978. *Homosexualities: A Study of Diversity among Men and Women.* New York: Simon and Schuster.

Bell, D. 1980. Desert politics: Choices in the "marriage market." In *Women and Colonization,* ed. Mona Etienne and Eleanor Leacock. New York: Praeger.

Bell, S. G., ed. 1973. *Women: From the Greeks to the French Revolution.* Stanford: Stanford Univ. press.

Benbow, C. P., and J. C. Stanley. 1980. Sex differences in mathematical ability: Fact or artifact. *Science* 210:1234–36.

—. 1983. Sex differences in mathematical reasoning ability: More facts. *Science* 222:1029–31.

Benderly, B. L. 1987. *The Myth of Two Minds: What Gender Means and Doesn't Mean.* New York: Doubleday.

—. 1989. Don't believe everything you read: A case study of how the politics of sex differences research turned a small finding into a major media flap. *Psychology Today,* Nov. 63–66.

Benshoof, L., and R. Thornhill. 1979. The evolution of monogamy and concealed ovulation in humans. *Journal of Social and Biological Structures* 2:95–106.

Berger, J. 1986. *Wild Horses of the Great Basin: Social Competition and Population Size.* Chicago: Univ. Chicago Press.

Berggren, W. A., and C. D. Hollister. 1977. Plate tectonics and paleocirculation—Commotion in the ocean. *Tectonophysics* 38:11–48.

Bernard, J. 1964. The adjustment of married mates. In *Handbook of Marriage and the Family,* ed. H. I. Christensen. Chicago: Rand McNally.

Berndt, C. H. 1981. Interpretations and "facts" in aboriginal Australia. In *Woman the Gatherer,* ed. F. Dahlberg. New Haven: Yale Univ. Press.

Bernor, R. L. 1985. Neogene palaeoclimatic events and continental mammalian response: Is there global synchroneity? *South African Journal of Science* 81:261.

Berremann, G. 1962. Pahari polyandry: A comparison. *American Anthropologist* 64:60–75.

Bertram, B. C. R. 1975. Social factors influencing reproduction in wild lions. *Journal of Zoology* 177:463–82.

Betzig, L. L. 1982. Despotism and differential reproduction: A cross-cultural correlation of conflict asymmetry, hierarchy and degree of polygyny. *Ethology and Sociobiology* 3:209–21.

—. 1986. *Despotism and Differential Reproduction: A Darwinian View of History.* Hawthorne, N.Y.: Aldine.

—. 1989. Causes of conjugal dissolution: A cross-cultural study. *Current Anthropology* 30:654–76.

Betzig, L., A. Harrigan, and P. Turke. 1989. Childcare on Ifaluk. *Zeitschrift für Ethnologie* 114:161–77.

Bieber, I., H. J. Dain, P. R. Dince, M. G. Drellich, H. G. Grand, R. H. Gundlach, M. W. Kremer, A. H. Rifkin, C. B. Wilbur, and T. B. Bieber. 1962. *Homosexuality: A Psychoanalytic Study of Male Homosexuals.* New York: Basic Books.

Binford, L. R. 1981. *Bones: Ancient Men and Modern Myths.* New York: Academic Press.

—. 1985. Human ancestors: Changing views of their behavior. *Journal of Anthropological Archaeology* 4:292–327.

—. 1987. The hunting hypothesis: Archaeological methods and the past. *Yearbook of Physical Anthropology* 30:1–9.

Birdsell, J. B. 1968. Some predictions for the Pleistocene based on equilibrium systems among recent hunter-gatherers. In *Man the Hunter,* ed. R. B. Lee and I. DeVore. New York: Aldine.

—. 1979. Ecological influences on Australian aborginal social organization. In *Primate Ecology and Human Origins,* ed. I. S. Bernstein and E. O. Smith. New York: Garland STPM Press.

Bischof, N. 1975a. A systems approach toward the functional connections of attachment and fear. *Child Development* 46:801–17.

—. 1975b. Comparative ethology of incest avoidance. In *Biosocial Anthropology,* ed. R. Fox. London: Malaby Press.

Blake, J. 1989a. *Family Size and Achievement.* Berkeley: Univ. California Press.

—. 1989b. Number of siblings and educational attainment. *Science* 245:32–36.

Blumenschine, R. J. 1986. *Early Hominid Scavenging Opportunities: Implications for Carcass Availability in the Serengeti and Ngorongoro Ecosystems.* British Archaeological Reports International Series, no. 283. Oxford: BAR.

—. 1987. Characteristics of an early hominid scavenging niche. *Current Anthropology* 28:383–407.

——. 1989. A landscape taphonomic model of the scale of prehistoric scavenging opportunities. *Journal of Human Evolution* 18:345–71.

Blumler, M. A., and R. Byrne. 1991. The ecological genetics of domestication and the origins of agriculture. *Current Anthropology* 32:23–54.

Blumstein, P., and P. Schwartz. 1983. *American Couples: Money, Work, Sex.* New York: William Morrow.

Blurton-Jones, N. G. 1984. A selfish origin for human sharing: Tolerated theft. *Ethology and Sociobiology* 5:1–3.

Boesch, C., and A. Boesch. 1984. Mental map in wild chimpanzees: An analysis of hammer transports for nut cracking. *Primates* 25:160–70.

Bohannan, P. 1985. *All the Happy Families: Exploring the Varieties of Family Life.* New York: McGraw-Hill.

Bonnefille, R. 1985. Evolution of the continental vegetation: The palaeobotanical record from East Africa. *South African Journal of Science* 81:267–70.

Borgerhoff Mulder, M. 1990. Kipsigis women's preferences for wealthy men: Evidence for female choice in mammals? *Behavioral Ecology and Sociobiology* 27:255–64.

Botwin, C. 1988. *Men Who Can't Be Faithful.* New York: Warner Books.

Bower, B. 1984. Fossil find may be earliest known hominid. *Science News* 125:230.

——. 1985. A mosaic ape takes shape. *Science News* 127:26–27.

——. 1986. The math gap: Puzzling sex differences. *Science News* 130:357.

——. 1988a. Ancient human ancestors got all fired up. *Science News* 134:372.

——. 1988b. Retooled ancestors. *Science News* 133:344–45.

——. 1989. Conflict enters early European farm life. *Science News* 136:165.

——. 1990. Average attractions: Psychologists break down the essence of physical beauty. *Science News* 137:298–99.

——. 1991. Darwin's minds. *Science News* 140:232–34.

Bowlby, J. 1969. *Attachment and Loss. Vol. 1, Attachment.* New York: Basic Books.

Brain, C. K. 1981. *The Hunters or the Hunted? An Introduction to African Cave Taphonomy.* Chicago: Univ. of Chicago Press.

Brain, C. K., and A. Sillen. 1988. Evidence from the Swartkrans cave for the earliest use of fire. *Nature,* 336:464–66.

Brandwein, N., J. MacNeice, and P. Spiers. 1982. *The Group House Handbook: How to Live with Others (and love it)*. Reston, Va.: Acropolis Books.

Bray, O. E., J. J. Kennelly, and J. L. Guarino. 1975. Fertility of eggs produced on territories of vasectomized red-winged blackbirds. *Wilson Bulletin* 87:187–95.

Briggs, J. L. 1970. *Never in Anger: Portrait of an Eskimo Family*. Cambridge: Harvard Univ. Press.

Brink, A. S. 1957. The spontaneous fire-controlling reactions of two chimpanzee smoking addicts. *South African Journal of Science* 53:241–47.

Brod, H. 1987. Who benefits from male involvement in wife's pregnancy? *Marriage and Divorce Today* 12 (no. 46): 3.

Bromage, T. G. 1987. The biological and chronological maturation of early hominids. *Journal of Human Evolution* 16:257–72.

Brown, E. 1987. The hidden meaning: An analysis of different types of affairs. *Marriage and Divorce Today* 12 (no. 44): 1.

Brown, F., et al. 1985. Early *Homo erectus* skeleton from West Lake Turkana, Kenya. *Nature* 316:788–92.

Brown, P. 1988. *The Body and Society: Men, Women and Sexual Renunciation in Early Christianity*. New York: Columbia Univ. Press.

Bullough, V. L. 1976. *Sexual Variance in Society and History*. Chicago: Univ. of Chicago Press.

Bullough, V. L., and B. Bullough. 1987. *Women and Prostituition: A Social History*. Buffalo: Prometheus Books.

Bunn, H. T., and E. M. Kroll. 1986. Systematic butchery by Plio/Pleistocene hominids at Olduvai Gorge, Tanzania. *Current Anthropology* 27:431–53.

Burch, E. S., Jr., and T. C. Correll. 1972. Alliance and conflict: Interregional relations in north Alaska. In *Alliance in Eskimo Society*, ed. L. Guemple. Seattle: Univ. of Washington Press.

Burgess, E. W., and L. S. Cottrell. 1939. *Predicting Success and Failure in Marriage*. New York: Prentice-Hall.

Burleson, M. H., and W. R. Trevathan. 1990. Non-ovulatory sexual activity: Possible physiological effects on women's lifetime reproductive success. Paper presented at the annual meeting of the Human Behavior and Evolution Society, Los Angeles.

Burley, N. 1979. The evolution of concealed ovulation. *American Naturalist* 114:835–58.

Burns, G. 1990. In *Newsweek Special Edition,* winter/spring, 10.

Burton, F. D. 1971. Sexual climax in female *Macaca mulatta.* In *Proceedings of the Third International Congress of Primatology, Zurich 1970,* 3:180–91. Basel: Karger.

Buss, D. M. 1989. Sex differences in human mate preferences: Evolutionary hypotheses tested in 37 cultures. *Behavioral and Brain Sciences* 12:1–49.

Bygott, J. D. 1974. Agonistic behavior and dominance in wild chimpanzees. Ph.D. thesis, Univ. of Cambridge.

—. 1979. Agonistic behavior, dominance and social structure in wild chimpanzees of the Gombe National Park. In *The Great Apes,* ed. D. A. Hamburg and E. R. McCown. Menlo Park, Calif.: Benjamin/Cummings.

Byrne, G. 1989. Overhaul urged for math teaching. *Science* 243:597.

Campbell, B., ed. 1972. *Sexual Selection and the Descent of Man, 1871–1971.* Chicago: Aldine.

Cant, J. G. H. 1981. Hypothesis for the evolution of human breasts and buttocks. *American Naturalist* 117:199–204.

Capellanus, A. 1959. *The Art of Courtly Love.* Trans. J. Parry. New York: Ungar.

Carcopino, J. 1973. The emancipation of the Roman matron. In *Women: From the Greeks to the French Revolution.* ed. S. G. Bell. Stanford: Stanford Univ. Press.

Carneiro, R. L. 1958. Extra-marital sex freedom among the Kuikuru Indians of Mato Grosso. *Revista do Museu Paulista* (São Paulo) 10:135–42.

—. 1981. The chiefdom: Precursor of the state. In *The Transition to Statehood in the New World,* ed. G. D. Jones and R. R. Kautz. New York: Cambridge Univ. Press.

—. 1987. Cross-currents in the theory of state formation. *American Ethnologist* 14:756–70.

—. 1991. The nature of the chiefdom as revealed by evidence from the Cauca valley of colombia. In *Profiles in Cultural Evolution.* ed. A. T. Rambo and K. Gillogly. Anthropology Papers, Museum of Anthropology, University of Michigan, no. 85:167–90.

Cavallo, J. A. 1990. Cat in the human cradle. *Natural History,* Feb., 53–60.

Cavallo J. A., and R. Blumenschine. 1989. Tree stored leopard kills: Expanding the hominid scavenging niche. *Journal of Human Evolution* 18:393–99.

Cetron, M., and O. Davies. 1989. *American Renaissance: Our Life at the Turn of the 21st Century.* New York: St. Martin's Press.

Chagnon, N. 1982. Sociodemographic attributes of nepotism in tribal populations: Man the rule breaker. In *Current Problems in Sociobiology,* ed. B. Bertram. Cambridge: Cambridge Univ. Press.

Chance, M. R. A. 1962. Social behavior and primate evolution. In *Culture and the Evolution of Man,* ed. M. F. A. Montagu. New York: Oxford Univ. Press.

Chance, N. A. 1966. *The Eskimo of North Alaska.* New York: Holt, Rinehart and Winston.

Chase, P. G., and H. L. Dibble. 1987. Middle Paleolithic symbolism: A review of current evidence and interpretations. *Journal of Anthropological Archaeology* 6:263–96.

Cherlin, A. J. 1978. Women's changing roles at home and on the job. *Proceedings of a conference on the national longitudinal surveys of mature women in cooperation with the employment and training administration.* Department of Labor Special Report, no. 26.

—. 1981. *Marriage, Divorce, Remarriage.* Cambridge: Harvard Univ. Press.

—. 1987. Women and the family. In *The American Woman, 1987–88,* ed. S. E. Rix. New York: W. W. Norton.

Chesters, K. I. M. 1957. The Miocene flora of Rusinga Island, Lake Victoria, Kenya. *Palaeontographica* 101B:30–67.

Chin, P. 1978. *The Family.* Trans. S. Shapiro. Peking: Foreign Languages Press.

Chivers, D. J. 1978. Sexual behavior of the wild siamang. In *Recent Advances in Primatology.* Vol. 1, *Behavior,* ed. D. J. Chivers and J. Herbert. New York: Academic Press.

Chute, M. 1949. *Shakespeare of London.* New York: E. P. Dutton.

Ciochon, R. L., and J. G. Fleagle. 1987. Part V: *Ramapithecus* and human origins. In *Primate Evolution and Human Origins,* ed. R. L. Ciochon and J. G. Fleagle. New York: Aldine de Gruyter.

Clark, G. 1980. *Mesolithic Prelude.* Edinburgh: Edinburgh Univ. Press.

Cohen, M. N. 1977. *The Food Crisis in Prehistory: Overpopulation and the Origins of Agriculture.* New Haven: Yale Univ. Press.

—. 1980. Speculations on the evolution of density measurement and population regulation in *Homo sapiens*. In *Biosocial Mechanisms of Population Regulation*, ed. M. N. Cohen, R. S. Malpass, and H. G. Klein. New Haven: Yale Univ. Press.

—. 1989. *Health and the Rise of Civilization*. New Haven: Yale Univ. Press.

Cohen, R. 1971. *Dominance and Defiance: A Study of Marital Instability in an Islamic African Society*. Washington, D.C: American Anthropological Association.

Cohen, Y. A. 1964. *The Transition from Childhood to Adolescence: Cross-Cultural Studies of Initiation Ceremonies, Legal Systems, and Incest Taboos*. Chicago: Aldine.

Collier, J. F. 1988. *Marriage and Inequality in Classless Societies*. Stanford: Stanford Univ. Press.

Conkey, M. W. 1983. On the origins of Paleolithic art: A review and some critical thoughts. In *The Mousterian Legacy*, ed. E. Trinkaus. Oxford: British Archaeological Reports.

—. 1984. To find ourselves: Art and social geography of prehistoric hunter gatherers. In *Past and Present in Hunter Gatherer Societies*, ed. C. Schrire. New York: Academic Press.

Conoway, C. H., and C. B. Koford. 1964. Estrous cycles and mating behavior in a free-ranging band of rhesus monkeys. *Journal of Mammalogy*. 45:577–88.

Conroy, G. E., M. W. Vannier, and P. V. Tobias. 1990. Endocranial features of *Australopithecus africanus* revealed by 2 and 3-D computed tomography. *Science* 247:838–41.

Constantine, L. L., and J. N. Constantine. 1973. *Group Marriage: A Study of Contemporary Multilateral Marriage*. New York: Macmillan.

Coolidge, H. J. 1933. *Pan paniscus*, pygmy chimpanzee from south of the Congo River. *American Journal of Physical Anthropology* 18:1–59.

Corruccini, R. S., R. L. Ciochon, and H. M. McHenry. 1976. The postcranium of Miocene hominoids: Were Dryopithecines merely "dental apes"? *Primates* 17:205–23.

Corruccini, R. S., and H. M. McHenry. 1979. Morphological affinities of *Pan paniscus*. *Science* 204:1341–42.

Cowan, A. L. 1989. Women's gains on the job: Not without a heavy toll. *New York Times*, Aug. 2.

Cronin, J. E. 1983. Apes, humans and molecular clocks: A reappraisal. In *New Interpretations of Ape and Human Ancestry,* ed. R. L. Ciochon and R. S. Corruccini. New York: Plenum Press.

Crook, J. H., and S. J. Crook. 1988. Tibetan polyandry: Problems of adaptation and fitness. In *Human Reproductive Behaviour,* ed. L. Betzig, M. B. Mulder, and P. Turke. Cambridge: Cambridge Univ. Press.

Cutler, W. B., G. Preti, A. Krieger, G. R. Huggins, C. R. Garcia, and H. J. Lawley. 1986. Human axillary secretions influence women's menstrual cycles: The role of donor extract from men. *Hormones and Behavior* 20:463–73.

Dahlberg, F., ed. 1981. *Woman the Gatherer.* New Haven: Yale Univ. Press.

Daly, M. 1978. The cost of mating. *American Naturalist* 112:771–74.

Daly, M., and M. Wilson, 1978. *Sex, Evolution, and Behavior: Adaptations for Reproduction.* North Scituate, Mass.: Duxbury Press.

—. 1983. *Sex, Evolution, and Behavior.* Boston: Willard Grant Press;

—. 1988. *Homicide.* New York: Aldine de Gruyter.

Damon, W. 1988. *The Moral Child: Nurturing Children's Natural Moral Growth.* New York: Free Press.

Daniels, D. 1983. The evolution of concealed ovulation and self-deception. *Ethology and Sociobiology* 4:69–87.

Darwin, C. 1859. *The Origin of Species.* New York: Modern Library.

—. 1871. *The Descent of Man and Selection in Relation to Sex.* New York: Modern Library.

—. [1872] 1965. *The Expression of the Emotions in Man and Animals.* Chicago: Univ. of Chicago Press.

Davis, D. E. 1964. The physiological analysis of aggressive behavior. In *Social Behavior and Organization among Vertebrates,* ed. W. Etkin. Chicago: Univ. of Chicago Press.

Davis, E. 1971. *The First Sex.* Harmondsworth, England: Penguin Books.

Dawkins, R. 1976. *The Selfish Gene.* Oxford: Oxford University Press.

Degler, C. N. 1991. *In Search of Human Nature: The Decline and Revival of Darwinism in American Social Thought.* New York: Oxford Univ. Press.

de Lacoste-Utamsing, C., and R. L. Holloway. 1982. Sexual dimorphism in the human corpus callosum. *Science* 216:1431–32.

Delson, E., ed. 1985. *Ancestors: The Hard Evidence.* New York: Alan R. Liss.

De Rougemont, D. 1983. *Love in the Western World.* New York: Schocken Books.

De Vos, G. J. 1983. Social behavior of black grouse: An observational and experimental field study. *Ardea* 71:1–103.

De Waal, F. 1982. *Chimpanzee Politics: Power and Sex among Apes.* New York: Harper & Row.

——. 1987. Tension regulation and nonreproductive functions of sex in captive bonobos *(Pan paniscus). National Geographic Research* 3:318–35.

——. 1989. *Peacemaking among Primates.* Cambridge: Harvard Univ. Press.

Diamond, M. 1980. The biosocial evolution of human sexuality. Reply to Precis of *The evolution of human sexuality,* by Donald Symons. *Behavioral and Brain Sciences* 3:171–214.

Diana, L. n.d. Extra-marital sex in Italy: A family responsibility. Social Science Program, Virginia Commonwealth Univ.

Dickemann, M. 1979. The ecology of mating systems in hypergynous dowry societies. *Social Science Information* 18:163–95.

Dionne, E. J. 1989. Struggle for work and family fueling women's movement. *New York Times,* Aug. 22.

Dissanayake, E. 1988. *What is Art For?* Seattle: Univ. of Washington Press.

Donaldson, F. 1971. Emotion as an accessory vital system. *Perspectives in Biology and Medicine* 15:46–71.

Dougherty, E. G. 1955. Comparative evolution and the origin of sexuality. *Systematic Zoology* 4:145–69.

Douglas, C. 1987. The beat goes on. *Psychology Today,* Nov., 37–42.

Draper, P. 1985. Two views of sex differences in socialization. In *Male-Female Differences: A Bio-Cultural Perspective,* ed. R. L. Hall, P. Draper, M. E. Hamilton, D. McGuinness, C. M. Otten, and E. A. Roth. New York: Praeger.

Dupâquier, J., E. Hélin, P. Laslett, M. Livi-Bacci and S. Sogner. 1981. *Marriage and Remarriage in Populations of the Past.* New York: Academic Press.

Durden-Smith, J., and D. Desimone. 1983. *Sex and the Brain.* New York: Arbor House.

Dychtwald, K., and J. Flower. 1989. *Age Wave: The Challenges and Opportunities of an Aging America.* Los Angeles: Jeremy P. Tarcher.

East, R. 1939. *Akiga's Story: The Tiv Tribe as Seen by One of Its Members.* London: Oxford Univ. Press.

Easterlin, R. A. 1980. *Birth and Fortune: The Impact of Numbers on Personal Welfare.* New York: Basic Books.

Eberhard, W. G. 1985. *Sexual Selection and Animal Genitalia.* Cambridge: Harvard Univ. Press.

—. 1987. Runaway sexual selection. *Natural History,* Dec., 4–8.

—. 1990. Animal genitalia and female choice. *American Scientist* 87:134–41.

Eibl-Eibesfeldt, I. 1970. *Ethology: The Biology of Behavior.* New York: Holt, Rinehart and Winston.

—. 1989. *Human Ethology.* New York: Aldine de Gruyter.

Ekman, P. 1980. *The Face of Man.* New York: Garland STPM Press.

—. 1985. *Telling Lies: Clues to Deceit in the Marketplace, Politics, and Marriage.* New York: W. W. Norton.

Ekman, P. E., R. Sorenson, and W. V. Friesen. 1969. Pan-cultural elements in facial displays of emotion. *Science* 164:86–88.

Elkin, A. P. 1939. Introduction to *Aboriginal Woman: Sacred and Profane,* by P. M. Kaberry. London: Routledge and Kegan Paul.

Ellis, B., and D. Symons. 1990. Sex differences in sexual fantasy: An evolutionary psychological approach. Paper presented at the annual meeting of the Human Behavior and Evolution Society, Los Angeles.

Ember, M., and C. R. Ember. 1979. Male-female bonding: A cross-species study of mammals and birds. *Behavior Science Research* 14:37–56.

Emlen, S. T., and L. W. Oring. 1977. Ecology, sexual selection and the evolution of mating systems. *Science* 197:215–23.

Engels, F. [1884] 1954. *Origin of the Family, Private Property, and the State.* Trans. Ernest Untermann. Moscow: Foreign Languages Publishing House.

Epstein, C. 1988. *Deceptive Distinctions: Sex, Gender and the Social Order.* New York: Russell Sage.

Espenshade, T. J. 1985. Marriage trends in America: Estimates, implications, and underlying causes. *Population and Development Review* 11 (no. 2): 193–245.

Etienne, M., and E. Leacock, eds. 1980. *Women and Colonization: Anthropological Perspectives.* New York: Praeger.

Evans, M. S. 1987. Women in twentieth century America: An overview. In *The American Woman: 1987–88* ed. S. E. Rix. New York: W. W. Norton.

Eveleth, P. B. 1986. Timing of menarche: Secular trend and population differences. In *School-Age Pregnancy and Parenthood: Biosocial Dimensions,* ed. J. B. Lancaster and B. A. Hamburg. New York: Aldine de Gruyter.

Farah, M. 1984. *Marriage and Sexuality in Islam: A Translation of al-Ghazālī's* Book on the Etiquette of Marriage from the Ihyā. Salt Lake City: Univ. of Utah Press.

Fedigan, L. M. 1982. *Primate Paradigms: Sex Roles and Social Bonds.* Montreal: Eden Press.

Fehrenbacker, G. 1988. Moose courts cows, and disaster. *Standard-Times* (New Bedford, Mass.), Jan. 23.

Feinman, S., and G. W. Gill. 1978. Sex differences in physical attractiveness preferences. *Journal of Social Psychology* 105:43–52.

Feld, A., ed. 1990. How to stay married in the 90s. *Bride's* magazine, Dec., 126.

Fennema, E. 1990. Justice, equity and mathematics education. In *Mathematics and Gender,* ed. E. Fennema and G. C. Leder. New York: Teachers College Press.

Fennema, E. and G. C. Leder, eds. 1990. *Mathematics and Gender.* New York: Teachers College Press.

Field, T. M., et al. 1982. Discrimination and imitation of facial expressions by neonates. *Science* 218:179–81.

Finn, M. V., and B. S. Low. 1986. Resource distribution, social competition and mating patterns in human societies. In *Ecological Aspects of Social Evolution,* ed. D. I. Rubenstein and R. W. Wrangham. Princeton: Princeton Univ. Press.

Fisher, H. E. 1975. The loss of estrous periodicity in hominid evolution. Ph.D. diss., Univ. of Colorado, Boulder.

—. 1982. *The Sex Contract: The Evolution of Human Behavior.* New York: William Morrow.

—. 1987. The four-year itch. *Natural History,* Oct., 22–33.

—. 1989. Evolution of human serial pairbonding. *American Journal of Physical Anthropology* 78:331–54.

—. 1991. Monogamy, adultery and divorce in cross-species perspective. In *Man and Beast Revisited*, ed. M. H. Robinson and L. Tiger. Washington, D.C.: Smithsonian Institution Press.

—. In preparation. Human divorce patterns: An update.

Fishman, S. M., and D. V. Sheehan. 1985. Anxiety and panic: Their cause and treatment. *Psychology Today*, April, 26–32.

Flinn, M. V., and B. S. Low. 1986. Resource distribution, social competition and mating patterns in human societies. In *Ecological Aspects of Social Evolution*, ed. D. I. Rubenstein and R. W. Wrangham. Princeton: Princeton Univ. Press.

Fluehr-Lobban, C. 1979. A Marxist reappraisal of the matriarchate. *Current Anthropology* 20:341–60.

Foley, R. A., and P. C. Lee. 1989. Finite social space, evolutionary pathways, and reconstructing hominid behavior. *Science* 243:901–06.

Ford, C. S., and F. A. Beach. 1951. *Patterns of Sexual Behavior*. New York: Harper & Brothers.

Forsyth, A. 1985. Good scents and bad. *Natural History*, Nov., 25–32.

Fortune, R. 1963. *Sorcerers of Dobu*. New York: E. P. Dutton.

Fossey, D. 1979. Development of the mountain gorilla *(Gorilla gorilla beringei):* The first thirty-six months. In *The Great Apes*, ed. D. A. Hamburg and E. R. McCown. Menlo Park, Calif.: Benjamin/Cummings.

—. 1983. *Gorillas in the Mist*. Boston: Houghton Mifflin.

Foucault, M. 1985. *The History of Sexuality*. Vol 2, *The Use of Pleasure*. Trans. R. Hurley. New York: Pantheon Books.

Fouts, D. 1983. Louis tries his hand at surgery. *Friends of Washoe* 3, no. 4.

Fox, R. 1972. Alliance and constraint: Sexual selection in the evolution of human kinship systems. In *Sexual Selection and the Descent of Man*, ed. B. Campbell. Chicago: Aldine.

—. 1980. *The Red Lamp of Incest*. New York: E. P. Dutton.

Frank, R. 1985. *Choosing the Right Pond: Human Behavior and the Quest for Status*. New York: Oxford Univ. Press.

Frayer, D. W., and M. H. Wolpoff. 1985. Sexual Dimorphism. *Annual Review of Anthropology*. 14:429–73.

Frayser, S. 1985. *Varieties of Sexual Experience: An Anthropological Perspective on Human Sexuality.* New Haven: HRAF Press.

Frazer, J. G. [1922] 1963. *The Golden Bough.* New York: Macmillan.

Freud, S. 1918. *Totem and Taboo.* Trans. A. A. Brill. New York: Moffat, Yard.

Friedl, E. 1975. *Women and Men: An Anthropologist's View.* New York: Holt, Rinehart and Winston.

Frisch, R. E. 1978. Population, food intake and fertility. *Science* 199:22–30.

—. 1989. Body weight and reproduction. *Science* 246:432.

Frisch, R. E., and R. Revelle. 1970. Height and weight at menarche and a hypothesis of critical weights and adolescent events. *Science* 169:397–99.

Fuller, C. J. 1976. *The Nayars Today.* Cambridge: Cambridge Univ. Press.

Furstenberg, F. F., Jr. 1981. Remarriage and intergenerational relations. In *Aging: Stability and Changes in the Family.* ed. R. W. Fogel et al. New York: Academic Press.

Furstenberg, F. F., Jr., and G. B. Spanier. 1984. *Recycling the Family: Remarriage after Divorce.* Beverly Hills, Calif.: Sage Publications.

Gage, R. I. 1979. *Fox Family.* New York: Weatherhill/Heibonsha.

Galdikas, B. M. F. 1979. Orangutan adaptation at Tanjung Puting Reserve: Mating and ecology. In *The Great Apes,* ed. D. A. Hamburg and E. R. McCown. Menlo Park, Calif.: Benjamin/Cummings.

Galdikas, B. M. F., and J. W. Wood. 1990. Birth spacing patterns in humans and apes. *American Journal of Physical Anthropology* 83:185–91.

Gallup, G. G. 1982. Permanent breast enlargement in human females: A sociobiological analysis. *Journal of Human Evolution* 11:597–601.

Gargett, R. H. 1989. Grave shortcomings: The evidence for Neanderthal burial. *Current Anthropology* 30:157–90.

Gaulin, S. J., and J. Boster. 1985. Cross-cultural differences in sexual dimorphism: Is there any variance to be explained? *Ethology and Sociobiology* 6:219–25.

Gaulin, S. J., and R. W. FitzGerald. 1989. Sexual selection for spatial-learning ability. *Animal Behavior.* 37:322–31.

Gaulin, S. J., and M. J. Konner. 1977. On the natural diet of primates, including humans. In *Nutrition and the Brain.* Vol. 1, ed. R. and J. Wurtman. New York: Raven Press.

Gehlback, F. R. 1986. Odd couples of suburbia. *Natural History,* July, 56–66.

Geschwind, N. 1974. The anatomical basis of hemispheric differentiation. In *Hemispheric Function of the Human Brain,* ed. S. J. Dimond and J. G. Beaumont. New York: John Wiley.

Gibbons, A. 1990a. Our chimp cousins get that much closer. *Science* 250:376.

——. 1990b. Paleontology by bulldozer. *Science* 247:1407–9.

——. 1991. First hominid finds from Ethiopia in a decade. *Science* 251:1428.

Gibbs, H. L., et al. 1990. Realized reproductive success of polygynous red-winged blackbirds revealed by DNA markers. *Science* 250:1394–97.

Gibson, K. R. 1981. Comparative neuroontogeny, its implications for the development of human intelligence. In *Infancy and Epistemology,* ed. G. Butterworth. Brighton, England: Harvester Press.

Gies, F. and J. Gies. 1978. *Women in the Middle Ages.* New York: Barnes & Noble Books.

Giese, J. 1990. A communal type of life, and dinner's for everyone. *New York Times,* Sept. 27.

Gilligan C. 1982a. *In a Different Voice.* Cambridge: Harvard Univ. Press.

——. 1982b. Why should a woman be more like a man? *Psychology Today,* June, 70–71.

Gilligan, C., and G. Wiggins. 1988. The origins of morality in early childhood relationships. In *Mapping the Moral Domain,* ed. C. Gilligan et al. Cambridge: Harvard Univ. Press.

Gimbutas, M. A. 1989. *The Language of the Goddess.* San Francisco: Harper & Row.

Givens, D. B. 1983. *Love Signals: How to Attract a Mate.* New York: Crown.

——. 1986. The big and the small: Toward a paleontology of gesture. *Sign Language Studies* 51:145–70.

Gladkih, M. I., N. L. Kornieta, and O. Soffer. 1984. Mammoth-bone dwellings on the Russian plain. *Scientific American* 251 (no. 5):164–75.

Glenn, N., and M. Supancic. 1984. The social and demographic correlates of divorce and separation in the United States: An update and reconsideration. *Journal of Marriage and the Family* 46:563–75.

Glick, P. C. 1975. Some recent changes in American families. *Current Population Reports.* Social Studies Series P-23, no. 52. Washington, D.C.: U.S. Bureau of the Census.

Goldberg, S. 1973. *The Inevitability of Patriarchy.* New York: William Morrow.

Goldin, C. 1990. *Understanding the Gender Gap: An Economic History of American Women.* New York: Oxford Univ. Press.

——. 1991. A conversation with Claudia Goldin. *Harvard Gazette,* Feb. 1, pp. 5–6.

Goldizen, A. W. 1987. Tamarins and marmosets: Communal care of offspring. In *Primate Societies,* ed. B. B. Smuts, D. L. Cheney, R. M. Seyfarth, R. W. Wrangham, and T. T. Struhsaker. Chicago: Univ. of Chicago Press.

Goldstein, B. 1976. *Human Sexuality.* New York: McGraw-Hill.

Goldstein, M. 1976. Fraternal polyandry and fertility in a high Himalayan village in N. W. Nepal. *Human Ecology* 4 (no. 3): 223–33.

Goldstein, M. C. 1987. When brothers share a wife. *Natural History,* March, 39–49.

Goleman, D. 1981. The 7,000 faces of Dr. Ekman. *Psychology Today,* Feb., 43–49.

——. 1986. Two views of marriage explored: His and hers. *New York Times,* April 1.

——. 1989. Subtle but intriguing differences found in the brain anatomy of men and women. *New York Times,* April 11.

Goodale, J. C. 1971. *Tiwi Wives: A Study of the Women of Melville Island, North Australia.* Seattle: Univ. of Washington Press.

Goodall, J. 1968. The behavior of free-ranging chimpanzees in the Gombe Stream Reserve. *Animal Behavior Monographs* 1:161–311.

——. 1970. Tool-using in primates and other vertebrates. *Advanced Studies of Behavior* 3:195–249.

——. 1977. Watching, Watching, Watching. *New York Times,* Sept. 15.

——. 1986. *The Chimpanzees of Gombe: Patterns of Behavior.* Cambridge: Belknap Press/Harvard Univ. Press.

——. 1988. *In the Shadow of Man.* Rev. ed. Boston: Houghton Mifflin.

Goodall, J., A. Bandora, E. Bergmann, C. Busse, H. Matama, E. Mpongo, A. Pierce, and D. Riss. 1979. Intercommunity interactions in the chimpanzee population of the Gombe National Park. In *The Great Apes,* ed. D. A. Hamburg and E. R. McCown. Menlo Park, Calif.: Benjamin/Cummings.

Goodenough, W. H. 1970. *Description and Comparison in Cultural Anthropology.* Chicago: Aldine.

Goody, J. 1969. Inheritance, property, and marriage in Africa and Eurasia. *Sociology* 3:55–76.

—. 1983. *The Development of the Family and Marriage in Europe.* Cambridge: Cambridge Univ. Press.

Gorer, G. 1938. *Himalayan Village: An Account of the Lepchas of Sikkim.* London: M. Joseph.

Gough, E. K. 1968. The Nayars and the definition of marriage. In *Marriage, Family, and Residence,* ed. P. Bohannan and J. Middleton. Garden City, N.Y.: Natural History Press.

Gould, J. L. 1982. *Ethology: The Mechanisms and Evolution of Behavior.* New York: W. W. Norton.

Gould, J. L., and C. G. Gould. 1989. *The Ecology of Attraction: Sexual Selection.* New York: W. H. Freeman.

Gould, S. J. 1977. *Ontogeny and Phylogeny.* Cambridge: Harvard Univ. Press.

—. 1981. *The Mismeasure of Man.* New York: W. W. Norton.

—. 1987a. Freudian slip. *Natural History,* Feb., 14–19.

—. 1987b. Steven Jay Gould Replies to John Alcock's "Ardent Adaptationism." *Natural History,* April, 4.

Gove, C. M. 1989. Wife lending: Sexual pathways to transcendence in Eskimo culture. In *Enlightened Sexuality,* ed. G. Feuerstein. Freedom, Calif.: Crossing Press.

Graham, C. A., and W. C. McGrew. 1980. Menstrual synchrony in female undergraduates living on a coeducational campus. *Psychoneuroendocrinology* 5:245–52.

Gray, J. P., and L. D. Wolfe. 1983. Human female sexual cycles and the concealment of ovulation problem. *Journal of Social and Biological Structures* 6:345–52.

Greenfield, L. O. 1980. A late-divergence hypothesis. *American Journal of Physical Anthropology* 52:351–66.

—. 1983. Toward the resolution of discrepancies between phenetic and paleontological data bearing on the question of human origins. In *New Interpretations of Ape and Human Ancestry,* ed. R. L. Ciochon and R. S. Corruccini. New York: Plenum Press.

Gregersen, E. 1982. *Sexual Practices: The Story of Human Sexuality.* London: Mitchell Beazley.

Gregg, S. A. 1988. *Foragers and Farmers: Population Interaction and Agricultural Expansion in Prehistoric Europe.* Chicago: Univ. of Chicago Press.

Gregor, T. 1985. *Anxious Pleasures: The Sexual Lives of an Amazonian People.* Chicago: Univ. of Chicago Press.

Grine, F. E. 1989. *Evolutionary History of the Robust Australopithecines.* New York: Aldine de Gruyter.

Griffin, D. R. 1984. *Animal Thinking.* Cambridge: Harvard Univ. Press.

Gubernick, D. J. Department of Psychology, Univ. of Wisconsin, Madison. Personal communication.

Guttentag, M., and P. F. Secord. 1983. *Too Many Women? The Sex Ratio Question.* Beverly Hills, Calif.: Sage Publications.

Hall, E. T. 1959. *The Silent Language.* New York: Doubleday.

—. 1966. *The Hidden Dimension.* New York: Anchor Books.

—. 1976. *Beyond Culture.* New York: Doubleday/Anchor Press.

Hall, J. 1984. *Nonverbal Sex Differences.* Baltimore: Johns Hopkins Press.

Hall, J. A., R. Rosenthal, D. Archer, M. R. DiMatteo, and P. L. Rogers. 1977. The profile of nonverbal sensitivity. In *Advances in Psychological Assessment.* Vol. 4, ed. P. McReynolds. San Francisco: Jossey-Bass.

—. 1978. Decoding wordless messages. *Human Nature,* May, 68–75.

Hall, R. L. 1982. *Sexual Dimorphism in Homo Sapiens: A Question of Size.* New York: Preager.

Hall, T. 1987. Infidelity and women: Shifting patterns. *New York Times,* June 1.

Hames, R. B. 1988. The allocation of parental care among the Ye'kwana. In *Human Reproductive Behavior: A Darwinian Perspective.* ed. L. Betzig, M. Borgerhoff Mulder, and P. Turke. New York: Cambridge Univ. Press.

Hamilton, W. D. 1964. The genetical evolution of social behaviour: I. and II. *Journal of Theoretical Biology* 7:1–52.

—. 1980. Sex versus non-sex versus parasite. *Oikos* 35:282–90.

Hamilton, W. D., P. A. Henderson, and N. A. Moran. 1981. Fluctuation of environment and coevolved antagonist polymorphism as factors in the maintenance of sex. In *Natural Selection and Social Behavior*, ed. R. D. Alexander and D. W. Tinkle. New York: Chiron Press.

Harcourt, A. H. 1979. Social relationships between adult male and female mountain gorillas in the wild. *Animal Behavior* 27:325–42.

——. 1979. The social relations and group structure of wild mountain gorillas. In *The Great Apes*, ed. D. A. Hamburg and E. R. McCown. Menlo Park, Calif.: Benjamin/Cummings.

Harris, M. 1977. Why men dominate women. *New York Times Magazine*, Nov. 13, 46, 115–23.

——. 1981. *America Now: The Anthropology of a Changing Culture*. New York: Simon and Schuster.

Harrison, R. J. 1969. Reproduction and reproductive organs. In *The Biology of Marine Mammals*, ed. H. T. Andersen. New York: Academic Press.

Hart, C. W. M., and A. R. Pilling. 1960. *The Tiwi of North Australia*. New York: Holt, Rinehart and Winston.

Harwood, D. M. 1985. Late Neogene climate fluctuations in the southern high-latitudes: Implications of a warm Pliocene and deglaciated Antarctic continent. *South African Journal of Science* 81:239–41.

Hassan, F. 1980. The growth and regulation of human population in prehistoric times. In *Biosocial Mechanisms of Population Regulation*, ed. M. N. Cohen, R. S. Malpass, and H. G. Klein. New Haven: Yale Univ. Press.

Hausfater, G. and S. B. Hrdy. 1984. *Infanticide: Comparative and Evolutionary Perspectives*. New York: Aldine.

Hawkes, K., K. Hill, and J. F. O'Connell. 1982. Why hunters gather: Optimal foraging and the Ache of eastern Paraguay. *American Ethnologist* 9:379–98.

Hay, R. L., and M. D. Leakey. 1982. The fossil footprints of Laetoli. *Scientific American*, Feb., 50–57.

Heider, K. G. 1976. Dani sexuality: A low energy system. *Man* 11:188–201.

Henley, N. 1977. *Body Politics: Power, Sex and Nonverbal Communication*. Englewood Cliffs, N.J.: Prentice-Hall.

Henry, D. J. 1985. The little foxes. *Natural History*, Jan., 46–56.

Henry, J. 1941. *Jungle People*. Richmond: William Byrd.

Hess, E. H. 1975. *The Tell-Tale Eye*. New York: Van Nostrand Reinhold.

Hewlett, B., ed. 1992. *Father Child Relations*. New York: Aldine de Gruyter.

Hiatt, L. R. 1989. On Cuckoldry. *Journal of Social and Biological Structures.* 12:53–72.

Hite, S. 1981. *The Hite Report on Male Sexuality.* New York: Ballantine Books.

Hochschild, A., with A. Machung. 1989. *The Second Shift.* New York: Viking.

Holloway, R. L. 1985. The poor brain of *Homo sapiens neanderthalensis:* See what you please. . . . In *Ancestors: The Hard Evidence.* ed. E. Delson. New York: Alan R. Liss.

Hopson, J. L. 1979. *Scent Signals: The Silent Language of Sex.* New York: William Morrow.

—. 1980. Scent: Our hot-blooded sense. *Science Digest Special,* Summer, 52–53, 110.

Howell, J. M. 1987. Early farming in northwestern Europe. *Scientific American* 257:118–24, 126.

Howell, N. 1979. *Demography of the Dobe !Kung.* New York: Academic Press.

Hrdy, S. B. 1981. *The Woman That Never Evolved.* Cambridge: Harvard Univ. Press.

—. 1983. Heat loss. *Science 83,* Aug., 73–78.

—. 1986. Empathy, polyandry, and the myth of the coy female. In *Feminist Approaches to Science,* ed. R. Bleier. New York: Pergamon Press.

Hunt, M. M. 1959. *The Natural History of Love.* New York: Alfred A. Knopf.

—. 1974. *Sexual Behavior in the 1970s.* Chicago: Playboy Press.

Isaac, B. L., and W. E. Feinberg. 1982. Marital form and infant survival among the Mende of rural upper Bambara chiefdom, Sierra Leone. *Human Biology* 54:627–34.

James, S. R. 1989. Hominid use of fire in the Lower and Middle Pleistocene: A review of the evidence. *Current Anthropology* 30:1–26.

Jankowiak, W. 1992. *Sex, Death and Hierarchy in a Chinese City: An Anthropological Account.* New York: Columbia Univ. Press.

Jankowiak, W. R., and E. F. Fischer. 1992. A cross-cultural perspective on romantic love. *Ethnology* 31 (no.2):149–55.

Jarman, M. V. 1979. Impala social behavior: Territory, hierarchy, mating and use of space. *Fortschritte Verhaltensforschung* 21:1–92.

Jenni, D. A. 1974. Evolution of polyandry in birds. *American Zoology* 14:129–44.

Jespersen, O. [1922] 1950. *Language: Its Nature, Development and Origin.* London: George Allen and Unwin.

Jia, L., and H. Weiwen. 1990. *The Story of Peking Man: From Archaeology to Mystery.* New York: Oxford Univ. Press.

Johanson, D., and M. Edey. 1981. *Lucy: The Beginnings of Humankind.* New York: Simon and Schuster.

Johanson, D., and J. Shreeve. 1989. *Lucy's Child: The Discovery of a Human Ancestor.* New York: William Morrow.

Johanson, D. C., and T. D. White. 1979. A systematic assessment of early African hominids. *Science* 203:321–30.

Johnson, A. W., and T. Earle. 1987. *The Evolution of Human Societies: From Foraging Group to Agrarian State.* Stanford: Stanford Univ. Press.

Johnson, L. L. 1989. The Neanderthals and population as prime mover. *Current Anthropology* 30:534–35.

Johnson, R. A. 1983. *We: Understanding the Psychology of Romantic Love.* San Francisco: Harper & Row.

Johnson, S. C. 1981. Bonobos: Generalized hominid prototypes or specialized insular dwarfs? *Current Anthropology* 22:363–75.

Johnston, F. E., ed. 1982. Pliocene hominid fossils from Hadar, Ethiopia. *American Journal of Physical Anthropology* 57:373–19.

Jorgensen, W. 1980. *Western Indians.* San Francisco: W. H. Freeman.

Jost, A. 1972. A new look at the mechanisms controlling sex differentiation in mammals. *Johns Hopkins Medical Journal* 130:38–53.

Jungers, W. 1988. Relative joint size and hominoid locomotor adaptations. *Journal of Human Evolution* 17:247.

Kaberry, P. M. 1939. *Aboriginal Woman: Sacred and Profane.* London: Routledge and Kegan Paul.

Kagan, J., and S. Lamb, eds. 1987. *The Emergence of Morality in Young Children.* Chicago: Univ. of Chicago Press.

Kagan, J., J. S. Reznick, and N. Snidman. 1988. Biological Bases of Childhood Shyness. *Science* 240:167–71.

Kano, T. 1979. A pilot study on the ecology of pygmy chimpanzees, *Pan panis-cus.* In *The Great Apes,* ed. D. A. Hamburg and E. R. McCown. Menlo Park, Calif.: Benjamin/Cummings.

—. 1980. Social behavior of wild pygmy chimpanzees *(Pan paniscus)* of Wamba: A preliminary report. *Journal of Human Evolution* 9:243–260.

Kano, T., and M. Mulavwa. 1984. Feeding ecology of the pygmy chimpanzees *(Pan paniscus)* of Wamba. In *The Pygmy Chimpanzee,* ed. R. L. Susman. New York: Plenum Press.

Kantrowitz, B., and P. Wingert. 1990. Step by step. *Newsweek Special Edition,* Winter/Spring, 24–34.

Kay, R. F. 1981. The nut-crackers: A new theory of the adaptations of the Ramapithecinae. *American Journal of Physical Anthropology* 55:141–51.

Kimura, D. 1983. Sex differences in cerebral organization for speech and praxic functions. *Canadian Journal of Psychology* 37:19–35.

—. 1989. How sex hormones boost or cut intellectual ability. *Psychology Today,* Nov., 63–66.

Kinsey, A. C., W. B. Pomeroy, and C. E. Martin. 1948. *Sexual Behavior in the Human Male.* Philadelphia: W. B. Saunders.

Kinsey, A. C., W. B. Pomeroy, C. E. Martin, and P. H. Gebhard. 1953. *Sexual Behavior in the Human Female.* Philadelphia: W. B. Saunders.

Kinzey, W. G. 1987. Monogamous primates: A primate model for human mating systems. In *The Evolution of Human Behavior,* ed. W. G. Kinzey. Albany: State Univ. of New York Press.

Kirkendall, L. A., and A. E. Gravatt. 1984. Marriage and family: Styles and forms. In *Marriage and the Family in the Year 2000,* ed. L. A. Kirkendall and A. E. Gravatt. Buffalo: Prometheus Books.

Kleiman, D. G. 1977. Monogamy in mammals. *Quarterly Review of Biology* 52:39–69.

Kleiman, D. G., and J. F. Eisenberg. 1973. Comparisons of child and felid social systems from an evolutionary perspective. *Animal Behavior* 21:637–59.

Kleiman, D. G., and J. R. Malcolm. 1981. The evolution of male parental investment in mammals. In *Parental Care in Mammals,* ed. D. J. Gubernick and P. H. Klopfer. New York: Plenum Press.

Klein, L. 1980. Contending with colonization: Tlingit men and women in change. In *Woman and Colonization,* ed. M. Etienne and E. Leacock. New York: Praeger.

Kohlberg, L. 1969. Stage and sequence: The cognitive-developmental approach to socialization. In *Handbook of Socialization Theory and Research,* ed. D. A. Goslin. Chicago: Rand McNally.

Kohler, W. 1925. *The Mentality of Apes.* London: Routledge and Kegan Paul. Reprint. New York: Liveright, 1976.

Konner, M. J. 1982. *The Tangled Wing: Biological Constraints on the Human Spirit.* New York: Harper & Row.

——. 1988. Is orgasm essential? *Sciences,* March–April 4–7.

Konner, M., and C. Worthman. 1980. Nursing frequency, gonadal function, and birth spacing among !Kung hunter-gatherers. *Science* 207:788–91.

Krier, B. A. 1988. Why so many singles? *Los Angeles Times,* June 26.

Kristof, N. D. 1991. Love, the starry-eyed kind, casts spell on China. *New York Times,* March 6.

Kruuk, H. 1972. *The Spotted Hyena: A Study of Predation and Social Behavior.* Chicago: Univ. of Chicago Press.

Kummer, H. 1968. *Social Organization of Hamadryas Baboons* Chicago: Univ. of Chicago Press.

Kuroda, S. 1984. Interaction over food among Pygmy Chimpanzees. In *The Pygmy Chimpanzee,* ed. R. L. Susman. New York: Plenum Press.

Lacey, W. K. 1973. Women in democratic Athens. In *Women: From the Greeks to the French Revolution.* ed. S. G. Bell. Stanford: Stanford Univ. Press.

Lack, D. 1968. *Ecological Adaptations for Breeding in Birds.* London: Methuen.

Laitman, J. T., R. C. Heimbuch, and E. S. Crelin. 1979. The basicranium of fossil hominids as an indicator of their upper respiratory system. *American Journal of Physical Anthropology* 51:15–34.

Laitman, J. T. 1984. The anatomy of human speech. *Natural History,* Aug., 20–27.

Lampe, P. E., ed. 1987. *Adultery in the United States: Close Encounters of the Sixth (or Seventh) Kind.* Buffalo: Prometheus Books.

Lancaster, J. B. 1979. Sex and gender in evolutionary perspective. In *Human Sexuality,* ed. M. Katchadourian. Berkeley: Univ. of California Press.

——. 1986. Human adolescence and reproduction: An evolutionary perspective. In *School-Age Pregnancy and Parenthood,* ed. J. B. Lancaster and B. A. Hamburg. New York: Aldine de Gruyter.

——. In preparation. Parental investment and the evolution of the juvenile phase of the human life course. In *The Origins of Humanness,* ed. A. Brooks. Washington, D.C.: Smithsonian Institution Press.

Lancaster, J. B., and C. S. Lancaster, 1983. Parental investment: The hominid adaptation. In *How Humans Adapt: A Biocultural Odyssey,* ed. D. J. Ortner. Washington, D.C.: Smithsonian Institution Press.

Latimer, B. M., T. D. White, W. H. Kimbel, D. C. Johanson, and C. O. Lovejoy. 1981. The pygmy chimpanzee is not a living missing link in human evolution. *Journal of Human Evolution* 10:475–88.

Lawrence, R. J. 1989. *The Poisoning of Eros: Sexual Values in Conflict.* New York: Augustine Moore Press.

Lawson, A. 1988. *Adultery: An Analysis of Love and Betrayal.* New York: Basic Books.

Leacock, E. B., ed. 1972. *The Origins of the Family, Private Property and the State, By Frederick Engels with an Introduction by Eleanor Burke Leacock.* New York: International Publishers.

Leacock, E. B. 1980. Montagnais women and the Jesuit program for colonization. In *Women and Colonization,* ed. M. Etienne E. Leacock. New York: Praeger.

——. 1981. *Myths of Male Dominance.* New York: Monthly Review Press.

Leakey, M. D. 1971. *Olduvai Gorge.* Vol. 3. London: Cambridge Univ. Press.

Leakey, M. D., and R. L. Hay. 1979. Pliocene footprints in the Laetolil beds at Laetoli, northern Tanzania. *Nature* 278:317–23.

Leakey, M. D., R. L. Hay, G. H. Curtis, R. E. Drake, M. K. Jackes, and T. D. White. 1976. Fossil hominids from the Laetolil Beds. *Nature* 262:460–66.

LeBoeuf, B. J. 1974. Male-male competition and reproductive success in elephant seals. *American Zoologist* 14:163–76.

Le Clercq, C. 1910. *New relation of Gaspesia,* ed. W. F. Ganong. Toronto: Champlain Society.

Leder, G. C. 1990. Gender differences in mathematics: An overview. In *Mathematics and Gender,* ed. E. Fennema and G. C. Leder. New York: Teachers College Press.

Lee, R. B. 1968. What hunters do for a living, or, How to make out on scarce resources. In *Man the Hunter,* ed. R. B. Lee aand I. DeVore. New York: Aldine.

——. 1980. Lactation, ovulation, infanticide, and women's work: A study of hunter-gatherer population regulation. In *Biosocial Mechanisms of Population Regulation,* ed. M. N. Cohen, R. S. Malpass, and H. G. Klein. New Haven: Yale Univ. Press.

Lehrman, N. S. 1962. Some origins of contemporary sexual standards. *Journal of Religion and Health* 1:362–86.

——. 1963. Moses, monotheism and marital fidelity. *Journal of Religion and Health* 3:70–89.

Leroi-Gourhan, A. 1975. The flowers found with Shanidar IV: A Neanderthal burial in Iraq. *Science* 190:562–64.

Lévi-Strauss, C. 1985. *The View from Afar.* New York: Basic Books.

Levinger, G. 1968. Marital cohesiveness and dissolution: An integrative review. In *Selected Studies in Marriage and the Family,* ed. R. R. Winch and L. L. Goodman. 3d ed. New York: Holt, Rinehart and Winston.

Levitan, S. A., R. S. Belous, and F. Gallo. 1988. *What's Happening to the American Family?* Baltimore: Johns Hopkins Univ. Press.

Lewin, R. 1982. How did humans evolve big brains? *Science* 216:840–41.

——. 1983a. Fossil Lucy grows younger, again. *Science* 219:43–44.

——. 1983b. Is the orangutan a living fossil? *Science* 222:1222–23.

——. 1985. Surprise findings in the Taung child's face. *Science* 228:42–44.

——. 1987a. Africa: Cradle of modern humans. *Science* 237:1292–95.

——. 1987b. Four legs bad, two legs good. *Science* 235:969–71.

——. 1988a. A revolution of ideas in agricultural origins. *Science* 240:984–86.

——. 1988b. Conflict over DNA clock results. *Science* 241:1598–1600.

——. 1988c. DNA clock conflict continues. *Science* 241:1756–59.

——. 1988d. Subtleties of mating competition. *Science* 242:668.

——. 1989. Species questions in modern human origins. *Science* 243:1666–67.

Lewis, H. T. 1989. Reply to Hominid use of fire in the Lower and Middle Pleistocene: A review of the evidence, by S. R. James. *Current Anthropology* 30:1–26.

Lewis, R. A., and G. B. Spanier. 1979. Theorizing about the quality and stability of marriage. In *Contemporary Theories about the Family,* ed. W. Burr, R. Hill, F. Nye, And I Reiss. New York: Free Press.

Lieberman, P. 1984. *The Biology and Evolution of Language.* Cambridge: Harvard Univ. Press.

Liebowitz, M. R. 1983. *The Chemistry of Love.* Boston: Little, Brown.

Lindburg, D. G. 1982. Primate obstetrics: The biology of birth. *American Journal of Primatology.* Supplement. 1:193–99.

Lloyd, H. G. 1980. *The Red Fox.* London: Batsford.

Lloyd, P. 1968. Divorce among the Yoruba. *American Anthropologist* 70:67–81.

London, K. A., and B. Foley Wilson. 1988. D-i-v-o-r-c-e. *American Demographics,* Oct., 22–26.

Lovejoy, C. O. 1981. The origin of man. *Science* 211:341–50.

Low, B. S. 1979. Sexual selection and human ornamentation. In *Evolutionary Biology and Human Social Behavior,* ed. N. A. Chagnon and W. Irons. North Scituate, Mass.: Duxbury Press.

Low, B. S., R. D. Alexander, and K. M. Noonan. 1987. Human hips, breasts and buttocks: Is fat deceptive? *Ethology and Sociobiology* 8 (no. 4): 249–58.

Lucretius. 1965. *On the Nature of the Universe.* New York: Frederick Ungar.

Maccoby, E. E., and C. N. Jacklin. 1974. *The Psychology of Sex Differences.* Stanford: Stanford Univ. Press.

Mace, D., and V. Mace. 1959. *Marriage: East and West.* Garden City, N.Y.: Dolphin Books, Doubleday.

MacKinnon, J. 1979. Reproductive behavior in wild orangutan populations. In *The Great Apes,* ed. D. A. Hamburg and E. R. McCown. Menlo Park, Calif.: Benjamin/Cummings.

MacLean, P. D. 1973. *A Triune Concept of the Brain and Behaviour.* Toronto: Toronto Univ. Press.

Maglio, V. J. 1978. Patterns of faunal evolution. In *Evolution of African Mammals,* ed. V. J. Maglio and H. B. S. Cooke. Cambridge: Harvard Univ. Press.

Malinowski, B. 1965. *Sex and Repression in Savage Society.* New York: World.

Mansperger, M. C. 1990. The precultural human mating system. *Journal of Human Evolution* 5:245–59.

Marks, J. 1989. The hominin clad. *Science* 246:1645.

Marriage and Divorce Today. 1987. The hidden meaning: An analysis of different types of affairs. June 1, pp. 1–2.

—. 1986. May 12, p. 1.

Martin, M. K., and B. Voorhies. 1975. *Female of the Species.* New York: Columbia Univ. Press.

Martin, R. D. 1982. Human brain evolution in an ecological context. Fifty-second James Arthur Lecture on the Evolution of the Human Brain, American Museum of Natural History, New York.

Mascia-Lees, F. E., J. H. Relethford, and T. Sorger. 1986. Evolutionary perspectives on permanent breast enlargement in human females. *American Anthropologist* 88:423–29.

Maxwell, M. 1984. *Human Evolution: A Philosophical Anthropology.* New York: Columbia Univ. Press.

Maynard Smith, J. 1978. *The Evolution of Sex.* Cambridge: Cambridge Univ. Press.

McClintock, M. K. 1971. Menstrual synchrony and suppression. *Nature* 229: 244–45.

McCorriston, J., and F. Hole. 1991. The ecology of seasonal stress and the origins of agriculture in the Near East. *American Anthropologist* 93:46–69.

McGinnis, P. R. 1979. Sexual behavior in free-living chimpanzees: Consort relationships. In *The Great Apes,* ed. D. A. Hamburg and E. R. McCown. Menlo Park, Calif.: Benjamin/Cummings.

McGrew, W. C. 1974. Tool use by wild chimpanzees in feeding upon driver ants. *Journal of Human Evolution* 3:501–8.

—. 1979. Evolutionary implications of sex differences in chimpanzee predation and tool use. In *The Great Apes,* ed. D. A. Hamburg and E. R. McCown. Menlo Park, Calif.: Benjamin/Cummings.

—. 1981. The female chimpanzee as a human evolutionary prototype. In *Woman the Gatherer,* ed. F. Dahlberg. New Haven: Yale Univ. Press.

McGuiness, D. 1976. Perceptual and cognitive differences between the sexes. In *Explorations in Sex Differences,* B. Lloyd and J. Archer. New York: Academic Press.

—. 1979. How schools discriminate against boys. *Human Nature,* Feb., 82–88.

—. 1985. Sensory biases in cognitive development. In *Male-Female Differences: A Bio-Cultural Perspective.* ed. R. L. Hall, P. Draper, M. E. Hamilton, D. McGuinness, C. M. Otten, and E. A. Roth. New York: Praeger.

McGuinness, D., and K. H. Pribram. 1979. The origin of sensory bias in the development of gender differences in perception and cognition. In *Cognitive Growth and Development*, ed. M. Bortner. New York: Brunner/Mazel.

McGuire, M. M. Raleigh, and G. Brammer. 1982. Sociopharmacology. *Annual Review of Pharmacology and Toxicology* 22:643–61.

McHenry, H. M. 1986. The first bipeds. *Journal of Human Evolution* 15:177.

McHenry, H. M., and C. J. O'Brien. 1986. Comment on H. T. Bunn and E. M. Kroll, "Systematic butchery by Plio/Pleistocene hominids at Olduvai Gorge, Tanzania." *Current Anthropology* 27:431–53.

McMillan, V. 1984. Dragonfly monopoly. *Natural History*, July, 33–38.

McWhirter, N., and R. McWhirter. 1975. *Guinness Book of World Records*. New York: Sterling.

Mead, M. 1935. *Sex and Temperament in Three Primitive Societies*. New York: William Morrow.

—. 1949. *Male and Female*. New York: William Morrow.

—. 1966. Marriage in two steps. *Redbook*, July, 47–49, 84, 86.

Mealey, L. 1985. The relationship between social status and biological success: A case study of the Mormon religious hierarchy. *Ethology and Sociobiology* 6:249–57.

Meggitt, M. J. 1962. *Desert People: A Study of the Walbiri Aborigines of Central Australia*. Chicago: Univ. of Chicago Press.

Mellars, P. 1989. Major issues in the emergence of modern humans. *Current Anthropology* 30:349–85.

Mellen, S. L. W. 1981. *The Evolution of Love*. San Francisco: W. H. Freeman.

Michod, R. E. 1989. What's love got to do with it? *The Sciences*, May–June, 22–28.

Michod, R. E., and B. R. Levin, eds. 1987. *The Evolution of Sex: An Examination of Current Ideas*. Sunderland, Mass.: Sinauer.

Miller, J. A. 1983. Masculine/feminine behavior: New views. *Science News* 124:326.

Mitterauer, M. and R. Sieder. 1982. *The European Family: Patriarchy to Partnership from the Middle Ages to the Present*. Chicago: Univ. of Chicago Press.

Miyamoto, M. M., J. L. Slightom, and M. Goodman. 1987. Phylogenetic relations of humans and African apes from DNA sequences in the ψ7-globin region. *Science* 238:369–72.

Mock, D. W., and M. Fujioka. 1990. Monogamy and long-term pair bonding in vertebrates. *Trends in Ecology and Evolution* 5 (no. 2): 39–43.

Moir, A., and D. Jessel. 1989. *Brain Sex: The Real Differences between Men and Women.* London: Michael Joseph.

Moller, A. P. 1988. Ejaculate quality, testes size and sperm competition in primates. *Journal of Human Evolution* 17:479.

Money, J. 1980. *Love and Love Sickness: The Science of Sex, Gender Difference, and Pair-Bonding.* Baltimore: Johns Hopkins Univ. Press.

——. 1986. *Lovemaps: Clinical Concepts of Sexual/Erotic Health and Pathology, Paraphilia, and Gender Transposition in Childhood, Adolescence and Maturity.* New York: Irvington Publishers.

Money, J., and A. A. Ehrhardt. 1972. *Man and Woman, Boy and Girl: The Differentiation and Dimorphism of Gender Identity from Conception to Maturity.* Baltimore: Johns Hopkins Univ. Press.

Montagu, A. 1937. *Coming into Being among the Australian Aborigines.* London: Routledge.

——. 1961. Neonatal and infant immaturity in man. *Journal of the American Medical Association* 178:56–57.

——. 1971. *Touching: The Human Significance of the Skin.* New York: Columbia Univ. Press.

——. 1981. *Growing Young.* New York: McGraw-Hill.

Morgan, L. H. 1877. *Ancient Society.* New York: World.

Morris, D. 1967. *The Naked Ape.* New York: McGraw-Hill.

——. 1971. *Intimate Behavior.* New York: Bantam Books.

Morrison, P. 1987. Review of *Dark caves, bright visions: Life in Ice Age Europe*, by Randall White. *Scientific American* 256 (no. 3):26–27.

Moss, C. 1988. *Elephant Memories: Thirteen Years in the Life of an Elephant Family.* New York: William Morrow.

Murdock, G. P. 1949. *Social Structure.* New York: Free Press.

——. 1965. Family stability in non-European culture. In *Culture and Society*, ed. G. P. Murdock. Pittsburgh: Univ. of Pittsburgh Press.

——. 1967. *Ethnographic Atlas.* Pittsburgh: Univ. of Pittsburgh Press.

Murdock, G. P., and D. R. White. 1969. Standard cross-cultural sample. *Ethnology* 8:329–69.

Nadel, S. F. 1942. *A Black Byzantium: The Kingdom of Nupe in Nigeria.* London: Oxford Univ. Press.

Nadler, R. D. 1975. Sexual cyclicity in captive lowland gorillas. *Science* 189: 813–14.

——. 1988. Sexual aggression in the great apes. In *Human Sexual Aggression,* ed. R. A. Prentky and V. L. Quinsey. Annals of the New York Academy of Sciences, vol. 528:154–61. New York: NYAS.

Nimuendaju, C. 1946. *The Eastern Timbira.* Trans. R. H. Lowie. Univ. of California Publications in American Archaeology and Ethnology, vol. 41. Berkeley: Univ. of California Press.

Nishida, T. 1979. The social structure of chimpanzees of the Mahali Mountains. In *The Great Apes,* ed. D. A. Hamburg and E. R. McCown. Menlo Park, Calif.: Benjamin/Cummings.

Nissen, H. J. 1988. *The Early History of the Ancient Near East, 9000–2000 B.C.* Chicago: Univ. of Chicago Press.

Oakley, K. P. 1956. Fire as a Paleolithic tool and weapon. *Proceedings of the Prehistoric Society* 21:36–48.

O'Brien, E. M. 1984. What was the acheulean hand ax? *Natural History,* July, 20–24.

Okonjo, K. 1976. The dual-sex political system in operation: Igbo women and community politics in midwestern Nigeria. In *Women in Africa: Studies in Social and Economic Change,* ed. N. J. Hafkin and E. G. Bay. Stanford: Stanford Univ. Press.

Orians, G. H. 1969. On the evolution of mating systems in birds and mammals. *American Naturalist* 103:589–603.

Ortner, S. B., and H. Whitehead. 1981. Introduction: Accounting for sexual meanings. In *Sexual Meanings,* ed. S. B. Ortner and H. Whitehead. Cambridge: Cambridge Univ. Press.

Otten, C. M. 1985 Genetic effects on male and female development and on the sex ratio. In *Male-Female Differences: A Bio-Cultural Perspective.* ed. R. H. Hall, P. Draper, M. E. Hamilton, D. McGuinness, C. M. Otten, and E. A. Roth. New York: Praeger.

Pagels, E. 1988. *Adam, Eve and the Serpent.* New York: Vintage Books.

Parker, G. A., R. R. Baker, and V. G. F. Smith. 1972. The origin and evolution of gamete dimorphism and the male-female phenomenon. *Journal of Theoretical Biology* 36:529–53.

Pavelka, M. S., and L. M. Fedigan. 1991. Menopause: A comparative life history perspective. *Yearbook of Physical Anthropology* 34:13–38.

Peck, J. R., and M. W. Feldman. 1988. Kin selection and the evolution of monogamy. *Science* 240:1672–74.

People magazine. 1986. Unfaithfully Yours: Adultery in America. Aug. 18, 85–95.

Perper, T. 1985. *Sex Signals: The Biology of Love.* Philadelphia: ISI Press.

Pfeiffer, J. E. 1982. *The Creative Explosion: An Inquiry into the Origins of Art and Religion.* New York: Harper & Row.

Phillips, R. 1988. *Putting Asunder: A History of Divorce in Western Society.* Cambridge: Cambridge Univ. press.

Pilbeam, D. 1985. Patterns of hominoid evolution. In *Ancestors: The Hard Evidence.* ed. E. Delson. New York: Alan R. Liss.

Pittman, F. 1989. *Private Lies: Infidelity and the Betrayal of Intimacy.* New York: W. W. Norton.

Plooij, F. X. 1978. Tool-use during chimpanzee's bushpig hunt. *Carnivore* 1:103–6.

Potts, R. 1984. Home bases and early hominids. *American Scientist* 72:338–47.

——. 1988. *Early Hominid Activities at Olduvai.* New York: Aldine de Gruyter.

——. 1991. Untying the knot: Evolution of early human behavior. In *Man and Beast Revisited,* ed. M. H. Robinson and L. Tiger. Washington, D.C.: Smithsonian Institution Press.

Power, E. 1973. The position of women. In *Women: From the Greeks to the French Revolution.* ed. S. G. Bell. Stanford: Stanford Univ. Press.

Preti, G., W. B Cutler, C. R. Garcia, G. R. Huggins, and H. J. Lawley. 1986. Human axillary secretions influence women's menstrual cycles: The role of donor extract of females. *Hormones and Behavior* 20:474–82.

Price, D., and J. A. Brown, eds. 1985. *Prehistoric Hunter-Gatherers: The Emergence of Cultural Complexity.* New York: Academic Press.

Pusey, A. E. 1979. Intercommunity transfer of chimpanzees in Gombe National Park. In *The Great Apes,* ed. D. A. Hamburg and E. R. McCown. Menlo Park, Calif.: Benjamin/Cummings.

——. 1980. Inbreeding avoidance in chimpanzees. *Animal Behavior* 28:543–52.

Quadagno, D. M., H. E. Shubeita, J. Deck, and D. Francoeur. 1981. Influence of male social contacts, exercise and all-female living conditions on the menstrual cycle. *Psychoneuroendocrinology* 6:239–44.

Queen, S. A., and R. W. Habenstein. 1974. *The Family in Various Cultures.* Philadelphia: J. B. Lippincott.

Radcliffe-Brown, A. R. 1922. *The Andaman Islanders.* Cambridge: Cambridge Univ. Press.

Raleigh, M. et al. In press. Serotonergic mechanisms promote dominance acquisition in adult male vervet monkeys. *Brain Research.*

Rancourt-Laferriere, D. 1983. Four adaptive aspects of the female orgasm. *Journal of Social and Biological Structures,* 6:319–33.

Rawson, B. ed. 1986. *The Family in Ancient Rome: New Perspectives.* Ithaca: Cornell Univ. Press.

Reichard, G. S. 1950. *Navaho Religion.* New York: Bollingen Foundation.

Reiter, R. R. 1975. Introduction. In *Toward an Anthropology of Women,* ed. R. R. Reiter. New York: Monthly Review Press.

—, ed. 1975. *Toward an Anthropology of Women.* New York: Monthly Review Press.

Repenning C. A., and O. Fejfar. 1982. Evidence for early date of Ubeidiya, Israel, hominid site. *Nature* 299:344–47.

Retallack, G. J., D. P. Dugas, and E. A. Bestland. 1990. Fossil soils and grasses of the Middle Miocene East African grassland. *Science* 247:1325.

Roberts, L. 1988. Zeroing in on the sex switch. *Science* 239:21–23.

Rodman, P. S. 1988. Orangutans. *Institute of Human Origins Newsletter* 6 (no. 1): 5.

Rogers, S. C. 1975. Female forms of power and the myth of male dominance: A model of female/male interaction in peasant society. *American Ethnologist* 2:727–56.

Rohrlich-Leavitt, R. B. Sykes, and E. Weatherford. 1975. Aboriginal woman: Male and female, anthropological perspectives. In *Toward an Anthropology of Women,* ed. R. R. Reiter. New York: Monthly Review Press.

Rosaldo, M. Z. 1974. Woman, culture, and society: A theoretical overview. In *Woman, Culture, and Society,* ed. M. Z. Rosaldo and L. Lamphere. Stanford: Stanford Univ. Press.

Rosaldo, M. Z., and L. Lamphere, eds. 1974. *Women, Culture, and Society.* Stanford: Stanford Univ. Press.

Rose, M. D. 1983. Miocene hominoid postcranial morphology: monkey-like, ape-like, neither, or both? In *New Interpretations of Ape and Human Ancestry*, ed. R. L. Ciochon and R. S. Corruccini. New York: Plenum Press.

Rose, R. M., J. W. Holaday and I. S. Bernstein. 1971. Plasma testosterone, dominance rank and aggressive behavior in male rhesus monkeys. *Nature* 231: 366–68.

Rose, R. M., I. S. Bernstein, T. P. Gordon, and S. F. Catlin. 1974. Androgens and aggression: A review and recent findings in primates. *Primate Aggression, Territoriality, and Xenophobia*, ed. R. L. Holloway. New York: Academic Press.

Rosenblum, A. 1976. *The Natural Birth Control Book*. Philadelphia: Aquarian Research Foundation.

Rossi, A. 1984. Gender and parenthood. *American Sociological Review* 49:1–19.

Rowell, T. E. 1972. Female reproductive cycles and social behavior in primates. In *Advances in the Study of Behavior*, Vol 4, ed. D. S. Lehrman, R. A. Hinde, and E. Shaw. New York: Academic Press.

Rue, L. L. 1969. *The World of the Red Fox*. Philadelphia: J. B. Lippincott.

Ruse, M. 1988. *Homosexuality: A Philosophical Inquiry*. Oxford: Basil Blackwell.

Russell, M. J. 1976. Human olfactory communication. *Nature* 260:520–22.

Russett, C. E. 1989. *Sexual Science: The Victorian Construction of Womanhood*. Cambridge: Harvard Univ. Press.

Rutberg, A. T. 1983. The evolution of monogamy in primates. *Journal of Theoretical Biology* 104:93–112.

Ryan, A. S., and D. C. Johanson. 1989. Anterior dental microwear in *Australopithecus afarensis:* Comparisons with human and nonhuman primates. *Journal of Human Evolution* 18:235–68.

Ryder, N. B. 1974. The family in developed countries. *Scientific American*, March, 123–32.

Sabelli, H. C. 1991. Rapid treatment of depression with selegiline-phenylalanine combination. Letter to the editor. *Journal of Clinical Psychiatry* 52:3.

Sabelli, H. C., L. Carlson-Sabelli, and J. I. Javaid. 1990. The thermodynamics of bipolarity: A bifurcation model of bipolar illness and bipolar character and its psychotherapeutic applications. *Psychiatry* 53:346–68.

Sacks, K. 1971. Comparative notes on the position of women. Paper delivered at the annual meeting of the American Anthropological Association, Washington, D.C.

——. 1979. *Sisters and Wives: The Past and Future of Sexual Equality.* Urbana: Univ. of Illinois Press.

Sade, D. S. 1968. Inhibition of son-mother mating among free-ranging rhesus monkeys. *Science and Psychoanalysis* 12:18–37.

Sahlins, M. 1972. *Stone Age Economics.* New York: Aldine.

Sanday, P. R. 1974. Female status in the public domain. In *Woman, Culture, and Society,* ed. M. Z. Rosaldo and L. Lamphere. Stanford: Stanford Univ. Press.

——. 1981. *Female Power and Male Dominance: On the Origins of Sexual Inequality.* Cambridge: Cambridge Univ. Press.

Sapolsky, R. M. 1983. Endocrine aspects of social instability in the olive baboon. *American Journal of Primatology* 5:365–76.

Sarich, V. M., and A. C. Wilson. 1967a. Immunological time scale for hominid evolution. *Science* 158:1200–1203.

——. 1967b. Rates of albumin evolution in primates. *Proceedings of the National Academy of Sciences* 58:142–48.

Sarich, V. M., and J. E. Cronin. 1976. Molecular systematics of the primates. In *Molecular Anthropology,* ed. M. Goodman and R. E. Tashian. New York: Plenum Press.

Savage-Rumbaugh, E. S., and B. J. Wilkerson. 1978. Socio-sexual behavior in *Pan paniscus* and *Pan troglodytes:* A comparative study. *Journal of Human Evolution* 7:327–44.

Schaller, G. B. 1972. *The Serengeti Lion: A Study of Predator-Prey Relations.* Chicago: Univ. of Chicago Press.

Schaller, G. B., and G. R. Lowther. 1969. The relevance of carnivore behavior to the study of early hominids. *Southwestern Journal of Anthropology* 25:307–41.

Schlegel, A. 1972. *Male Dominance and Female Autonomy: Domestic Authority in Matrilineal Societies.* New Haven: HRAF Press.

Schneider, H. K. 1971. Romantic love among the Turu. In *Human Sexual Behavior,* ed. D. S. Marshall and R. C. Suggs. Englewood Cliffs, N.J.: Prentice Hall.

Schrire, C., ed. 1984. *Past and Present in Hunter-Gatherer Societies.* New York: Academic Press.

Seligman, J. 1990. Variations on a theme. *Newsweek Special Edition,* Winter/ Spring, 38–46.

Service, E. R. 1978. The Arunta of Australia. In *Profiles in Ethnology,* ed. E. R. Service. 3d ed. York: Harper & Row.

Sexuality Today. 1988. Approaching the male of the species. March 7, p. 5.

Shepher, J. 1971. Mate selection among second generation kibbutz adolescents and adults: Incest avoidance and negative imprinting. *Archives of Sexual Behavior* 1:293–307.

—. 1983. *Incest—A Biosocial View.* New York: Academic Press.

Sherfey, M. J. 1972. *The Nature and Evolution of Female Sexuality.* New York: Vintage Books.

Sherman, J. 1978. *Sex-Related Cognitive Differences: An Essay on Theory and Evidence.* Springfield, Ill.: Charles C. Thomas.

Shipman, P. 1984. Scavenger Hunt. *Natural History,* April, 20–27.

—. 1986. Scavenging or hunting in early hominids: Theoretical framework and tests. *American Anthropologist* 88:27–43.

—. 1987. Studies of hominid-faunal interaction at Olduvai Gorge. *Journal of Human Evolution* 15:691–706.

Shorey, H. H. 1976. *Animal Communication by Pheromones.* New York: Academic Press.

Short, R. V. 1976. The evolution of human reproduction. *Proceedings of the Royal Society,* ser. B, 195:3–24.

—. 1977. Sexual selection and descent of man. In *Reproduction and Evolution,* ed. J. H. Calaby and C. Tyndale-Biscoe. Canberra: Australian Academy of Science.

—. 1984. Breast feeding. *Scientific American,* April, 35–41.

Shostak. M. 1981. *Nisa: The Life and Words of a !Kung Woman.* New York: Random House.

Sibley, C., and J. Ahlquist. 1984. The phylogeny of hominoid primates, as indicted by DNA-DNA hybridization. *Journal of Molecular Evolution* 20:2–11.

Silverman, I., and M. Beals. 1990. Sex differences in spatial abilities: Evolutionary theory and data. Paper delivered at the annual meeting of the Human Behavior and Evolution Society, Los Angeles.

Silverstein, C. 1981. *Man to Man: Gay Couples in America.* New York: William Morrow.

Simons, E. L. 1985. Origins and characteristics of the first hominoids. In *Ancestors: The Hard Evidence.* ed. E. Delson. New York: Alan R. Liss.

—. 1989. Human origins. *Science* 245:1343–50.

Simpson-Hebert, M., and S. L. Huffman. 1981. The contraceptive effect of breastfeeding. In *Breastfeeding.* ed. E. C. Baer and B. Winikoff. Special Issue of *Studies in Family Planning* 12 (no. 4):125–33.

Sinclair, A. R. E., M. D. Leakey, and M. Norton-Griffiths. 1986. Migration and Hominid bipedalism. *Nature* 324:307.

Slocum, S. 1975. Woman the gatherer: Male bias in anthropology. In *Toward an Anthropology of Women,* ed. R. R. Reiter. New York: Monthly Review Press.

Small, M. F. 1988. Female primate sexual behavior and conception: Are there really sperm to spare? *Current Anthropology* 29:81–100.

Smith, B. H. 1986. Dental development in *Australopithecus* and early *Homo. Nature* 323:327.

Smith, R. L. 1984. Human sperm competition. In *Sperm Competition and the Evolution of Mating Systems,* ed. R. L. Smith. New York: Academic Press.

Smuts, Barbara B. 1985. *Sex and Friendship in Baboons.* New York: Aldine de Gruyter.

—. 1987. What are friends for? *Natural History,* Feb., 36–44.

—. 1992. Male-infant relationships in nonhuman primates: Parental investment or mating effort? In *Father Child Relations,* ed. B. Hewlett. New York: Aldine de Gruyter.

Solecki, R. S. 1971. *Shanidar: The First Flower People.* New York: Knopf.

—. 1989. On the evidence for Neanderthal burial. *Current Anthropology* 30:324.

Solway, J. S., and R. B. Lee. 1990. Foragers, genuine or spurious? *Current Anthropology* 31:109–46.

Sostek, A. J., and R. J. Wyatt. 1981. The chemistry of crankiness. *Psychology Today,* Oct., 120.

Spencer, R. F. 1959. *The North Alaskan Eskimo: A Study in Ecology and Society.* Washington, D.C.: Smithsonian Institution Press.

Spiro, M. E. 1958. *Children of the Kibbutz.* Cambridge: Harvard Univ. Press.

Springer, S. P., and G. Deutsch. 1985. *Left Brain, Right Brain.* Rev. ed. San Francisco: W. H. Freeman.

Stendhal. [1822] 1975. *Love.* Trans. G. Sale and S. Sale. Harmondsworth, England: Penguin Books.

Stephens, W. N. 1963. *The Family in Cross-Cultural Perspective.* New York: Holt, Rinehart and Winston.

Stoehr, T., ed. 1979. *Free Love in America: A Documentary History.* New York: AMS Press.

Stone, L. 1990. *Road to Divorce: England, 1530–1987.* New York: Oxford Univ. Press.

Strassman, B. I. 1981. Sexual selection, parental care, and concealed ovulation in humans. *Ethology and Sociobiology* 2:31–40.

Straus, L. G. 1989. On early hominid use of fire. *Current Anthropology* 30:488–89.

Stringer, C. B., and P. Andrews, 1988. Genetic and fossil evidence for the origin of modern humans. *Science* 239:1263–68.

Strum, S. 1990. *Almost Human: A Journey into the World of Baboons.* New York: W. W. Norton.

Suggs, R. C., and D. S. Marshall. 1971. Anthropological perspectives on human sexual behavior. In *Human Sexual Behavior,* ed. D. S. Marshall and R. C. Suggs. Englewood Cliffs, N.J.: Prentice-Hall.

Susman, R. L. 1984. The locomotor behavior of *Pan paniscus* in the Lomako Forest. In *The Pygmy Chimpanzee,* ed. R. L. Susman. New York: Plenum Press.

—. 1989. New hominid fossils from the Swartkrans formation excavations (1979–1986): Postcranial specimens. *American Journal of Physical Anthropology* 79:451–74.

—. 1990. Evidence for tool behavior in the earliest hominids. Paper delivered at the Anthropology Section of the New York Academy of Sciences, Nov. 19.

Susman, R. L., J. T. Stern, Jr., and W. L. Jungers. 1985. Locomotor adaptations in the Hadar hominids. In *Ancestors: The Hard Evidence.* ed. E. Delson. New York: Alan R. Liss.

Symons, D. 1979. *The Evolution of Human Sexuality.* New York: Oxford Univ. Press.

Symons, D. 1982. Another woman that never existed. *Quarterly Review of Biology* 57:297–300.

Symons, D., and B. Ellis. 1989. Human male-female differences in sexual desire. In *The Sociobiology of Sexual and Reproductive Strategies,* ed. A. E. Rasa, C. Vogel, and E. Voland. New York: Chapman and Hall.

Tanner, N. M. 1981. *On Becoming Human.* Cambridge: Cambridge Univ. Press.

Tanner, N. M., and A. L. Zihlman. 1976. Women in evolution. Part I: Innovation and selection in human origins. *Signs: Journal of Women in Culture and Society* 1:585–608.

Tavris, C., and S. Sadd. 1977. *The Redbook Report on Female Sexuality.* New York: Delacorte Press.

Teleki, G. 1973a. *The Predatory Behavior of Wild Chimpanzees.* Lewisburg: Bucknell Univ. Press.

—. 1973b. The omnivorous chimpanzee. *Scientific American,* Jan., 3–12.

Tennov, D. 1979. *Love and Limerence: The Experience of Being in Love.* New York: Stein and Day.

Textor, R. B. 1967. *A Cross-Cultural Summary.* New Haven: HRAF Press.

Thomas, H. 1985. The Early and Middle Miocene land connection of the Afro-Arabian plate and Asia: A major event for hominoid dispersal? In *Ancestors: The Hard Evidence.* ed. E. Delson. New York: Alan R. Liss.

Thompson-Handler, N., R. K. Malenky, and N. Badrian. 1984. Sexual behavior of *Pan paniscus* under natural conditions in the Lomako Forest, Equateur, Zaire. In *The Pygmy Chimpanzee,* ed. R. L. Susman. New York: Plenum Press.

Thornhill, R., and J. Alcock. 1983. *The Evolution of Insect Mating Systems.* Cambridge: Harvard Univ. Press.

Tiger, L. 1992. *The Pursuit of Pleasure,* Boston: Little, Brown.

Tobias, P. V. 1991. *Olduvai Gorge.* Vol. 4, *The Skulls, Endocasts and Teeth of Homo habilis.* New York: Cambridge Univ. Press.

Tofler, A. 1980. *The Third Wave.* New York: William Morrow.

Torrence, R., ed. 1989. *Time, Energy and Stone Tools.* New York: Cambridge Univ. Press.

Trevathan, W. R. 1987. *Human Birth: An Evolutionary Perspective.* New York: Aldine de Gruyter.

Trivers, R. L. 1972. Parental investment and sexual selection. In *Sexual Selection and the Descent of Man, 1871–1971,* ed. B. Campbell. Chicago: Aldine.

—. 1985. *Social Evolution.* Menlo Park, Calif.: Benjamin/Cummings.

Tunnell, G. G. 1990. Systematic scavenging: Minimal energy expenditure at Olare Orok in the Serengeti ecosystem. In *Problem Solving in Taphonomy,* ed. S. Solomon, I. Davidson, and D. Watson. Santa Lucia, Queensland, Australia: Univ. of Queensland Press.

Turke, P. W. 1984. Effects of ovulatory concealment and synchrony on protohominid mating systems and parental roles. *Ethology and Sociobiology* 5:33–44.

Turnbull, C. M. 1981. Mbuti womanhood. In *Woman the Gatherer,* ed. F. Dahlberg. New Haven: Yale Univ. Press.

Tutin, C. E. G. 1979. Mating patterns and reproductive strategies in a community of wild chimpanzees (*Pan troglodytes schweinfurthii*). *Behavioral Ecology and Sociobiology* 6:39–48.

Tutin, C. E. G., and R. McGinnis. 1981. Chimpanzee reproduction in the wild. In *Reproductive Biology of the Great Apes,* ed. C. E. Graham. New York: Academic Press.

Tuttle, R. H. 1990. The pitted pattern of Laetoli feet. *Natural History,* March, 61–64.

Tylor, E. B. 1889. On a method of investigating the development of institutions: Applied to laws of marriage and descent. *Journal of the Royal Anthropological Institute* 18:245–69.

Udry, J. R., and N. M. Morris. 1977. The distribution of events in the human menstrual cycle. *Journal of Reproductive Fertility* 51:419–25.

United Nations. Statistical Office, Department of Economic and Social Affairs. 1955. Divorce rates per 1000 married couples, 1935–53 *Demographic Yearbook: 1954.* Chart 35. New York: United Nations.

—. 1958. Technical Notes. *Demographic Yearbook: 1954.* New York: United Nations.

—. 1984. *Demographic Yearbook: 1982.* New York: United Nations.

U.S. Bureau of the Census. 1986. *Statistical Abstract of the United States.* Washington D.C. 1985. Chart 124.

Van Allen, J. 1976. "Aba Riots" or Igbo Women's War? Ideology, Stratification, and the Invisibility of Women. In *Women in Africa,* ed. N. J. Hafkin and E. G. Bay. Stanford: Stanford Univ. Press.

Van Couvering, J. A., and J. A. H. Van Couvering. 1975. African isolation and the Tethys seaway. In *Proceedings of the VI Congress of the Regional Committee on Mediterranean Neogene Stratigraphy.* Bratislava: Slovak Academy of Science.

Van Couvering, J. A. H. 1980. Community evolution and succession in East Africa during the Late Cenozoic. In *Bones in the Making,* ed. A. Hill and K. Berensmeyer. Chicago: Univ. of Chicago Press.

van den Berghe, P. L. 1979. *Human Family Systems: An Evolutionary View* Westport, Conn.: Greenwood Press.

Vandiver, P., O. Soffer, B. Klima, and J. Svoboda. 1989. The origins of ceramic technology at Dolni Vestonice, Czechoslovakia. *Science* 246:1002–8.

Van Gulik, R. 1974. *Sexual Life in Ancient China: A Preliminary Survey of Chinese Sex and Society from Ca. 1500 BC until 1644 AD.* Leiden: E. J. Brill.

Van Hooff, J. A. R. A. M. 1971. *Aspects of the Social Behavior and Communication in Human and Higher Non-Human Primates.* Rotterdam: Bronder-Offset.

Van Valen, L. 1973. A new evolutionary law. *Evolutionary Theory* 1:1–30.

Veit, P. G. 1982. Gorilla society. *Natural History,* March, 48–58.

Velle, W. 1982. Sex, hormones and behavior in animals and man. *Perspectives in Biology and Medicine* 25:295–315.

Verner, J., and M. F. Willson. 1966. The influence of habitats on mating systems of North American passerine birds. *Ecology* 47:143–47.

Vital Statistics of the United States, 1960. 1964. Vol. 3. Washington, D.C.: National Center for Health Statistics. Table 4-7.

—. *1970.* 1974. Vol. 3. Rockville, Md.: National Center for Health Statistics. Table 2-4.

—. *1977.* 1981. Vol. 3. Hyattsville, Md.: National Center for Health Statistics. Table 2-17.

—. *1979.* 1984. Vol. 3. Hyattsville, Md.: National Center for Health Statistics. Table 2-22.

—. *1981.* 1985. Vol. 3. Hyattsville, Md: National Center for Health Statistics. Table 2-13.

——. *1983*. 1987. Vol. 3. Hyattsville, Md.: National Center for Health Statistics. Table 2-10.

——. *1986*. 1990. Vol. 3. Hyattsville, Md.: National Center for Health Statistics. Table 2-29.

Vrba, E. S. 1985. African Bovidae: Evolutionary events since the Miocene. *South African Journal of Science* 81:263–66.

Wagner, J., ed. 1982. *Sex Roles in Contemporary American Communes.* Bloomington: Indiana Univ. Press.

Washburn, S. L., and C. S. Lancaster, 1968. The evolution of hunting. In *Man the Hunter,* ed. R. B. Lee and I. DeVore. New York: Aldine.

Washburn, S. L., and R. Moore. 1974. *Ape into Man: A Study of Human Evolution.* Boston: Little, Brown.

Watanabe, H. 1985. *Why Did Man Stand Up?: An Ethnoarchaeological Model for Hominization.* Tokyo: Univ. of Tokyo Press.

Weiner, A. B. 1976. *Women of Value, Men of Renown: New Perspective in Trobriand Exchange.* Austin: Univ. of Texas Press.

Weisman, S. R. 1988. Broken marriage and brawl test a cohesive cast. *New York Times,* Feb. 21.

Weiss, R. 1987. "How dare we? Scientists seek the sources of risk-taking behavior. *Science News* 132:57–59.

——. 1988. Women's skills linked to estrogen levels. *Science News* 134:341.

Weiss, R. S. 1975. *Marital Separation.* New York: Basic Books.

Werner, D. 1984. Paid sex specialists among the Mekranoti. *Journal of Anthropological Research* 40:394–405.

Westermarck, E. 1922. *The History of Human Marriage.* 5th ed. New York: Allerton.

——. 1934. Recent theories of exogamy. *Sociological Review* 26:22–44.

Westneat, D. F., P. W. Sherman, and M. L. Morton. 1990. The ecology and evolution of extra-pair copulations in birds. In *Current Ornithology.* Vol. 7, ed. D. M. Power. New York: Plenum Press.

White, J. M. 1987. Premarital cohabitation and marital stability in Canada. *Journal of Marriage and the Family* 49:641–47.

White, R. 1986. *Dark Caves, Bright Visions: Life in Ice Age Europe.* New York: American Museum of Natural History.

—. 1989a. Visual thinking in the Ice Age. *Scientific American* July, 92–99.

—. 1989b. Production complexity and standardization in Early Aurignacian bead and pendant manufacture: Evolutionary implications, In *The Human Revolution*, ed. P. Mellars and C. B. Stringer. Vol. 1. Edinburgh: Edinburgh Univ. Press.

White. T. D. 1977. New fossil hominids from Laetoli, Tanzania. *American Journal of Physical Anthropology* 46:197–229.

—. 1980. Additional fossil hominids from Laetoli, Tanzania: 1976–1979 specimens. *American Journal of Physical Anthropology* 53:487–504.

—. 1985. The hominids of Hadar and Laetoli: An element-by-element comparison of the dental samples. In *Ancestors: The Hard Evidence.* ed. E. Delson. New York: Alan R. Liss.

Whiting, B. 1965. Sex identity conflict and physical violence: A comparative study. *American Anthropologist* 67:123–40.

Whiting, B. B., and J. W. M. Whiting. 1975. *Children in Six Cultures.* Cambridge: Harvard Univ. Press.

Whitten, R. G. 1982. Hominid promiscuity and the sexual life of proto-savages: Did *Australopithecus* swing? *Current Anthropology* 23:99–101.

Whyte, M. K. 1978. *The Status of Women in Preindustrial Societies.* Princeton: Princeton Univ. Press.

—. 1990. *Dating, Mating, and Marriage.* New York: Aldine de Gruyter.

Wickler, W. 1976. *The Ethological Analysis of Attachment.* Berlin: Verlag Paul Parey.

Williams, G. C. 1975. *Sex and Evolution.* Princeton: Princeton Univ. Press.

Wilmsen. E. N. 1989. *Land Filled with Flies: A Political Economy of the Kalahari.* Chicago: Univ. of Chicago Press.

Wilmsen, E. N., and J. R. Denbow. 1990. Paradigmatic history of San-speaking peoples and current attempts at revision. *Current Anthropology* 31:489–524.

Wilson, E. O. 1975. *Sociobiology: The New Synthesis.* Cambridge: Belknap Press/Harvard Univ. Press.

Wilson, H. C. 1988. Male axillary secretions influence women's menstrual cycles: A critique. *Hormones and Behavior* 22:266–71.

Wilson, M., and M. Daly. 1991. The man who mistook his wife for a chattel. In *The Adapted Mind: Evolutionary Psychology and the Generation of Culture,* ed. J. H. Barkow, L. Cosmides, and J. Tooby. New York: Oxford Univ. Press.

Wittenberger, J. F., and R. L. Tilson. 1980. The evolution of monogamy: Hypotheses and evidence. *Annual Review of Ecology and Systematics* 11:197–232.

Wolfe, L. 1981. *Women and Sex in the 80s: The Cosmo Report.* New York: Arbor House.

Wolpoff, M. H. 1980. *Paleo-Anthropology.* New York: Alfred A. Knopf.

——. 1982. Ramapithecus and hominid origins. *Current Anthropology* 23:501–22.

——. 1984. Evolution of *Homo erectus:* The question of stasis. *Paleobiology* 10:389–406.

——. 1989. Multiregional evolution: The fossil alternative to Eden. In *The Human Revolution,* ed. P. Mellars and C. B. Stringer. Vol. 1. Edinburgh: Edinburgh Univ. Press.

Wolpoff, M. H., J. N. Spuhler, F. H. Smith, J. Radovcic, G. Pope, D. W. Frayer, R. Eckhardt, and G. Clark. 1988. Modern human origins. *Science* 241:772–74.

Woodburn, J. 1968. An introduction to Hadza ecology. In *Man the Hunter,* ed. R. B. Lee and I. DeVore. New York: Aldine.

Wrangham, R. W. 1977. Feeding behavior of chimpanzees in Gombe National Park, Tanzania. In *Primate Ecology,* ed. T. H. Clutton-Brock. London: Academic Press.

——. 1979a. On the evolution of ape social systems. *Social Science Information* 18:335–68.

——. 1979b. Sex differences in chimpanzee dispersion. In *The Great Apes,* ed. D. A. Hamburg and E. R. McCown. Menlo Park, Calif.: Benjamin/Cummings.

WuDunn, S. 1991. Romance, a novel idea, rocks marriages in China. *New York Times,* April 17.

Yerkes, R. M., and J. H. Elder. 1936. Oestrus, receptivity and mating in the chimpanzee. *Comparative Psychology Monographs* 13:1–39.

Zihlman, A. L. 1979. Pygmy chimpanzee morphology and the interpretation of early hominids. *South African Journal of Science* 75:165–68.

——. 1981. Women as shapers of the human adaptation. In *Woman the Gatherer,* ed. F. Dahlberg. New Haven: Yale Univ. Press.

Zihlman, A. L., and N. Tanner. 1978. Gathering and hominid adaptation. In *Female Hierarchies,* ed. L. Tiger and H. Fowler. Chicago: Beresford Book Service.!

Zihlman, A. L., J. E. Cronin, D. L. Cramer, and V. M. Sarich. 1987. Pygmy chimpanzee as a possible prototype for the common ancestor of humans, chimpanzees and gorillas. In *Interpretations of Ape and Human Ancestry,* ed. R. L. Ciochon and R. S. Corruccini. New York: Plenum Press.

Zimen, E., ed. 1980. *The Red Fox: Symposium on Behavior and Ecology.* The Hague: Junk.

Zuckerman, M. 1971. Dimensions of sensation seeking. *Journal of Consulting and Clinical Psychology* 36:45–52.

Zuckerman, M., M. S. Buchsbaum, and D. L. Murphy. 1980. Sensation seeking and its biological correlates. *Psychological Bulletin* 88:187–214.

Zuckerman, M., J. A. Hall, S. W. DeFrank, and R. Rosenthal. 1976. Encoding and decoding of spontaneous and posed facial expressions. *Journal of Personality and Social Psychology* 34:966–77.

Zuckerman, Sir S. 1932. *The Social Life of Monkeys and Apes.* London: Butler and Turner.

Index

Page numbers beginning with 313 refer to notes.

Industrial Revolution, divorce and, 106–7, 290, 294–95, 309
infancy, duration of, 141, 153–54, 157, 159, 160, 232, 234
infanticide, 92, 127
infants, 30, 48, 103, 172, 178, 196, 249, 252, 270, 299, 315, 317, 338
    altricial, *see* altriciality
    baboon, 155
    breast-feeding of, 153, 154, 157, 179–80, 335, 336
    chimpanzee, 92, 133
    gender differences in, 192, 194, 197
    hominid, 141, 149, 153–54, 156, 160, 164, 187, 195, 203
    incipient morality in, 255–56
    newborn, 41, 231–32, 255, 346
    precocial, 335
    smiling of, 25
    weaning of, 121, 122, 153, 154, 160, 185, 232, 233, 260
    see also children
infatuation, 12, 36, 37–58, 72, 73–74, 98–99, 109, 120, 144, 162, 163–66, 167, 173, 174, 231
    brain chemistry of, 51–56, 57, 62, 87, 163, 165, 171, 306, 316, 317
    characteristics of, 38–40
    crystallization vs. idealization in, 39
    cultural influence on, 55–58
    duration of, 56–57, 111, 163
    enhanced by barriers, 48, 49, 56, 163
    individual variation in experience of, 56
    intrusive thinking in, 38–39
    love at first sight in, 12, 49–51, 73
    love blindness vs., 56
    love maps in, 44–47, 49, 55, 316
    mystery and, 47–48, 49
    pheromones in, 40–44, 49, 55, 181, 186, 315
    physical sensations of, 39–40
    of romance junkies, 53–54
    similarity and, 48, 49
    teenage, 261, 263
    timing in, 48, 49
    see also attachment
infertility, 102, 154, 279, 315, 324
infidelity, *see* adultery
initiation rituals, 240–42, 262
    of Australian aborigines, 241–42
    cave paintings and, 240–41, 242, 249
insects, 19, 28, 41, 136, 139, 251, 319–20
    courtship feeding by, 34–35, 94

pair-bonding of, 149–50
sperm competition and, 177–78
intelligence, 189–90, 198, 229, 262, 346
intention cues, 28
interactional body synchrony, 30
In the Shadow of Man (Goodall), 11
intimacy, 204–5
intrusive thinking, 38–39
intuition, 195, 198, 199, 203, 342
Inuit (Eskimo), 78, 79, 153, 214–15, 216, 219
Iran, 249, 278
Iraq, 244, 278
Iroquois, 282, 325, 344
Islam, 280, 290
    divorce in, 98–100, 108, 110, 116, 361
    veil mandated by, 92
Ismail, Moulay, the Bloodthirsty, 66
Israel, 278
    ancient, 288
    kibbutzim of, 47–48, 250–51
    Sea of Galilee in, 237
Italy, 75–76, 79, 290

Jankoviak, William, 50
Japan, 20, 25, 44, 150, 196, 218, 280, 290, 325
    adultery in, 79–80
    double suicide *(shin ju)* in, 49
    marriage in, 73, 115–16
Java, 235, 237
jealousy, 89, 102, 167–69, 249–50, 265, 268, 269, 270, 321
    polygamy as cause of, 67, 70, 108, 128, 168, 261, 263
Jespersen, Otto, 36
Jesus, 83, 106, 289, 290
jewelry, 248, 249
Jilimi, 212
Johanson, Donald, 140
Johnson, Samuel, 103
Josephine, Empress of France, 41
Judaism, 73, 81–82, 83, 92
Jung, Carl, 37
jus primae noctis, 78

Kaingang, 321, 325
Kama Sutra (Vatsya), 49
Kant, Immanuel, 239
Kanuri, 116
Kenya, 196, 206–7, 229, 230, 319, 344
kevutza, 251